Diseases of Blood and Skin

Robert Gniadecki • Minakshi Taparia
Jean Deschenes • Jori Hardin
Etienne Mahe
Editors

Diseases of Blood and Skin

A Dermatologic Correlation of Hematologic Disorders

Springer

Editors
Robert Gniadecki
Department of Dermatology
University of Alberta
Edmonton, AB, Canada

Minakshi Taparia
Department of Hematology
University of Alberta Hospital
Edmonton, AB, Canada

Jean Deschenes
Department of Pathology and
Laboratory Medicine
Cross Cancer Institute
Edmonton, AB, Canada

Jori Hardin
Department of Dermatology
University of Calgary
Calgary, AB, Canada

Etienne Mahe
Division of Hematology, Department of
Pathology & Laboratory Medicine, and
Hematology & Hematological
Malignancies,
University of Calgary
Calgary, AB, Canada

ISBN 978-3-031-65291-2 ISBN 978-3-031-65292-9 (eBook)
https://doi.org/10.1007/978-3-031-65292-9

This Springer imprint is published by the registered company Springer Nature Switzerland AG
The registered company address is: Gewerbestrasse 11, 6330 Cham, Switzerland

Preface

For more than half a century, geographers, in an attempt to understand the complex system that is the Earth, acknowledged that *everything is related to everything else, but near things are more related than distant things.*[1] Yet, in the realm of medicine, dealing with the equally complex system of the human body, we tended to ignore the vital interconnectedness between different tissues and focused on organ-specific diseases in isolation.

Dermatology and hematology are no exception. While the origins of both specialties lie in internal medicine, dermatology and hematology have diverged along distinct trajectories, leading to a chasm between the two disciplines. The vernacular of dermatology remains opaque to hematologists, and vice versa, hindering the interdisciplinary collaboration necessary for a comprehensive understanding of disease processes.

The idea of this book emerged from discussions at multidisciplinary tumor boards, where perplexing cases involving both blood and skin disorders were dissected. When we reviewed patients' symptoms and signs alongside what we saw under the microscope, diseases metamorphosed from static, lifeless entities into dynamic processes. This clinical experience proved invaluable, enabling us to effectively convey the essence of diseases to patients and involve them more actively in therapeutic decisions. It also significantly enhanced our understanding of clinical–pathological correlations while overall improving the quality of diagnostic results. Throughout this book, our goal has been to capture this interdisciplinary spirit.

Richard Feynman, the genius physicist, Nobel Prize winner, and brilliant educator, understood the importance of simplicity, focusing on what is well understood rather than delving into the speculative. In the introduction to his lectures on quantum electrodynamics, he wrote[2]:

> *What I'd like to talk about is a part of physics that is known, rather than a part that is unknown. People are always asking for the latest developments of the unification of this theory with that theory, and they don't give us a chance to tell them about the theories that we know pretty well. They always want to know things we don't know. So, rather than confound you with a lot of half-cooked, partially analyzed theories, I would like to tell you about a subject that has been very thoroughly analyzed.*

---

[1]Tobler WR. A computer movie simulating urban growth in the Detroit region. *Econ Geogr*. 1970;46: 234.

[2]Feynman RP. *QED: The Strange Theory of Light and Matter*. Princeton University Press; 2014.

While we do not possess Feynman's genius in distilling complex concepts or his eloquent prose, we have endeavored to extract pertinent information and present it in a manner relevant to patient care. This is not an exhaustive academic treatise but rather a concise, pragmatic guide tailored to clinicians—dermatologists and hematologists—confronted with patients exhibiting skin manifestations of blood diseases and seeking a concise introduction to this specialized field of medicine. It may also be valuable for surgical pathologists, hematopathologists, and dermatopathologists who have come to fully appreciate the importance of clinical correlations and proactive differential diagnostic thinking to establish a sound pathological diagnosis. Drawing on the analogy of geography, we perceive this book as a navigational tool to assist clinicians and diagnosticians in traversing the challenging terrain between dermatology and hematology to achieve optimal outcomes for their patients.

As with any scholarly endeavor, we acknowledge the impermanence of knowledge in the face of evolving scientific inquiry. The landscape of medicine is ever-shifting, with new discoveries reshaping our understanding and challenging our assumptions. Thus, we have refrained from delving into the minutiae of disease pathogenesis and therapy, recognizing the transient nature of such knowledge. On that account, we urge clinicians to rely on the latest evidence and their clinical judgment when navigating the complexities of patient care, understanding that no textbook can offer immutable truths in the ever-changing landscape of medicine.

Edmonton, AB, Canada — Robert Gniadecki
Edmonton, AB, Canada — Minakshi Taparia
Edmonton, AB, Canada — Jean Deschenes
Calgary, AB, Canada — Jori Hardin
Calgary, AB, Canada — Etienne Mahe
February 2024

Contents

Abbreviations

AD	Atopic dermatitis
AESOP	Adenopathy and extensive skin patch overlying a plasmacytoma
aGvHD	Acute GvHD
AITL	Angioimmunoblastic T-cell lymphoma
ALCL	Anaplastic large cell lymphoma
ALHE	Angiolymphoid hyperplasia with eosinophilia
ALK	Anaplastic lymphoma kinase
ALL	Lymphoblastic leukemia/lymphoma
alloHSCT	Allogeneic hematopoietic stem cell transplantation
AML	Acute myeloid leukemia
ANCA	Anti-neutrophil cytoplasmic antibody
APECED	Autoimmune polyendocrinopathy with candidiasis and ectodermal dystrophy
ASM	Aggressive systemic mastocytosis (ASM)
ATCLL	Adult T-cell leukemia/lymphoma
AXG	Adult xanthogranuloma
B-ALL	B-lymphoblastic leukemia/lymphoma
BPDCN	Blastic plasmacytoid dendritic cell neoplasm
CD	Castleman disease
CGD	Chronic granulomatous disease
cGvHD	Chronic GvHD
CLH	Cutaneous lymphoid hyperplasia
CLL	Chronic lymphocytic leukemia
CM	Cutaneous mastocytosis
CML	Chronic myelogenous leukemia
CMML	Chronic myelomonocytic leukemia
CMV	Cytomegalovirus
CTCL	Primary cutaneous T-cell lymphoma
CVID	Common variable immunodeficiency
DLI	Donor lymphocyte infusion
EBER	Epstein-Barr-encoded RNA
EBV	Epstein-Barr virus
ECD	Erdheim Chester disease
ECMM	Extramedullary cutaneous multiple myeloma
ECP	Extracorporeal photopheresis
EDHM	Eosinophilic dermatosis of hematological malignancy

EED	Erythema elevatum diutinum
FCL	Follicular lymphoma
FDG	Fluorodeoxyglucose
fMF	Folliculotropic MF
GEH	Generalized eruptive histiocytosis
gMF	Granulomatous mycosis fungoides
GSS	Granulomatous slack skin disease
GvHD	Graft-versus-host disease
HCDD	Heavy chain deposition disease
HDACi	Inhibitors of histone deacetylases
HES	Hypereosinophilic syndrome
HIES	Hyper IgE syndrome
HLH	Hemophagocytic lymphohistiocytosis
HPV	Human papilloma virus
HSCT	Hematopoietic stem cell transplantation
HαT	Hereditary alpha tryptasemia
IgG4-RD	IgG4-related disease
IgH	Immunoglobulin heavy chain
IHC	Immunohistochemistry
I-HE	Idiopathic hypereosinophilia
IL	Interleukin
ISM	Indolent systemic mastocytosis (ISM)
IV-LBCL	Intravascular large B-cell lymphoma
IVLPD	Intravascular lymphoproliferative disorders
LC	Leukemia cutis
LCDD	Light chain deposition disease
LCH	Langerhans cell histiocytosis
LCT	Large cell transformation
LDH	Lactate dehydrogenase
LHCDD	Mixed (heavy and light chain) deposition disease
L-HES	Lymphocyte variant HES
LLP-IDD	Lymphomas and lymphoid proliferations associated with immune deficiency and dysregulation
LP	Lymphoplasmacytic lymphoma
LyG	Lymphomatoid granulomatosis
LyP	Lymphomatoid papulosis
MAPK	Mitogen-activated protein kinase
MCAD	Mast cell activation disorders
MCAS	Mast cell activation syndrome
mCD	Idiopathic multicentric Castleman's disease
mCD	Multicentric Castleman disease
MCL	Mast cell leukemia (MCL)
MCS	Mast cell sarcoma
MDS	Myelodysplastic syndrome
MF	Mycosis fungoides
MGUS	Monoclonal gammopathy of undetermined significance
MIDD	Monoclonal immunoglobulin deposition disease

MLN-eo-TK	Myeloid-lymphoid neoplasms with eosinophilia and tyrosine kinase gene fusion
MM	Multiple myeloma
MPO	Myeloperoxidase
MRC	Multicentric reticulohistiocytosis
MRI	Magnetic resonance imaging
NGS	Next-generation sequencing
NOS	Not otherwise specified
NXG	Necrobiotic xanthogranuloma
PAS	Periodic acid-Schiff
pcALCL	Primary cutaneous anaplastic large cell lymphoma
pcCD30-IVLPD	Primary cutaneous benign $CD30^+$ intravascular lymphoproliferative disease
pcCD4-LPD	Primary cutaneous $CD4^+$ small medium pleomorphic T-cell lymphoproliferative disease
pcCD8-AECTCL	Primary cutaneous $CD8^+$ aggressive epidermotropic cytotoxic T-cell lymphoma
pcDLBCL-LT	Primary cutaneous diffuse large B-cell lymphoma, leg type
pcFCL	Primary cutaneous follicle center (follicular) lymphoma
pcGDTCL	Primary cutaneous gamma-delta T-cell lymphoma
pcMZL/LPD	Primary cutaneous marginal zone lymphoma/lymphoproliferative disease
PCR	Polymerase chain reaction
pcSPTCL	Subcutaneous panniculitis-like T-cell lymphoma
PET/CT	Positron emission tomography/computed tomography scan
PG	Pyoderma gangrenosum
PNH	Progressive nodular histiocytosis
POEMS	Polyneuropathy, organomegaly, endocrinopathy, monoclonal protein, and skin changes
PTCL-NOS	Peripheral T-cell Lymphoma, not otherwise specifies
PTLD	Post-transplant lymphoproliferative disorder
PUVA	Psoralen ultraviolet A therapy
RDD	Rosai–Dorfman disease
SAA	Serum amyloid A protein
SCP	Solitary cutaneous plasmacytoma
SIgAD	Selective IgA deficiency
SLL	Small lymphocytic lymphoma
SM	Systemic mastocytosis
SM-ANH	Systemic mastocytosis with an associated hematologic neoplasm
SPD	Subcorneal pustular dermatosis
SS	Sezary syndrome
SSM	Smoldering systemic mastocytosis (SSM)
T-ALL	T-lymphoblastic leukemia/lymphoma
TCL	T-cell lymphoma
TCR	T-cell receptor

TEMPI	Telangiectasia, elevated erythropoietin and erythrocytosis, monoclonal gammopathy, perinephric fluid collections, intrapulmonary shunting
TEN	Toxic epidermal necrolysis
T_{FH}	T follicular helper cell
TMEP	Telangiectasia macularis eruptiva perstans
T-PLL	T-cell prolymphocytic leukemia
TSEB	Total skin electron beam radiation therapy
uCD	Unicentric Castleman's disease
UVA	Ultraviolet A
UVB	Ultraviolet B
VEXAS	Vacuoles, E1 enzyme, X-linked autoinflammatory, Somatic syndrome
VZV	Varicella zoster virus
WM	Waldenstrom's macroglobulinemia
XD	Xanthoma disseminatum
γδMF	MF expressing γδ T-cell receptor (MF)

1 Malignant Infiltrations of the Skin in Hematological Cancers

Robert Gniadecki, Minakshi Taparia, Jean Deschenes, Jori Hardin, and Etienne Mahe

Malignant infiltrations of the skin manifest when malignant cells from systemic leukemia or lymphoma display dermotropism, secondarily infiltrating the skin and giving rise to an array of clinically observable lesions (Fig. 1.1 and Table 1.1). The classification of these secondary malignant skin infiltrations reflects the corresponding systemic process giving rise to them, including leukemia cutis (characterized by the presence of leukemic cells in the skin) and secondary skin infiltrates seen in patients with malignant lymphomas or plasma cell neoplasms. Some patients with hematological cancers will experience cutaneous extramedullary hematopoiesis (CEMH); however, the pathophysiology of this process is still unclear and hence it will be dealt with in Sect. 18.3. Neoplastic histiocytic disorders also frequently involve the skin.

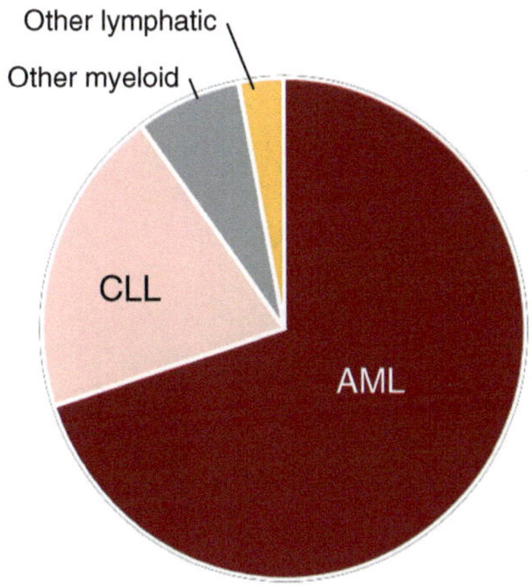

Fig. 1.1 Relative frequency of hematologic cancers producing malignant infiltrations in the skin

R. Gniadecki (✉)
Division of Dermatology, University of Alberta, Edmonton, AB, Canada
e-mail: r.gniadecki@ualberta.ca

M. Taparia
Division of Hematology, University of Alberta Hospital, Edmonton, AB, Canada

J. Deschenes
Department of Pathology and Laboratory Medicine, Cross Cancer Institute, Edmonton, AB, Canada
e-mail: Jean.Deschenes@albertaprecisionlabs.ca

J. Hardin
Division of Dermatology, University of Calgary, Calgary, AB, Canada
e-mail: Jori.hardin@albertahealthservices.ca

E. Mahe
Department of Pathology & Laboratory Medicine, and Hematology & Hematological Malignancies, University of Calgary, Calgary, AB, Canada
e-mail: etienne.mahe@albertaprecisionlabs.ca

R. Gniadecki et al. (eds.), *Diseases of Blood and Skin*, https://doi.org/10.1007/978-3-031-65292-9_1

Table 1.1 Malignant infiltrations of the skin in hematological cancers

Condition	Hematological disease
Leukemia cutis (Chaps. 2 and 3)	Myeloid (Chap. 2)
	Acute myeloid leukemia (AML) and related leukemias (acute myelomonocytic leukemia, acute monoblastic/monocytic leukemia)
	Chronic myelogenous leukemia (CML), chronic myelomonocytic leukemia (CMML)
	Myelodysplastic syndromes
	Blastic plasmacytoid dendritic cell neoplasm (BPDCN)
	Lymphoproliferative (Chap. 3)
	Chronic lymphocytic leukemia (CLL)
	Adult T-cell leukemia/lymphoma (ATCLL)
	T-cell prolymphocytic leukemia (T-PLL)
	B-lymphoblastic leukemia/lymphoma (B-ALL)
	T-lymphoblastic leukemia/lymphoma (T-ALL)
	Hairy cell leukemia
Secondary lymphomatous infiltrates in the skin (Chap. 3)	Mantle cell lymphoma
	Follicular lymphoma
	Intravascular lymphoma
	Lymphomatoid granulomatosis
	Hodgkin lymphoma
Plasma cell infiltrates (Chap. 4)	Multiple myeloma
	Waldenström macroglobulinemia
Other	Histiocytoses (Chap. 12)
	Mastocytosis (Chap. 14)

2 Myeloid Leukemia Cutis

Robert Gniadecki, Minakshi Taparia,
Jean Deschenes, Jori Hardin, and Etienne Mahe

2.1 Practice Essentials

- Leukemia cutis is the infiltration of the skin by malignant myeloid cells, most commonly due to underlying acute myeloid leukemia (AML).
- Leukemia cutis can predate the manifestation of systemic leukemia (aleukemic leukemia cutis) or develop concurrently with bone marrow involvement (synchronous leukemia cutis). Patients with aleukemic leukemia cutis invariably develop systemic disease.
- Leukemia cutis may be the first sign of disease relapse after allogeneic hematopoietic stem cell transplant.
- Clinical manifestations of leukemia cutis are protean and comprise a wide range of skin lesions, from mild macular rash to ulcerated tumors.
- The diagnosis should be made using clinicalopathological correlation. Histology alone is often non-specific or misleading, simulating many benign and malignant skin diseases. Diagnosis needs to be informed by ancillary techniques, such as immunohistochemistry. There may be discordance of phenotype and cytogenetic aberrations in leukemia cutis relative to leukemic cells in bone marrow.
- No consensus management guidelines exist, although systemic treatment is usually required. Radiotherapy may be an effective skin-directed palliative therapy.

2.2 Leukemia Cutis: Definition

Leukemia cutis (LC) is characterized by the infiltration of the skin by leukemic cells, giving rise to clinically recognizable skin lesions [1]. LC represents an instance of extramedullary leukemia localized within the skin. This condition may precede the onset of systemic leukemia (referred to as aleukemic or metachronous LC) or occur concurrently with clinically mani-

R. Gniadecki (✉)
Division of Dermatology, University of Alberta, Edmonton, AB, Canada
e-mail: r.gniadecki@ualberta.ca

M. Taparia
Division of Hematology, University of Alberta Hospital, Edmonton, AB, Canada

J. Deschenes
Department of Pathology and Laboratory Medicine, Cross Cancer Institute, Edmonton, AB, Canada
e-mail: Jean.Deschenes@albertaprecisionlabs.ca

J. Hardin
Division of Dermatology, University of Calgary, Calgary, AB, Canada
e-mail: Jori.hardin@albertahealthservices.ca

E. Mahe
Department of Pathology & Laboratory Medicine, and Hematology & Hematological Malignancies, University of Calgary, Calgary, AB, Canada
e-mail: etienne.mahe@albertaprecisionlabs.ca

R. Gniadecki et al. (eds.), *Diseases of Blood and Skin*, https://doi.org/10.1007/978-3-031-65292-9_2

fest leukemia involving the blood and bone marrow. A relatively common scenario is LC following a diagnosis of acute leukemia, now in apparent remission, the skin lesions indicating relapse.

Various terms have been employed interchangeably to describe LC associated with acute myeloid leukemia (AML). The World Health Organization (WHO) 2017 classification of myeloid neoplasms introduced the term "myeloid sarcoma" to denote any tissue infiltration featuring myeloid blasts outside the bone marrow [2, 3]. Consequently, many leukemia cutis can be categorized as a subtype of myeloid sarcoma occurring in the skin. Some older but still relevant terms include "chloroma" (derived from the Greek word "chloros," signifying green, a color produced by the oxidation of myeloperoxidase within the granules of immature myeloid precursors), "primary extramedullary leukemia" or "granulocytic sarcoma."

LC encompasses any infiltration of the skin by malignant leukemic cells, regardless of their cellular origin (myeloid, lymphocytic, plasma cells, etc.). However, in clinical practice, the term "leukemia cutis" is often used narrowly in reference to myeloid neoplasms, particularly AML, since this constitutes the majority of cases, which is the convention we will adopt here.

2.3 Incidence and Risk Factors

Synchronous leukemia cutis, which manifests either concurrently with or following the diagnosis of myeloid disorders, is the predominant presentation, accounting for approximately 60% and 25% of cases, respectively. Conversely, metachronous leukemia cutis, occurring before the diagnosis of myeloid disorders, constitutes a minority of cases, representing less than 5% [4, 5].

Leukemia cutis (LC) is most frequently associated with acute myeloid leukemia (AML), accounting for approximately 50–60% of all cases of LC [4–7], with acute lymphoid leukemia (ALL) a distant second, accounting for approximately 10% of cases [8] (Table 2.1).

Table 2.1 Leukemia cutis in different myeloid neoplasms. The overall probability of skin involvement is approximately 10%, with a higher risk of congenital and pediatric leukemias

Condition	Probability of clinically apparent skin involvement[a]
AML (including acute myelomonocytic leukemia and acute monoblastic/monocytic leukemia)	++ (2.5–9.1%, up to 15%) Higher incidence in AML with t(8,21) Higher incidence in AMMoL and AMoL
BPDCN	+++ (90%)
Chronic myeloid and myelomonocytic leukemias (CML, CMML)	+ (CML) to ++ (CMML)
Myelodysplastic syndrome	+

[a] Strength of association: + occasional <4%, ++ frequent 5–20%, +++ very frequent >20%

In contrast, cutaneous involvement by chronic lymphoid leukemia/small lymphocytic lymphoma (CLL/SLL, estimated at 6% of cases of LC), chronic myelomonocytic leukemia (CMML, estimated at 5% of cases of LC, occasionally in the setting of blastic transformation, to be excluded), and chronic myeloid leukemia (CML) (estimated to represent 3% of cases) is far less common [9]. Myelodysplastic syndromes (MDS) are associated with less than 5% of cases of LC, often in the setting of evolution to a more aggressive process.

Mature T-cell lymphoproliferative disorders (such as T-cell prolymphocytic leukemia, T-PLL, or adult T-cell leukemia lymphoma, ATLL) may also quite commonly demonstrate secondary skin involvement during their clinical course, but they are a rare cause of LC in clinical practice. Plasma cell neoplasms are a rare cause of LC.

Of note, blastic plasmacytoid dendritic cell neoplasm (BPDCN) almost invariably presents with skin involvement, which led to its previous classification as a primary cutaneous lymphoma. Unlike AML, BPDCN typically exhibits either metachronous skin involvement, preceding bone marrow and blood-related manifestations, or presents with skin involvement as the initial sign of the disease alongside bone marrow involvement.

Predicting the occurrence of leukemia cutis for a given hematological neoplasm is difficult. Overall, 10–15% of patients with AML will develop LC, and among those, the incidence of LC is highly variable. For example, up to 50% of patients with acute myelomonocytic (AMMoL) and monocytic (AMoL) types of AML will experience LC, while this is vanishingly rare in patients with erythroid differentiation [10, 11]. LC is less common in patients with chronic MPN and with MDS, but patients with chronic myelomonocytic leukemia (CMML) have a higher tendency to develop LC, compared to CML patients [7, 12–15]. In patients with ALL and plasma cell neoplasm, only a small fraction develop leukemia cutis [5] (see Chap. 3). The frequency of LC is higher in children with leukemia (AML or ALL), compared with adult AML or ALL patients, as 25–30% of infants suffering from congenital leukemia will develop skin lesions [16].

Some clinical risk factors have also been identified. In AML, leukemia cutis appears to be more prevalent in patients with a median age of 56–59 years (slightly younger than the median age of 68 years without leukemia cutis), in males (constituting 52–59% of cases). It may be more common in patients with the chromosomal translocation t(8,21) [1, 11, 17]. Leukemia cutis in AML patients also occurs more frequently following allogeneic hematopoietic stem cell transplantation (alloHSCT), typically emerging 6–12 months post-transplant and comprising approximately 20% of all post-alloHSCT relapses [18–21]. Notably, in contrast to the primary disease, the majority (around 70%) of post-alloHSCT leukemia cutis cases are aleukemic.

Regarding lymphocytic leukemias, skin involvement has been described in less than 20% of patients with CLL/SLL. By contrast, mature T-cell leukemia (the rare T-PLL, ATLL, and Sézary syndrome) is often accompanied by skin involvement (in up to 70% of patients [16, 22–24]); however, as noted above, because of their overall rarity they represent a very limited subset of LC patients, lymphoid lesions infiltrating the skin will be further addressed in the next chapter.

2.4 Clinical Presentation (Figs. 2.1 and 2.2)

Less than one in ten cases present before systemic leukemia was ever diagnosed. This is usually an AML, with no manifest or obvious bone marrow or peripheral blood involvement, for which LC represents the first clinical sign of leukemia (so-called "aleukemic leukemia cutis"). Among the remaining LC patients, leukemia has

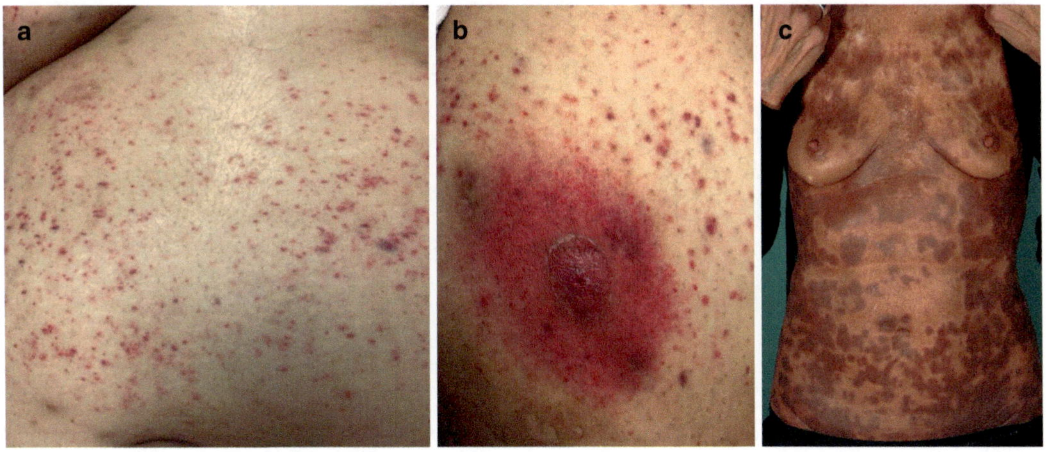

Fig. 2.1 Leukemia cutis in a patient with acute myeloid leukemia (AML). Note numerous papular lesions imitating purpura (**a**) and a larger infiltrated plaque with central necrosis (**b**). The patient in (**c**) presented with violaceous confluent plaques, demonstrating the heterogeneity of the clinical manifestations of myeloid leukemia cutis

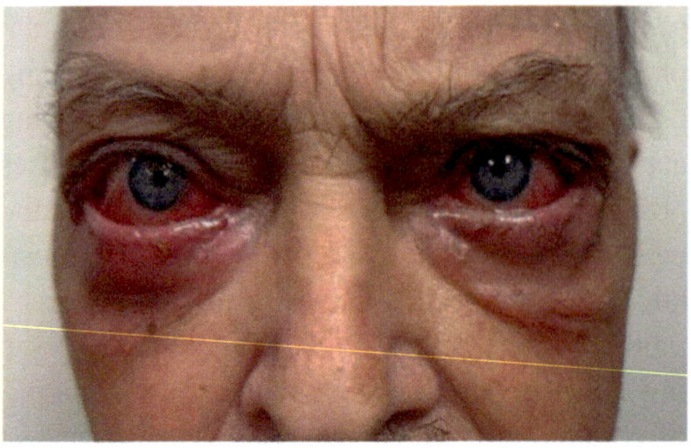

Fig. 2.2 Myeloid leukemia cutis in a patient with AML manifesting as infiltration of the skin of the eyelids and ectropion

been diagnosed, and some have concurrent active systemic leukemia, representing about one-third of all LC patients [25, 26]. This leaves the majority (about 60%) of LC patients presenting with LC in apparent isolation after a diagnosis of systemic leukemia was previously established, but no concomitant systemic disease is clinically manifest at the time LC is diagnosed.

The clinical presentations of leukemia cutis are diverse and lack specificity for the underlying leukemia (Figs. 2.1, 2.2, and 2.3). Typically, patients present with either a solitary tumor or multiple nodules characterized by a distinctive

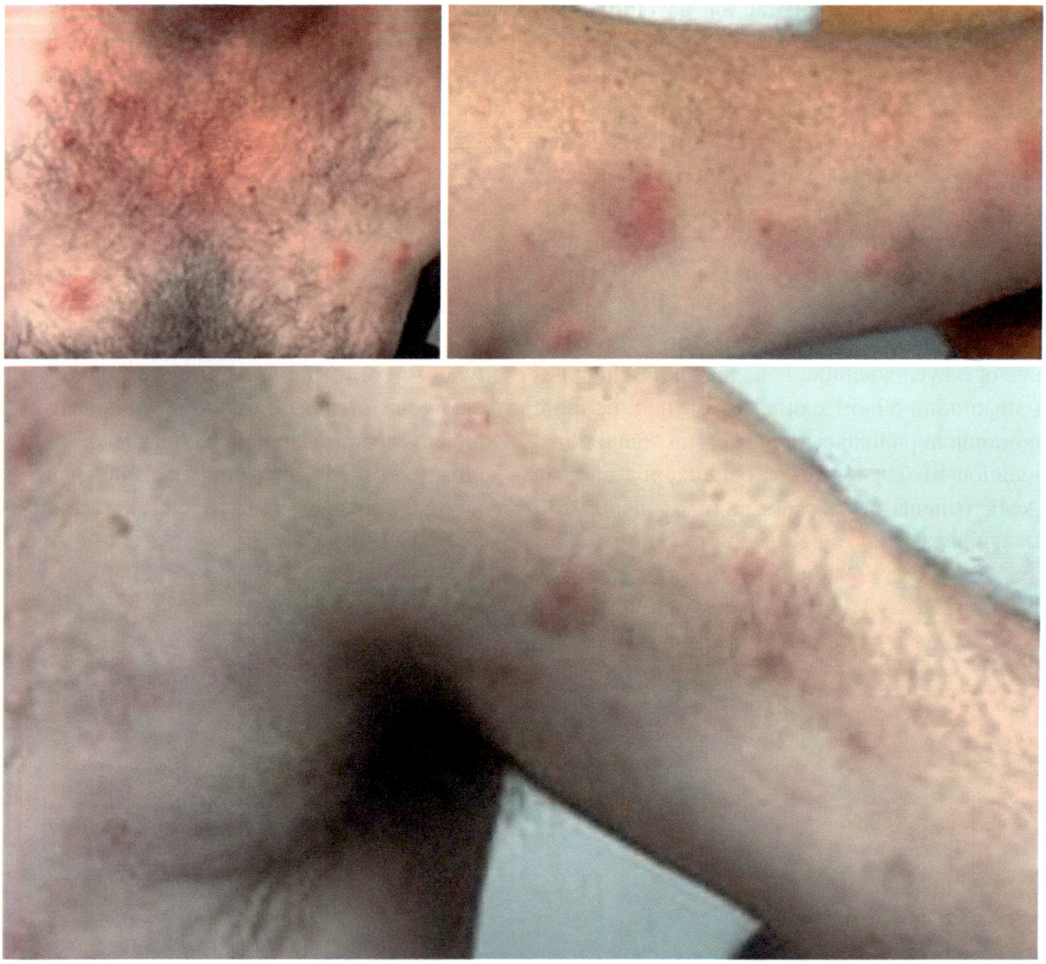

Fig. 2.3 Aleukemic leukemia cutis preceding myeloid leukemia. This is a 40-year-old male patient who presented with a 6-month history of dozens of painful nodules throughout his body and progressive severe pain in his abdomen and joints. A repeated punch biopsy showed a perivascular lymphoid infiltrate with some atypia and positivity for CD4, CD45, CD43, CD123, and MPO stains. CD56, CD3, CD61, CD99, CD34, CD138, CD8, CD117, IgG4, and TdT stains were negative. Detailed case description is in [33]

dark-red to violaceous color, often displaying hemorrhagic features or necrosis [5, 27]. These lesions tend to appear preferentially at sites of prior trauma (such as catheter or needle insertion points) or previous inflammation (e.g., herpes zoster), but they can arise anywhere on the skin. The most common locations for these lesions include the lower extremities, followed by the upper extremities, back, trunk, and face.

Other presentations encompass a range of manifestations, including small asymptomatic papules, a macular and/or papular rash, or widespread skin infiltration, ulceration, and even erythroderma [4, 27, 28]. Leukemia cutis can mimic various benign conditions, such as venous leg ulcers, dyshidrotic eczema, cutaneous vasculitis, Jessner lymphocytic infiltration, granuloma annulare, or rosacea [4, 5, 11, 28]. In some instances, deep leukemia cutis may be confused with lipomas [29].

Myeloid sarcoma involving the breast and leukemic gingival hyperplasia are rare but distinctive clinical manifestations of AML. Breast involvement typically occurs in patients experiencing a relapse after alloHSCT and typically presents as a palpable breast mass [30]. In women with breast implants, distinguishing it from breast implant-associated anaplastic lymphoma or even an inflammatory reaction around the implant can be exceptionally challenging.

Gingival hyperplasia has only been observed in AML-related leukemia cutis and in cases of blastic plasmacytoid dendritic cell neoplasm [27]. Approximately 2% of all cases of gingival hyperplasia may be indicative of AML [20], and 3% of leukemia cutis cases manifest as gum hyperplasia [31, 32]. Diagnosing gingival hyperplasia as myeloid sarcoma can be exceedingly difficult due to often non-specific histopathological findings that do not consistently reveal the presence of leukemic cells [32].

Leukemias may also manifest with leukemids, i.e., paraneoplastic cutaneous symptoms not directly related to the presence of malignant cells in the skin (Chap. 18). These nonleukemic cutaneous manifestations are more prevalent than leukemia cutis, occurring in over 40% of leukemia patients [5]. They primarily result from cytopenias and drug reactions associated with the underlying hematologic condition.

Petechiae and purpura are small red or purple, usually non-palpable macules caused by minor bleeding from capillaries in thrombocytopenic patients. Ecchymoses (bruises) may also develop due to compromised blood clotting. Leukocytoclastic vasculitis, an inflammatory condition affecting small blood vessels, leads to palpable purpura. Neutrophilic dermatoses, such as Sweet's syndrome, characterized by fever and painful skin lesions, and pyoderma gangrenosum, featuring rapidly progressing, painful skin ulcers, are notable cutaneous presentations (Chap. 18).

Opportunistic infections further contribute to leukemids. Thrush, a fungal infection causing white patches on the tongue and oral mucosa, disseminated herpes zoster with widespread skin lesions, and severe or atypical presentations of herpes simplex virus are common infectious complications.

2.5 Diagnostic Workup

Leukemia cutis always signifies the presence of concurrent or impending systemic leukemia. Therefore, the detection of leukemia cutis in a patient without a known systemic leukemia (referred to as asynchronous leukemia cutis) should trigger the standard diagnostic systemic evaluation in accordance with local guidelines. This evaluation aims to determine the extent of involvement in the bone marrow, blood, and other organs.

A skin biopsy of the lesion is imperative to establish a diagnosis and is typically the initial diagnostic step. In myeloid neoplasms, skin infiltration typically occurs both superficially and deeply and comprises proliferating blastoid, atypical mononuclear cells [34]. The histomorphology may resemble other entities such as B- or T-cell lymphomas or extramedullary hematopoiesis [35–37]. Approximately 40% of leukemia cutis cases are initially misdiagnosed as they mimic a wide range of both benign and malignant conditions. The infiltrate may be subtle and resemble non-specific dermatitis, granuloma annulare, histiocytoid Sweet's syndrome, vasculitis, or multicentric reticulohistiocytosis [4, 11, 38, 39]. Diagnosing leukemia cutis can be challenging, and if the pathological description does not align with the clinical presentation, a repeat biopsy may be necessary.

Since the histopathological findings may be misleading, specimens suspected to represent LC should be further assessed by the immunohistochemical method using a panel of carefully selected antibodies. Multi-parametric flow cytometry analysis (FCM) is a useful diagnostic adjunct. However, as an adequate sampling of fresh tissue for FCM is rarely done or feasible (due to technical limitations on small skin samples and/or lack of clinical suspicion, preventing a small sample from being segregated and sent to the flow lab before fixation of the biopsy material), the practical benefits of FCM are limited. This panel should include: myeloperoxidase (MPO), lysozyme, CD3, CD34, CD4, CD20, CD43, CD56, CD68, CD117, and CD123, the combination of which can accurately identify myeloid leukemia cutis in the majority of cases [40]. Among these, CD68 is often the most sensitive, being present in more than 90% of cases [35]. Leukemia cutis typically exhibits a high proliferation rate (Ki-67 between 50% and 95%) [35]. CD10 and TdT are useful, especially if one suspects acute lymphoblastic leukemia, rather than myeloid LC. CD117 and MPO immunostaining are negative in monoblastic skin infiltrates and in cases of BPDCN [4, 11, 34]. The latter is diagnosed based on the expression of plasmacytoid dendritic cell markers (including CD4, CD56, CD123, CD303 [BDCA2]), an absence of lysozyme or MPO expression, and is usually also positive for TCL1 and BCL-2. Exclusion of other potential differential diagnoses such as B- and T-cell lymphoproliferative disorders may also require the use of B cell markers (such as PAX5 and CD20), additional T cell markers (such as CD5)) and more specific antibodies (such as CD23, CD25, TCL1, Cyclin D1, LEF1), see next chapter for details.

The diagnosis should always be based on the integrated combination of immunophenotypic, morphological, and clinical data and will benefit from integrating other laboratory data (e.g., molecular or cytogenetic findings).

Cytogenetic abnormalities are found in up to 50% of cases, and cytogenetic studies should be conducted in all instances [35]. While cytogenetic aberrations have not been systematically studied in leukemia cutis, it is presumed that the molecular features observed in myeloid sarcomas in other locations are also present in the skin [1, 28, 35, 41]. Molecular genetic techniques may also be of utility: LC cases of myeloid derivation would be expected to demonstrate germline configuration immunoglobulin and/or T-cell receptor gene rearrangement assays. Variants in genes commonly interrogated in the setting of marrow-based myeloid neoplasms may also be detected in LC (e.g., FLT3, NPM1, etc.). It is important to recognize that the immune profile and cytogenetic features of leukemia cutis may differ from those of leukemic cells in the peripheral blood or bone marrow. These disparities likely reflect the distinct subclonal evolution of malignant cells in various anatomical compartments [40, 42]. It has been argued that comprehensive immunohistochemical and cytogenetic profiling should be conducted for skin biopsies with leukemia cutis, as it may uncover new features of potential prognostic or therapeutic significance. For instance, FMS-related tyrosine kinase 3 gene (FLT3) mutations, associated with an unfavorable prognosis, may exhibit discordant mutation status between the bone marrow and the myeloid sarcoma [43].

In cases of leukemic infiltrates in chronic lymphocytic leukemia (CLL), the condition comprises small monomorphous lymphocytes with an abnormal marker pattern ($CD20^+$, $CD79a^+$, $LEF1^+$, $CD5^+$ $CD23^+$) in a lichenoid, perivascular, or nodular pattern [6]. Demonstrating a monoclonal B cell population characterized by a specific rearrangement of the immunoglobulin heavy chain (IgH) genes may serve as a useful diagnostic aid in selected cases.

Regarding imaging, the question of whether the presence of synchronous leukemia cutis in a patient with an established AML diagnosis should prompt further imaging remains a subject of debate. The presence of leukemia cutis does not appear to be directly correlated with the risk of extramedullary leukemia involvement in other tissues. It is believed that the migration of leukemic cells to the skin is primarily mediated by the expression of specific chemokines and chemokine receptors that facilitate the homing of malignant cells to the skin (e.g., CCL3, CXCR4, CXCR7, CCR [44–46]). However, certain guidelines (e.g., NCCN guidelines) recommend FDG-PET/CT imaging for all patients with myeloid sarcoma, regardless of the anatomical site. This recommendation is based on observations suggesting that patients with myeloid sarcomas may have a higher risk of brain involvement, although such a correlation has not been conclusively established for leukemia cutis.

2.6 Differential Diagnoses

Because of the lack of specificity of skin lesions, the differential diagnosis is mostly based on the histopathological features in the skin biopsy (Table 2.2).

Table 2.2 Pathological differential diagnosis of myeloid leukemia cutis

Acute lymphoblastic leukemia/ lymphoma	Positive for B- or T-cell markers and negative for myeloid markers. Positive for TdT and CD10
Diffuse large B-cell lymphoma	Positive for B-cell markers
Histiocytosis	Chapter 12 Positive for histiocyte markers (CD68, CD163, CD1a, S100). Often BRAF V600E positive. Negative for myeloperoxidase
Extramedullary hematopoiesis	Trilineage hematopoiesis with maturation
Histiocytoid Sweet syndrome	Chapter 18 Clinical course is similar to the classic Sweet syndrome, acute and relapsing. Skin biopsy with edema and foamy, histiocyte-like cells believed to be immature neutrophils. Histiocytoid Sweet's syndrome is associated with myeloid neoplasms
Mature plasmacytoid dendritic cell tumor	CD123, TCL1, and CD303 positive but CD56, CD1a, and S100 negative. Accompanies clinical CMML [9]
Blastic plasmacytoid dendritic cell neoplasm	Positive for CD56, CD4, CD123, CD303, TCL1; negative MPO, CD117, CD34, and lysozyme

2.7 Prognostic Importance

The prognostic significance of leukemia cutis remains unclear and has yielded conflicting findings in various studies. Some research has suggested that the presence of leukemia cutis does not significantly impact the 5-year survival of patients with AML [7], while other studies have associated it with a notably poorer survival, both in cases of AML and chronic myelomonocytic leukemia (CMML) [39, 47]. Interestingly, the t(8;21) translocation (AML1:ETO fusion) and inv.(16) (CBFB:MYH1), which are generally linked to a better prognosis in AML, have also been associated with the risk of myeloid sarcomas. However, it remains uncertain whether such a correlation specifically exists for leukemia cutis [1, 28, 35, 41]. In patients with chronic myeloid leukemia (CML) and CMML, skin involvement may indicate disease progression and blast-phase transformation; this has to be carefully excluded by histopathological assessment of the skin lesions. Most guidelines and experts consider leukemia cutis as a negative prognostic marker.

2.8 Therapy

The choice of therapy depends on the clinical context, with treatment typically guided by the underlying leukemia. In many cases, specialists may opt to intensify the chemotherapy regimen for patients with leukemia cutis. It is worth noting that skin lesions may at times respond less effectively to chemotherapy compared to the disease in the bone marrow or blood, which may necessitate considering skin-targeted modalities.

Leukemia cutis consistently demonstrates sensitivity to radiotherapy. Depending on the location of the lesions, both photon and electron beam therapies are highly effective skin-directed treatment options. Different treatment centers may employ varying dosing and fractionation regimens, but a total dose of approximately 20 Gy is generally suitable for most patients [48, 49]. Local control can be expected in over 90% of patients treated with radiotherapy. However, it is important to note that radiotherapy does not influence prognosis and overall survival [50, 51].

Leukemia cutis that develops after allogeneic hematopoietic stem cell transplantation (allo-HCT) tends to be responsive to the graft-versus-leukemia effect. Reports have indicated the efficacy of approaches such as tapering of immunosuppressive medications and donor lymphocyte infusion [48]. Conventional AML-type chemotherapy is usually administered, either with or without skin-directed radiotherapy, in these cases.

References

1. Shallis RM, Gale RP, Lazarus HM, Roberts KB, Xu ML, Seropian SE, et al. Myeloid sarcoma, chloroma, or extramedullary acute myeloid leukemia tumor: a tale of misnomers, controversy and the unresolved. Blood Rev. 2021;47:100773.
2. Campo E, Harris NL, Pileri SA, Jaffe ES, Stein H, Thiele J. WHO classification of tumours of haematopoietic and lymphoid tissues. IARC; 2017.
3. Döhner H, Estey E, Grimwade D, Amadori S, Appelbaum FR, Büchner T, et al. Diagnosis and management of AML in adults: 2017 ELN recommendations from an international expert panel. Blood. 2017;129:424–47.
4. Bénet C, Gomez A, Aguilar C, Delattre C, Vergier B, Beylot-Barry M, et al. Histologic and immunohistologic characterization of skin localization of myeloid disorders: a study of 173 cases. Am J Clin Pathol. 2011;135:278–90.
5. Cho-Vega JH, Medeiros LJ, Prieto VG, Vega F. Leukemia cutis. Am J Clin Pathol. 2008;129:130–42.
6. Cerroni L, Zenahlik P, Höfler G, Kaddu S, Smolle J, Kerl H. Specific cutaneous infiltrates of B-cell chronic lymphocytic leukemia: a clinicopathologic and prognostic study of 42 patients. Am J Surg Pathol. 1996;20:1000–10.
7. Agis H, Weltermann A, Fonatsch C, Haas O, Mitterbauer G, Müllauer L, et al. A comparative study on demographic, hematological, and cytogenetic findings and prognosis in acute myeloid leukemia with and without leukemia cutis. Ann Hematol. 2002;81:90–5.
8. Findakly D. Leukemia cutis: a systematic review. Blood. 2020;136:1–1.
9. Vitte F, Fabiani B, Bénet C, Dalac S, Balme B, Delattre C, et al. Specific skin lesions in chronic myelomonocytic leukemia: a spectrum of myelomonocytic and dendritic cell proliferations: a study of 42 cases. Am J Surg Pathol. 2012;36:1302–16.
10. Horlick HP, Silvers DN, Knobler EH, Cole JT. Acute myelomonocytic leukemia presenting as a benign-appearing cutaneous eruption. Arch Dermatol. 1990;126:653–6.
11. Kaddu S, Zenahlik P, Beham-Schmid C, Kerl H, Cerroni L. Specific cutaneous infiltrates in patients with myelogenous leukemia: a clinicopathologic study of 26 patients with assessment of diagnostic criteria. J Am Acad Dermatol. 1999;40:966–78.
12. Dyachenko P, Rozenman D, Bennett M. Unusual skin and testicular lesions in a patient with CMML. Eur J Intern Med. 2006;17:290–1.
13. Copplestone JA, Oscier DG, Mufti GJ, Hamblin TJ. Monocytic skin infiltration in chronic myelomonocytic leukaemia. Clin Lab Haematol. 1986;8:115–9.
14. Braga D, Manganoni AM, Boccaletti V, Pancera C, Marocolo D, Facchetti F, et al. Specific skin infiltration as first sign of chronic myelomonocytic leukemia with an unusual phenotype. J Am Acad Dermatol. 1996;35:804–7.
15. Elenitoba-Johnson K, Hodges GF, King TC, Wu CD, Medeiros LJ. Extramedullary myeloid cell tumors arising in the setting of chronic myelomonocytic leukemia. A report of two cases. Arch Pathol Lab Med. 1996;120:62–7.
16. Resnik KS, Brod BB. Leukemia cutis in congenital leukemia. Analysis and review of the world literature with report of an additional case. Arch Dermatol. 1993;129:1301–6.
17. Tallman MS, Hakimian D, Shaw JM, Lissner GS, Russell EJ, Variakojis D. Granulocytic sarcoma is associated with the 8;21 translocation in acute myeloid leukemia. J Clin Oncol. 1993;11:690–7.
18. Harris AC, Kitko CL, Couriel DR, Braun TM, Choi SW, Magenau J, et al. Extramedullary relapse of acute myeloid leukemia following allogeneic hematopoietic stem cell transplantation: incidence, risk factors and outcomes. Haematologica. 2013;98:179–84.
19. Solh M, DeFor TE, Weisdorf DJ, Kaufman DS. Extramedullary relapse of acute myelogenous leukemia after allogeneic hematopoietic stem cell transplantation: better prognosis than systemic relapse. Biol Blood Marrow Transplant. 2012;18:106–12.
20. Yoshihara S, Ando T, Ogawa H. Extramedullary relapse of acute myeloid leukemia after allogeneic hematopoietic stem cell transplantation: an easily overlooked but significant pattern of relapse. Biol Blood Marrow Transplant. 2012;18:1800–7.
21. Sakellari I, Gavriilaki E, Batsis I, Mallouri D, Gavriilaki M, Apostolou C, et al. Isolated extramedullary relapse as a poor predictor of survival after allogeneic hematopoietic cell transplantation for acute leukemia. Biol Blood Marrow Transplant. 2019;25:1756–60.
22. Siegel RS, Gartenhaus RB, Kuzel TM. Human T-cell lymphotropic-I-associated leukemia/lymphoma. Curr Treat Options Oncol. 2001;2:291–300.
23. Dosaka N, Tanaka T, Miyachi Y, Imamura S, Kakizuka A. Examination of HTLV-I integration in the skin lesions of various types of adult T-cell leukemia

(ATL): independence of cutaneous-type ATL confirmed by Southern blot analysis. J Invest Dermatol. 1991;96:196–200.
24. Magro CM, Morrison CD, Heerema N, Porcu P, Sroa N, Deng AC. T-cell prolymphocytic leukemia: an aggressive T cell malignancy with frequent cutaneous tropism. J Am Acad Dermatol. 2006;55:467–77.
25. Su WP. Clinical, histopathologic, and immunohistochemical correlations in leukemia cutis. Semin Dermatol. 1994;13:223–30.
26. Baer MR, Barcos M, Farrell H, Raza A, Preisler HD. Acute myelogenous leukemia with leukemia cutis. Eighteen cases seen between 1969 and 1986. Cancer. 1989;63:2192–200.
27. Hirner JP, O'Malley JT, LeBoeuf NR. Blastic plasmacytoid dendritic cell neoplasm: the dermatologist's perspective. Hematol Oncol Clin North Am. 2020;34:501–9.
28. Aboutalebi A, Korman JB, Sohani AR, Hasserjian RP, Louissaint A Jr, Le L, et al. Aleukemic cutaneous myeloid sarcoma. J Cutan Pathol. 2013;40:996–1005.
29. Huang YYM, Liu M, Ruth JS, Potenziani S, Hsu S. Precursor-B-cell-ALL leukemia cutis resembling lipomas: an atypical presentation of a rare entity and a review of the literature. Dermatol Online J. 2017;23:13030/qt6bs2d542.
30. Huang C, Fei S, Yao J, Chen P, Luo J, Wang Y, et al. Breast myeloid sarcoma presenting as a palpable breast lump after allogeneic stem cell transplantation for acute myelomonocytic leukemia: a rare case report. World J Surg Oncol. 2021;19:289.
31. López-Valverde N, López-Valverde A, Gómez-de Diego R, Ramírez JM, Flores-Fraile J, Muriel-Fernández J. Gingival hyperplasia as an early manifestation of acute myeloid leukemia. A retrospective review. J Clin Exp Dent. 2019;11:e1139–42.
32. Dreizen S, McCredie KB, Keating MJ, Luna MA. Malignant gingival and skin "infiltrates" in adult leukemia. Oral Surg Oral Med Oral Pathol. 1983;55:572–9.
33. Du AX, Hung T, Surmanowicz P, Gniadecki R. Diagnostic challenge of aleukemic leukemia cutis preceding acute myelogenous leukemia: a case report. SAGE Open Med Case Rep. 2020;8:2050313X20919638.
34. Klco JM, Welch JS, Nguyen TT, Hurley MY, Kreisel FH, Hassan A, et al. State of the art in myeloid sarcoma. Int J Lab Hematol. 2011;33:555–65.
35. Pileri SA, Ascani S, Cox MC, Campidelli C, Bacci F, Piccioli M, et al. Myeloid sarcoma: clinicopathologic, phenotypic and cytogenetic analysis of 92 adult patients. Leukemia. 2007;21:340–50.
36. Neiman RS, Barcos M, Berard C, Bonner H, Mann R, Rydell RE, et al. Granulocytic sarcoma: a clinicopathologic study of 61 biopsied cases. Cancer. 1981;48:1426–37.
37. Byrd JC, Edenfield WJ, Shields DJ, Dawson NA. Extramedullary myeloid cell tumors in acute nonlymphocytic leukemia: a clinical review. J Clin Oncol. 1995;13:1800–16.
38. Paydaş S, Zorludemir S, Sahin B. Vasculitis and leukemia. Leuk Lymphoma. 2000;40:105–12.
39. Mathew RA, Bennett JM, Liu JJ, Komrokji RS, Lancet JE, Naghashpour M, et al. Cutaneous manifestations in CMML: indication of disease acceleration or transformation to AML and review of the literature. Leuk Res. 2012;36:72–80.
40. Cronin DMP, George TI, Sundram UN. An updated approach to the diagnosis of myeloid leukemia cutis. Am J Clin Pathol. 2009;132:101–10.
41. Bakst RL, Tallman MS, Douer D, Yahalom J. How I treat extramedullary acute myeloid leukemia. Blood. 2011;118:3785–93.
42. Welch JS, Ley TJ, Link DC, Miller CA, Larson DE, Koboldt DC, et al. The origin and evolution of mutations in acute myeloid leukemia. Cell. 2012;150:264–78.
43. Ansari-Lari MA, Yang C-F, Tinawi-Aljundi R, Cooper L, Long P, Allan RH, et al. FLT3 mutations in myeloid sarcoma. Br J Haematol. 2004;126:785–91.
44. Faaij CMJM, Willemze AJ, Révész T, Balzarolo M, Tensen CP, Hoogeboom M, et al. Chemokine/chemokine receptor interactions in extramedullary leukaemia of the skin in childhood AML: differential roles for CCR2, CCR5, CXCR4 and CXCR7. Pediatr Blood Cancer. 2010;55:344–8.
45. Burger JA, Bürkle A. The CXCR4 chemokine receptor in acute and chronic leukaemia: a marrow homing receptor and potential therapeutic target. Br J Haematol. 2007;137:288–96.
46. Petrella T, Meijer CJLM, Dalac S, Willemze R, Maynadié M, Machet L, et al. TCL1 and CLA expression in agranular CD4/CD56 hematodermic neoplasms (blastic NK-cell lymphomas) and leukemia cutis. Am J Clin Pathol. 2004;122:307–13.
47. Wang CX, Pusic I, Anadkat MJ. Association of leukemia cutis with survival in acute myeloid leukemia. JAMA Dermatol. 2019;155:826–32.
48. Bakst R, Wolden S, Yahalom J. Radiation therapy for chloroma (granulocytic sarcoma). Int J Radiat Oncol Biol Phys. 2012;82:1816–22.
49. Yamauchi K, Yasuda M. Comparison in treatments of nonleukemic granulocytic sarcoma: report of two cases and a review of 72 cases in the literature. Cancer. 2002;94:1739–46.
50. Tsimberidou A-M, Kantarjian HM, Estey E, Cortes JE, Verstovsek S, Faderl S, et al. Outcome in patients with nonleukemic granulocytic sarcoma treated with chemotherapy with or without radiotherapy. Leukemia. 2003;17:1100–3.
51. Lan T-Y, Lin D-T, Tien H-F, Yang R-S, Chen C-Y, Wu K. Prognostic factors of treatment outcomes in patients with granulocytic sarcoma. Acta Haematol. 2009;122:238–46.

3 Malignant Lymphoid Neoplasms Infiltrating the Skin

Robert Gniadecki, Minakshi Taparia, Jean Deschenes, Jori Hardin, and Etienne Mahe

3.1 Practice Essentials

- Malignant skin infiltration can occur in any lymphoid neoplasm. Chronic lymphocytic leukemia (CLL), T-cell prolymphocytic leukemia (T-PLL), adult T-cell leukemia lymphoma (ATLL), angioimmunoblastic T-cell lymphoma (AITL), intravascular large B-cell lymphoma (IV-LBCL), and lymphomatoid granulomatosis (LyG) have the highest incidence of skin involvement.
- Skin involvement is synchronous with systemic leukemia/lymphoma and often occurs late during the progression of hematological cancer. Exceptions are ATLL, anaplastic large cell lymphoma (ALCL), and follicular lymphoma (FCL) where skin may be the first clinical sign of the systemic disease.
- Skin infiltration in CLL, lymphoplasmacytic lymphoma/Waldenström's macroglobulinemia (LPL/WM), and FCL may be a manifestation of large-cell transformation.
- Clinical manifestations of neoplastic lymphoid skin involvement vary from solitary tumors and nodules to disseminated lesions and erythroderma.
- Diagnosis relies on skin and peripheral blood phenotyping and clinicopathological correlation.
- Radiotherapy or surgical excision can be used in addition to systemic therapy.

In this chapter, we will focus on skin infiltrations that occur due to the presence of malignant lymphocytic cells, which are secondary to nodal systemic lymphomas or lymphoid leukemias. It is important to distinguish these secondary infiltrations from the well-established category of primary cutaneous lymphomas, where the skin is considered the primary site of the disease, and systemic involvement is not detectable for at least 6 months after the onset of skin lesions (for more details, see Chap. 5). Simply having malignant lymphocytes present in the skin is not enough to

R. Gniadecki (✉)
Division of Dermatology, University of Alberta, Edmonton, AB, Canada
e-mail: r.gniadecki@ualberta.ca

M. Taparia
Division of Hematology, University of Alberta Hospital, Edmonton, AB, Canada

J. Deschenes
Department of Pathology and Laboratory Medicine, Cross Cancer Institute, Edmonton, AB, Canada
e-mail: Jean.Deschenes@albertaprecisionlabs.ca

J. Hardin
Division of Dermatology, University of Calgary, Calgary, AB, Canada
e-mail: Jori.hardin@albertahealthservices.ca

E. Mahe
Department of Pathology & Laboratory Medicine, and Hematology & Hematological Malignancies, University of Calgary, Calgary, AB, Canada
e-mail: etienne.mahe@albertaprecisionlabs.ca

R. Gniadecki et al. (eds.), *Diseases of Blood and Skin*, https://doi.org/10.1007/978-3-031-65292-9_3

make a diagnosis of secondary skin involvement. To qualify as a secondary skin infiltration, the detected malignant lymphocytes must exhibit infiltrative growth or disrupt the normal architecture of the skin, thus ruling out instances where small amounts of malignant cells merely pass through the skin without actively invading it.

Some experts consider secondary malignant infiltrations caused by lymphocytic leukemias as a subtype of leukemia cutis. However, as previously discussed in Chap. 2, in clinical parlance, we tend to reserve the term "leukemia cutis" for myeloid leukemias and instead use the term "leukemic/lymphomatous infiltration" when discussing lymphocytic neoplasms. Consequently, cutaneous myeloid leukemia infiltrates and lymphomatous infiltrations can be thought of as extramedullary leukemias and extranodal lymphomas localized within the skin, respectively.

3.2 Incidence and Disease Associations

Almost any lymphoid leukemia or lymphoma may secondarily colonize the skin; however, certain lymphoid neoplasms have a significantly higher tendency to involve the skin (Table 3.1) [3–6].

The risk of skin involvement is notably elevated in chronic lymphocytic leukemia (CLL), ranging from 4% to 20%. Additionally, there are two rare mature T-cell neoplasms—adult T-cell leukemia/lymphoma (ATLL), T-cell prolymphocytic leukemia (T-PLL), and one B-cell neoplasm, lymphomatoid granulomatosis (LyG)—where the risk of skin involvement is particularly high, ranging from 20% to 70%.

In contrast, in lymphocytic leukemias derived from precursor B or T cells such as T- or B-cell lymphoblastic leukemia/lymphoma (T-ALL or

Table 3.1 Secondary infiltrates in the skin by lymphoma or lymphoid leukemia

Condition	Probability of clinically apparent skin involvement[a]
Precursor leukemias: B- or T-ALL	+ (<3%)
Hodgkin lymphoma	+ (0.5–3.4%) [1, 2]
B-cell leukemias and lymphomas	
CLL	++ (4–20%)
Mantle cell lymphoma	+ (late-stage disease)
Follicular lymphoma	++
Intravascular large B-cell lymphoma (IV-LBCL)	+++
Lymphomatoid granulomatosis (LyG)	+++ (40–50% of patients)
Plasmablastic lymphoma	+ (4%)
Plasma cell neoplasms (Chap. 4)	Skin pathology due to paraproteinemia is reviewed in Chap. 4
Lymphoplasmacytic lymphoma/Waldenstrom's macroglobulinemia (LPL/WM)	+ (in WM with large cell transformation skin involvement is 12%)
Plasmacytoma	+
Plasma cell myeloma	+ (<2%, advanced disease)
T-cell and NK/T-cell lymphomas	
Anaplastic large cell lymphoma	++
Angioimmunoblastic lymphoma (AITL)	+ (paraneoplastic and reactive skin conditions are common)
Peripheral T-cell lymphoma NOS	+
ATLL	+++ (20–70%)
T-PLL	+++
Intravascular NK/T-cell lymphoma	+++
Extranodal NK/T cell lymphoma	+++ see Chap. 8

[a] Strength of association: + occasional <4%, ++ frequent 5–20%, +++ very frequent >20%

B-ALL), skin involvement is a rare phenomenon, occurring in 1–3% of patients with this disease [5].

It's important to note that unlike (myeloid) leukemia cutis, which can sometimes occur without evidence of systemic leukemia, the majority of secondary malignant lymphocytic infiltrations in the skin tend to be synchronous with the presence of lymph nodes or bone marrow involvement.

3.3 Clinical Presentation (Figs. 3.1, 3.2, 3.3, 3.4 and 3.5)

Skin lesions resulting from secondary malignant lymphocytic infiltrations exhibit a wide range of morphological characteristics and distribution patterns, similar to those seen in leukemia cutis. The most frequently encountered skin lesions include red plaques, papules, or nodules. However, they can also present as early-stage dermatitis, maculopapular rashes, or even erythroderma [1, 2, 7–13]. These lesions typically have minimal or no secondary changes such as scaling because secondary lymphocytic infiltrates tend to localize in the dermis and subcutis without affecting the epidermis. This is in contrast to many primary cutaneous lymphomas,

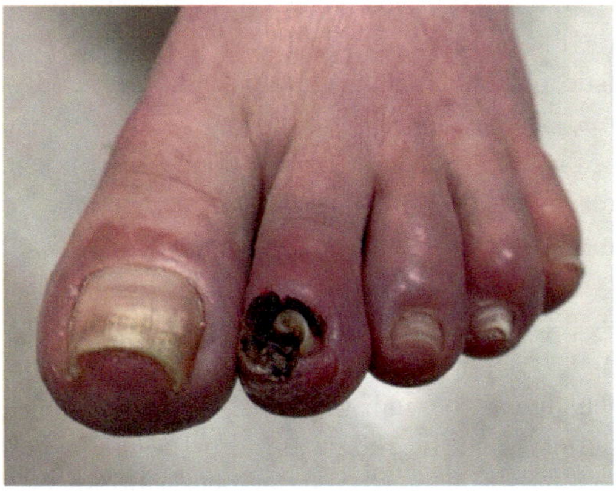

Fig. 3.1 Leukemic infiltrations of the toes in a patient with CLL, mimicking chilblains

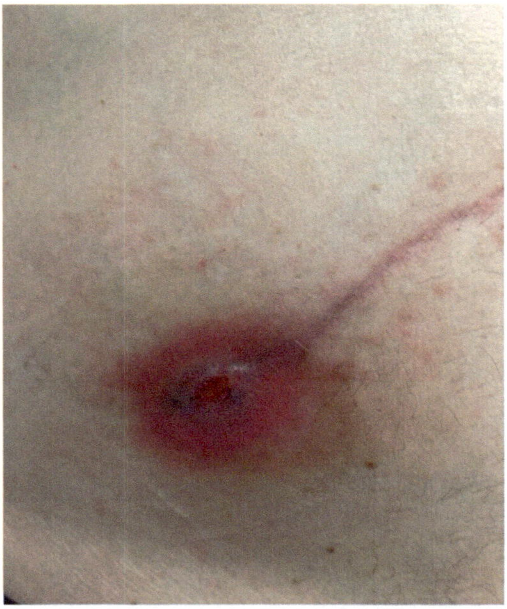

Fig. 3.2 Patient with nodal follicular B-cell lymphoma with skin involvement near a surgical scar. Clinically, there is a painful deep nodule with central necrosis

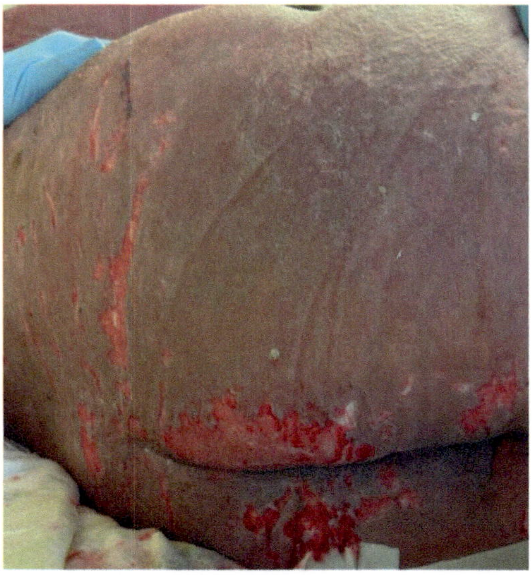

Fig. 3.3 Severe skin infiltration in a patient with advanced angioimmunoblastic lymphoma (AITL). Note dusky brown skin color, epidermal necrosis and ulcerations mimicking toxic epidermal necrolysis

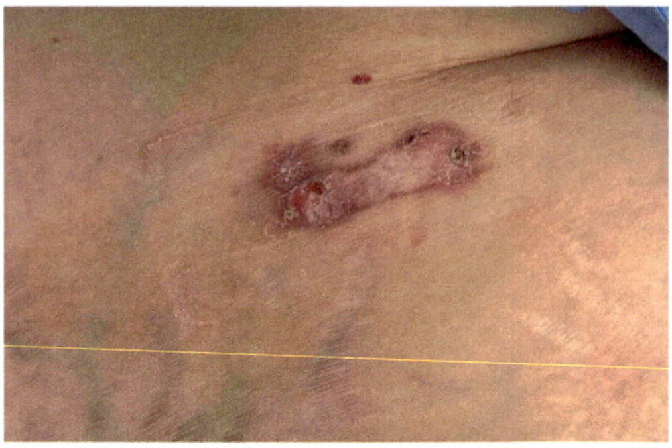

Fig. 3.4 A flat, fibrotic plaque with raised borders on the abdomen representing lymphomatous skin involvement in a patient with nodal anaplastic large cell lymphoma

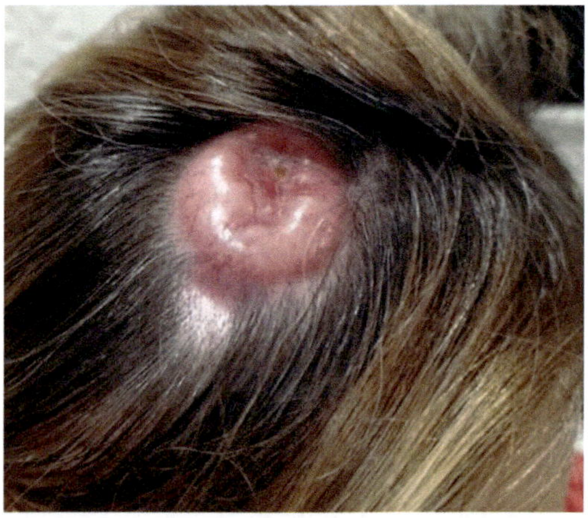

Fig. 3.5 Secondary skin infiltration by nodal follicular lymphoma. A 49-year-old woman developed a 3 cm pink tumor with telangiectasias and central ulceration on the parietal scalp. The biopsy of the lesion was obtained, which showed a B-cell follicular lymphoma with the phenotype $CD20^+$ $bcl\text{-}6^+$ $CD10^-$ with a patchy bcl-2 expression. The Ki67 was positive in approximately 40% of cells. IgH rearrangement was monoclonal. Note that skin infiltrates from nodal FCL are clinically indistinguishable from primary cutaneous FCL and both present with pink-red nodules and tumors, often on the scalp or upper trunk. CD10 staining does not discriminate between primary and secondary lymphomas with confidence and patchy bcl-2 positivity should raise a suspicion of a nodal lymphoma, even in patients with no clinically palpable lymph nodes. In this case, we performed total body PET-CT, which revealed ^{18}F-FDG uptake diffusely in the bone marrow and in retroperitoneal lymph nodes. Bone marrow biopsy confirmed the diagnosis of systemic FCL. The patient was treated with R-CHOP, which resulted in full remission of skin, lymph node, and bone marrow involvement

which often exhibit epidermotropism. Additionally, these secondary lesions are generally less hemorrhagic and necrotic compared to those seen in acute myeloid leukemia (AML).

Similar to myeloid leukemia cutis, lymphocytic infiltrates may mimic benign skin conditions such as rosacea, alopecia areata, Jessner lymphocytic infiltration, lupus erythematosus, granuloma annulare, or erythema multiforme. In such cases, clinicians should consider a low threshold for obtaining a skin biopsy [6].

3.3.1 Lymphomas and Leukemias with Common Skin Involvement: CLL, T-PLL, ATLL, LyG, Intravascular Lymphoma

Chronic lymphocytic leukemia (CLL) (Fig. 3.1): Skin infiltrates in CLL typically appear 3–4 years after the initial leukemia diagnosis. These lesions are often violaceous or dark-red plaques and nodules and tend to localize on the face, ears, and genitals. They also have a tendency to occur in areas affected by previous skin trauma, infections, or other skin conditions, such as actinic keratoses or keratinocyte carcinomas. Consequently, CLL infiltrates are occasionally discovered incidentally in skin cancer excision biopsies [6, 7, 14].

Adult T-cell leukemia/lymphoma (ATLL) (Fig. 3.3): Skin involvement is common early in the course of ATLL. In addition to the characteristic papular, nodular, tumoral, and erythrodermic lesions, skin purpura and ichthyosis-like scaling have been described. These lesions can resemble psoriasis, erythema multiforme, or mycosis fungoides (primary cutaneous T-cell lymphoma) and may be scaly and annular [15].

T-cell prolymphocytic leukemia (T-PLL): T-PLL is often associated with erythroderma, which can be indistinguishable from erythroderma seen in Sézary syndrome (SS). Skin involvement may also present with a diffuse, erythematous papular rash that evolves into purpuric and hemorrhagic lesions [4].

Lymphomatoid granulomatosis (LyG): This EBV-driven B-cell lymphoproliferative disease often affects individuals in middle age (40–60 years). More than 30% of patients with lymphomatoid granulomatosis have skin involvement, typically presenting as disseminated papules, nodules, or plaques [16].

Intravascular large B-cell lymphoma (IV-LBCL): Approximately 50% of patients with IV-LBCL develop skin lesions. These lesions are typically indurated, painful, and poorly demarcated, appearing as plaques, nodules, tumors, or deep panniculitic lesions, often with a violaceous color. Some patients may develop livedo racemosa and ulcerations due to vascular occlusion. While most cases involve disseminated lesions, there are reports of single lesions. Approximately 25% of patients present with the disease limited to the skin, referred to as the "cutaneous variant" of IV-LBCL, which has a better prognosis [17]. Patients with IV-LBCL are at risk for hemophagocytic lymphohistiocytosis (HLH), a hemophagocytic syndrome that manifests with multiorgan failure, hepatosplenomegaly, pancytopenia, accompanied by bone marrow infiltration and in a small number of cases CNS involvement. HLH in the setting of intravascular lymphoma has a median survival of 2–8 months [18].

Intravascular NK/T-cell lymphoma: This very rare, EBV-positive, aggressive lymphoma is not officially recognized as a distinct entity in current classifications of hematolymphoid neoplasms. It often affects the skin similarly to IV-LBCL. Clinical manifestations are similar, and differentiation between these entities relies on immunohistochemical markers [17, 19, 20] (Fig. 3.2).

In addition to these lymphomas and leukemias, there are other lymphomas with skin manifestations worth mentioning:

- In angioimmunoblastic lymphoma (AITL) (Fig. 3.3), direct skin infiltrations with leukemic cells are infrequent, but patients often develop various skin lesions representing paraneoplastic phenomena and autoimmune reactions [8, 21].
- Plasma cell neoplasms with coexisting monoclonal gammopathy rarely involve malignant plasma cell infiltrations in the skin, but skin manifestations due to paraproteinemia are common (see Chap. 4).
  Specifically, in multiple myeloma, plasma cell infiltrations forming violaceous plaques and tumors may occur in the late stage of the disease and have a poor prognosis. Some reports suggest that a solitary plasmacytoma of the bone can directly extend to the overlying skin, although reliable documentation of this phenomenon is lacking and might represent AESOP syndrome (adenopathy and extensive skin patch overlying a plasmacytoma [22]) rather than a true malignant plasma cell infiltration [9, 23].
- Waldenström's macroglobulinemia may manifest as lymphoplasmacytic infiltrates in the skin, appearing as violaceous plaques and nodules, often on the face and sometimes with striking symmetry resembling rosacea or lupus erythematosus [24].
- Skin involvement in Hodgkin lymphoma is very rare, and if it occurs at all, it does so in the advanced stages of the disease, with most patients experiencing a rapid decline in health following the development of skin lesions [1].
- In anaplastic large cell lymphoma (ALCL) and follicular lymphoma (FCL), skin involvement may be the initial sign of systemic disease. Proper differentiation from primary cutaneous ALCL/FCL is essential for appropriate management (discussed in Chap. 5) (Fig. 3.4).

3.4 Diagnostic Workup

Key diagnostic features that can help differentiate between different lymphoid neoplasms are summarized in Table 3.2.

Table 3.2 Key diagnostic phenotypic features of lymphoid malignant infiltrations of the skin

Underlying condition	Typical diagnostic morphological and phenotypic patterns
B-lymphoblastic leukemia/ lymphoma	CD19, CD22, PAX5, TdT, CD10, CD34, HLA-DR, CD79a, CD20, Negative for myeloperoxidase or lysozyme
T-lymphoblastic leukemia/ lymphoma	TdT, CD1a, cytoplasmic CD3, CD7, CD99, CD34, CD4, CD8 (double positive for CD4 and CD8 in 25% of cases), CD2, CD5, negative for myeloperoxidase or lysozyme
Hodgkin lymphoma	Reed-Sternberg cells in the skin are $CD30^{+}$, $CD15^{+}$, $MUM1^{+}$, $PAX5^{dim}$, $CD45^{-}$. Skin infiltrate phenotype does not always faithfully replicate the nodal disease (e.g., Negative CD15 in RS cells, in view of $CD15^{+}$ nodal disease) [13]
B-cell leukemias and lymphomas	
CLL	CD5 (but not CD3), CD23, CD43, CD200, LEF1
	Variable expression of B-cell markers CD19, CD20 (usually dim), CD79a. Negative for SOX11 and CD10; negative or minimal focal expression of Cyclin D1
Mantle cell lymphoma	CD19, CD20, CD5, SOX11, CD43, Cyclin D1
Follicular lymphoma	CD20, CD10 (90%), BCL6, CD23, BCL-2 (large fraction of grade 3 and cutaneous FL are BCL-2 negative)
	Negative for CD5, CD43, and Cyclin D1
Large B-cell lymphoma—intravascular type	Intravascular malignant lymphoid cells with occlusion and destruction of the vessel. Variable expression of B-cell markers CD20, CD79a, PAX5, BCL2, MUM1, subset positive for CD5 (approximately 30% of cases)
Lymphomatoid granulomatosis	Polymorphic infiltrate of atypical lymphoid cells, angiocentricity, angiodestruction, coagulative necrosis, larger cells are positive for CD20, CD30 (variable) and Epstein-Barr virus-encoded RNA by in situ hybridization (EBER-ISH) is positive. Background cells are $CD3^{+}$ T cells
T-cell lymphomas	
Anaplastic large cell lymphoma	Strong and diffuse CD30, EMA, ALK1, variable T-cell markers (CD2, CD4, CD5 more common), CD43, cytotoxic markers such as granzyme/TIA1 and perforin. Negative for PAX5, other B-cell markers, and EBER-ISH
AITL [25]	CD3, CD4, CD2, CD5, CD7, CXCL13, PD-1, CD10, Bcl-6
	Variable CD30 on immunoblastic cells
Peripheral T-cell lymphoma NOS	Variable expression of CD3, CD2, CD5, usually CD4 but may be CD8 and may demonstrate cytotoxic phenotype (TIA-1, granzyme, perforin)
ATLL	CD2, CD3, CD5, CD4, CD25, CD30 and CD52 variable; positive serology for HTLV-I/II
	CD8 usually negative but rare cases $CD4^{+}$ and $CD8^{+}$
	Negative for CD7, TdT, ALK1, TCL1, cytotoxic molecules
	May simulate MF, T-PLL and T-cell lymphoma, NOS (see below)
T-PLL	CD2, CD3, CD5, CD7, CD52, $TCL1^{+}$; CD30 is negative
	25%: $CD4^{+}$ and CD8; 60%: $CD4^{+}$ and $CD8^{-}$; 15%: $CD8^{+}$ and $CD4^{-}$
Disorders with plasmacytoid cells	
Lymphoplasmacytic/ Waldenström macroglobulinemia (LPL/WM) or marginal zone lymphoma	Subset of $CD20^{+}$/$PAX5^{+}$ small lymphocytes, which are usually negative for CD103, CD23 (not uncommonly positive), CD5 and CD10, accompanied by a subset of CD138/$CD45^{+}$ plasma cells which are negative for CD56, Cyclin D1 and may be $PAX5^{+}$/$MUM1^{+}$. Useful molecular testing, positive for the MYD88 L265P alteration in 95% of LPL/WM; no bony lytic lesions
Multiple myeloma	CD79a/$CD138^{+}$ plasmacytoid cells, with monotypic κ or λ immunoglobulin light chain expression, variably CD56, CD117 and cyclin D1 positive

3.4.1 Clinicopathological Correlations

The identification of a lymphocytic infiltrate in the skin can present considerable diagnostic challenges. Even in patients with a confirmed lymphoid malignancy, it is important to determine whether the skin lesion represents a reactive process or direct invasion by malignant cells. Clinicopathological correlation is essential in such cases. Furthermore, the phenotypic characteristics of malignant cells in the skin may not always precisely mirror those found in lymph nodes, which can raise questions about whether the skin lesion represents a secondary, coexisting lymphoma or a phenotypically distinct clone of the underlying malignancy. Below, we have outlined some common diagnostic issues:

1. **Incidental finding of CLL-like cells in a skin biopsy of a patient with normal blood counts.** Unlike myeloid leukemia cutis, which can precede the development of intramedullary acute myeloid leukemia (AML), CLL infiltrates in the skin typically indicate concurrent leukemia. However, CLL-like skin infiltrates have been reported in patients with CLL/SLL-type monoclonal B-cell lymphocytosis (MBL). This entity is characterized by the presence of a clonal B-cell population in the peripheral blood, showing a CLL/SLL-like phenotype, which does not exceed 5×10^9/L and is not accompanied by other signs of lymphoproliferative disease. In these cases, it is advisable to obtain peripheral blood for flow cytometry analysis to confirm the presence of a CLL-like population and precisely quantify them. Full staging should be considered to rule out concurrent small lymphocytic lymphoma, with secondary involvement of the skin. If the diagnosis of CLL/SLL-type MBL is confirmed (i.e., the lymph nodes are not abnormal and no evidence of soft tissue involvement is detected), and hence the skin appears to be the sole tissue involved by the abnormal population, the concept of "tissue (skin) MBL" may be considered. Systemic treatment is not usually necessary for MBL with limited skin involvement as the risk of progression to CLL is deemed to be low, and skin involvement does not predict aggressive disease [26–28]. However, such cases may rarely progress, hence clinical follow-up is recommended. The factors determining the risk of progression to lymphoma or CLL in this situation remain unclear, although the degree of infiltration has been proposed as a criterion to suggest a diagnosis of small lymphocytic lymphoma (SLL) rather than "MBL with skin involvement" when there is massive skin replacement by the abnormal population.
2. **Differentiation between Sézary's syndrome and systemic leukemia/lymphoma in patients with erythroderma** (Table 3.3). Primary cutaneous lymphoma, specifically Sézary's syndrome (SS), is the most common cause of erythroderma and is characterized by leukemic (usually $CD4^+$) T-cells in peripheral blood (see Chap. 7). However, erythroderma can also be associated with several systemic lymphomas, particularly adult T-cell leukemia/lymphoma (ATLL), T-cell prolymphocytic leukemia (T-PLL), and angioimmunoblastic T-cell lymphoma (AITL), all of which can lead to an increase in CD4/CD8 ratio and an absolute increase in CD4 cells. These diseases are most prevalent in males in their fifth and sixth decades of life. Skin biopsy results in erythrodermic cases may or may not reveal the presence of malignant cells, so diagnosis relies on the correlation between clinical signs, peripheral blood flow cytometry, and T-cell gene rearrangement analysis. Flow cytometry or immunohistochemistry can be particularly useful in distinguishing TCL1-positive T-PLL from TCL1-negative leukemias such as SS, ATLL, and leukemic peripheral T-cell lymphoma (PTCL) [29, 30].
3. **Skin nodule or tumor with plasma cell prominence in a patient with monoclonal gammopathy or hypergammaglobulinemia.** The differential diagnosis can be broad and is summarized in Table 3.4. An important distinguishing feature is whether the hypergammaglobulinemia is monoclonal or polyclonal, as the latter is typically secondary to another underlying process, which is generally non-neoplastic.

3.4.1.1 Differential Diagnosis of Intravascular Lymphoma

In the case of intravascular lymphoma, it's crucial to differentiate it from clinically benign lesions such as type E LyP (angiocentric) and CD30-positive intravascular lymphoproliferative disorders (IVLPD). Detailed examination and diagnostic tests are essential to make the distinction (see also Chap. 9). See Table 3.5.

Table 3.3 Differential diagnosis between malignant diseases causing erythroderma

Feature	SS	ATLL	T-PLL	AITL
B-symptoms	–	+/– (absent in smoldering and chronic types)	+	+
Hepatosplenomegaly	–	+/– (absent in smoldering and mild in chronic types)	+	+
Pleural effusions	–	+/– (absent in smoldering type)	+	+
Histopathological skin involvement	Changes may be subtle or nonspecific. Variable (often absent) epidermotropism. Phenotype mirrors peripheral blood Sézary cells	Epidermotropic infiltrate simulating SS both morphologically and phenotypically	Epidermotropic infiltrate simulating SS. Positive IHC for TCL1, positive for CD7	Subtle changes. Epidermotropism absent. Malignant cells with T_{FH} phenotype (see below), frequent EBER-ISH$^+$. CD30 may be positive in a subset of cells
Peripheral blood lymphocytes and related phenotype	Leukocyte count often normal	Chronic and acute variants have lymphocytosis	Leukocytosis	CD3^{dim} CD4$^+$ CD5$^+$, CD7$^+$, CD10$^+$ CXCL13$^+$, PD-1$^+$
	CD3$^+$ CD4$^+$ CD7$^-$ CD26$^-$ PD-1$^{+/-}$ CD4/CD8 ratio > 10	CD2$^+$, CD3$^+$, CD5$^+$, CD4$^+$ CD7$^-$ CD25$^+$ CD26$^-$, mostly CD8$^-$. Acute leukemic cases show typical "flower cells"	CD3^{dim} CD4$^+$ (occasionally CD8$^+$ or CD4$^+$8$^+$, see above) CD5$^+$ CD7$^+$ TCL1 rearrangement detected by FISH or demonstration of equivalent/related abnormal karyotype by conventional cytogenetics, CD52$^+$	CD4/CD8 ratio < 5
HTLV-1/2 serology or molecular detection of viral genome	–	+	–	–
TCR rearrangement	Monoclonal	Monoclonal	Monoclonal	Variable
Other	Lymphadenopathy and frequent pruritus	Hypercalcemia and elevated LDH frequent. Occasional lytic bone lesions	Diagnosis requires more than 5 × 10^9/L abnormal lymphocytes in peripheral blood, T-cell monoclonality and appropriate cytogenetics findings or surrogate abnormal IHC	Cutaneous lesions may be extremely difficult to diagnose as malignant
	Absence of systemic symptoms otherwise Some cases are preceded by mycosis fungoides (MF), designated as "SS preceded by MF"	Rare primary cutaneous type: no hypercalcemia, no lymphadenopathy nor hepatosplenomegaly, and no peripheral blood component		

Table 3.4 Differential diagnosis of skin nodules with plasma cell prominence

Disease	Clinical features	Paraprotein	Skin biopsy
LPL/WM	B-symptoms, lymphadenopathy, bleeding	Monotypic IgM (vast majority, rare cases with IgG or IgA)	Atypical B cells
Plasma cell myeloma	B-symptoms, bone pain. Skin involvement in late, advanced disease	Monotypic: IgG > IgA > light chain > IgD, IgE, IgM, and others	Atypical plasma cells
Cutaneous and systemic plasmacytosis (Chap. 4)	None or mild symptoms. Lymphadenopathy may be present	Polytypic/polyclonal light chain expression	Polyclonal, mature plasma cells without atypia
IgG4-related disease (Chap. 15)	Multiorgan involvement (lymph nodes, salivary glands, thyroid, retroperitoneum)	Polytypic/polyclonal light chain expression	Deep lymphoplasmacytic infiltrate, numerous IgG4$^+$ plasma cells without atypia
Multicentric Castleman disease (mCD) (Chap. 15)	Severe lymphadenopathy, constitutional symptoms, hepatomegaly, anemia, cytopenias. A subset of MCD is associated with the POEMS syndrome, showing cutaneous hyperpigmentation, hypertrichosis, glomeruloid angiomata, plethora, acrocyanosis, white nails, sclerodermoid changes and clubbing HHV8 may be positive in a subset of MCD, especially in immunosuppressed patients or with HIV infection	Polytypic light chains expression or apparent monotypic (IgM, λ) plasma cell phenotype; B and T cells are usually polyclonal, with rare exceptions (HIV$^+$ or immunosuppressed patients)	Reactive lymphoid follicular hyperplasia with numerous plasma cells without atypia

Table 3.5 Differential diagnosis of intravascular lymphoid lesions

	Intravascular large B-cell lymphoma	Intravascular NK/T-cell lymphoma	Lymphomatoid papulosis type E	Benign CD30$^+$ intravascular lymphoproliferative disease [31]
Lesions	Deep panniculitic infiltrates, livedo, ulcerations		Ulcerated papules, widespread or agminated	Prior inflammatory skin disease, area of trauma
Course, prognosis	Progressive, systemic dissemination, high mortality. Neurological manifestations are common. Better prognosis in "skin only" disease		Chronic, recurrent. Clinically benign	Incidental histopathological finding, benign lesion
Pathology	Lymphoma cells in vessel lumina. Large, anaplastic cells, centroblasts, immunoblasts		Large, atypical cells with angioinvasion, necrosis, and microhemorrhages, mostly in the dermis, occasionally in vessel lumen	Large blastoid cells in the lumen of the ectatic vessel in the upper dermis, no infiltration of vessel wall
Immunophenotype	CD20$^+$ CD79a$^+$ PAX5$^+$ BCL2$^+$ MUM1$^+$ CD10$^-$ CD30$^-$ BCL6$^-$	CD56$^+$ CD2$^+$, cytoplasmic CD3$^+$, TIA-1$^-$ EBER$^+$	CD30$^+$ CD3$^+$, CD8$^+$ (70%) variable expression of other T-cell markers [32]	CD30$^+$ CD4$^+$ CD3$^+$ CD2$^+$ CD5$^+$
TCR	Polyclonal	Usually polyclonal, occasionally monoclonal	Monoclonal	Polyclonal

3.5 Prognostic Importance

Regarding the prognostic significance of skin involvement, it remains largely unknown in many lymphomas, as skin involvement often occurs in advanced stages of the disease where the prognosis is already poor (e.g., in Hodgkin lymphoma, multiple myeloma, or mantle cell lymphoma). In chronic lymphocytic leukemia (CLL), skin involvement does not seem to significantly affect survival. However, it's worth noting that large cell transformation in CLL considerably increases the risk of skin involvement, which is associated with a poor prognosis. This parallels the poor prognosis seen in cases of large cell transformation in other lymphomas, such as Waldenström's macroglobulinemia or follicular lymphoma, where the presence of large blastic cells in the infiltrate is associated with a grave prognosis [6, 24, 33–35]. In ATLL, the type of cutaneous lesions correlates with prognosis, with worse survival observed in patients with tumors and erythroderma [36]. In intravascular large B-cell lymphoma, skin involvement is frequent and not typically associated with prognosis, except for the cutaneous variant of the disease, which generally has a better prognosis than the primary disseminated form.

3.6 Therapy

Treatment strategies for these cases primarily focus on addressing the underlying malignancy. While there are limited reports evaluating the efficacy of skin-directed therapy, lymphoid lesions are generally known to be radiosensitive. Adjuvant photon or electron beam therapy can be considered in certain cases. Total skin electron beam therapy (29 Gy) has shown success in the symptomatic treatment of disseminated CLL skin infiltrates. For solitary infiltrates, surgical excision has been performed in some patients, although systematic studies on the long-term efficacy of surgery are lacking [37, 38].

References

1. Smith JL Jr, Butler JJ. Skin involvement in Hodgkin's disease. Cancer. 1980;45:354–61.
2. White RM, Patterson JW. Cutaneous involvement in Hodgkin's disease. Cancer. 1985;55:1136–45.
3. Su WP. Clinical, histopathologic, and immunohistochemical correlations in leukemia cutis. Semin Dermatol. 1994;13:223–30.
4. Magro CM, Morrison CD, Heerema N, Porcu P, Sroa N, Deng AC. T-cell prolymphocytic leukemia: an aggressive T cell malignancy with frequent cutaneous tropism. J Am Acad Dermatol. 2006;55:467–77.
5. Cho-Vega JH, Medeiros LJ, Prieto VG, Vega F. Leukemia cutis. Am J Clin Pathol. 2008;129:130–42.
6. Cerroni L, Zenahlik P, Höfler G, Kaddu S, Smolle J, Kerl H. Specific cutaneous infiltrates of B-cell chronic lymphocytic leukemia: a clinicopathologic and prognostic study of 42 patients. Am J Surg Pathol. 1996;20:1000–10.
7. Fried LJ, Criscito MC, Stevenson ML, Pomeranz MK. Chronic lymphocytic leukemia and the skin: implications for the dermatologist. Int J Dermatol. 2022;61:519–31.
8. Balaraman B, Conley JA, Sheinbein DM. Evaluation of cutaneous angioimmunoblastic T-cell lymphoma. J Am Acad Dermatol. 2011;65:855–62.
9. Requena L, Kutzner H, Palmedo G, Calonje E, Requena C, Pérez G, et al. Cutaneous involvement in multiple myeloma: a clinicopathologic, immunohistochemical, and cytogenetic study of 8 cases. Arch Dermatol. 2003;139:475–86.
10. Geropoulos G, Psarras K, Vlachaki E, Kakos C, Vetsiou E, Vamvakis K, et al. Cutaneous manifestations of mantle cell lymphoma: an extensive literature review. Acta Dermatovenerol Alp Panonica Adriat. 2020;29:185–91.
11. Montes-Torres A, Llamas-Velasco M, Capusan TM, Aguado B, Adrados M. Cutaneous involvement as the first manifestation of T-lymphoblastic lymphoma and review of the literature. J Cutan Pathol. 2019;46:372–5.
12. Chimenti S, Fink-Puches R, Peris K, Pescarmona E, Pütz B, Kerl H, et al. Cutaneous involvement in lymphoblastic lymphoma. J Cutan Pathol. 1999;26:379–85.
13. Cerroni L, Beham-Schmid C, Kerl H. Cutaneous Hodgkin's disease: an immunohistochemical analysis. J Cutan Pathol. 1995;22:229–35.
14. Wee E, Goh MS, Estall V, Tiong A, Webb A, Mitchell C, et al. Retrospective audit of patients referred for further treatment following Mohs surgery for non-melanoma skin cancer. Australas J Dermatol. 2018;59:302–8.
15. Miyashiro D, Sanches JA. Cutaneous manifestations of adult T-cell leukemia/lymphoma. Semin Diagn Pathol. 2020;37:81–91.

16. Melani C, Jaffe ES, Wilson WH. Pathobiology and treatment of lymphomatoid granulomatosis, a rare EBV-driven disorder. Blood. 2020;135:1344–52.
17. Alegría-Landa V, Manzarbeitia F, Salvatierra Calderón MG, Requena L, Rodríguez-Pinilla SM. Cutaneous intravascular natural killer/T cell lymphoma with peculiar immunophenotype. Histopathology. 2017;71:994–1002.
18. Ponzoni M, Campo E, Nakamura S. Intravascular large B-cell lymphoma: a chameleon with multiple faces and many masks. Blood. 2018;132:1561–7.
19. Liao J-B, Hsieh P-P, Hwang Y-C, Lin S-L, Wu C-S. Cutaneous intravascular natural killer-cell lymphoma: a rare case and review of the literature. Acta Derm Venereol. 2011;91:472–3.
20. Alhumidi A. Cutaneous Intravascular NK/T-cell lymphoma mimic panniculitis clinically, case report and literature brief review. Diagn Pathol. 2015;10:107.
21. Botros N, Cerroni L, Shawwa A, Green PJ, Greer W, Pasternak S, et al. Cutaneous manifestations of angioimmunoblastic T-cell lymphoma: clinical and pathological characteristics. Am J Dermatopathol. 2015;37:274–83.
22. Lipsker D, Rondeau M, Massard G, Grosshans E. The AESOP (adenopathy and extensive skin patch overlying a plasmacytoma) syndrome: report of 4 cases of a new syndrome revealing POEMS (polyneuropathy, organomegaly, endocrinopathy, monoclonal protein, and skin changes) syndrome at a curable stage. Medicine. 2003;82:51–9.
23. Walsh NM, Kutzner H, Requena L, Cerroni L. Plasmacytic cutaneous pathology: a review. J Cutan Pathol. 2019;46:698–708.
24. Stien S, Durot E, Durlach A, Beylot-Barry M, Adamski H, Beltraminelli H, et al. Cutaneous involvement in Waldenström's macroglobulinaemia. Acta Derm Venereol. 2020;100:adv00225.
25. Xie Y, Jaffe ES. How I diagnose angioimmunoblastic T-cell lymphoma. Am J Clin Pathol. 2021;156:1–14.
26. Shanafelt TD, Kay NE, Rabe KG, Call TG, Zent CS, Maddocks K, et al. Brief report: natural history of individuals with clinically recognized monoclonal B-cell lymphocytosis compared with patients with Rai 0 chronic lymphocytic leukemia. J Clin Oncol. 2009;27:3959–63.
27. Strati P, Shanafelt TD. Monoclonal B-cell lymphocytosis and early-stage chronic lymphocytic leukemia: diagnosis, natural history, and risk stratification. Blood. 2015;126:454–62.
28. Slager SL, Lanasa MC, Marti GE, Achenbach SJ, Camp NJ, Abbasi F, et al. Natural history of monoclonal B-cell lymphocytosis among relatives in CLL families. Blood. 2021;137:2046–56.
29. Staber PB, Herling M, Bellido M, Jacobsen ED, Davids MS, Kadia TM, et al. Consensus criteria for diagnosis, staging, and treatment response assessment of T-cell prolymphocytic leukemia. Blood. 2019;134:1132–43.
30. Sun Y, Tang G, Hu Z, Thakral B, Miranda RN, Medeiros LJ, et al. Comparison of karyotyping, fluorescence in situ hybridisation and TCL1 immunohistochemistry in T cell prolymphocytic leukaemia. J Clin Pathol. 2018;71:309–15.
31. Fang H, Wang W, Zhang L, Shen Q, Yuan J, Reichard KK, et al. Reactive intralymphovascular immunoblastic proliferations mimicking aggressive lymphomas. Am J Surg Pathol. 2022;46:326–35.
32. Martinez-Cabriales SA, Walsh S, Sade S, Shear NH. Lymphomatoid papulosis: an update and review. J Eur Acad Dermatol Venereol. 2020;34:59–73.
33. Robak E, Robak T. Skin lesions in chronic lymphocytic leukemia. Leuk Lymphoma. 2007;48:855–65.
34. Martinez-Mera C, Herrero-Moyano M, López-Elzaurdia C, Loscertales J, Aragües M. Cutaneous involvement in a high grade B-cell lymphoma with rearrangement of MYC, BCL2, and BCL6 transformed from follicular lymphoma. Am J Dermatopathol. 2019;41:80–2.
35. Palacios-Álvarez I, Román-Curto C, García-Sancho AM, Santos-Briz Á, Santos-Durán JC, Fernández-López E. Cutaneous annular lesions as the first sign of transformation of follicular lymphoma into diffuse large B-cell lymphoma. Indian J Dermatol Venereol Leprol. 2015;81:495–7.
36. Sawada Y, Hino R, Hama K, Ohmori S, Fueki H, Yamada S, et al. Type of skin eruption is an independent prognostic indicator for adult T-cell leukemia/lymphoma. Blood. 2011;117:3961–7.
37. Robak E, Góra-Tybor J, Kordek R, Wawrzyniak E, Bartkowiak J, Bednarek A, et al. Richter syndrome first manifesting as cutaneous B-cell lymphoma clonally distinct from primary B-cell chronic lymphocytic leukaemia. Br J Dermatol. 2005;153:833–7.
38. Hauswald H, Zwicker F, Rochet N, Uhl M, Hensley F, Debus J, et al. Total skin electron beam therapy as palliative treatment for cutaneous manifestations of advanced, therapy-refractory cutaneous lymphoma and leukemia. Radiat Oncol. 2012;7:118.

4 Plasma Cell Neoplasms and Paraproteinemias: Cutaneous Manifestations and Their Benign Mimics

Robert Gniadecki, Minakshi Taparia, Jean Deschenes, Jori Hardin, and Etienne Mahe

Plasma cell disorders with skin manifestations can present a complex diagnostic and management challenge, given their mimicry of other skin conditions and the specific dermatopathological complications and associations related to paraproteins. These disorders generally fall into three overarching categories:

- Plasma cell neoplasms with direct skin involvement: These are uncommon but clinically significant conditions. They involve the direct infiltration of malignant plasma cells into the skin or can manifest as paraneoplastic dermatoses.
- Reactive plasma cell hyperplasias: These conditions are characterized by the presence of a polytypic, benign but florid plasma cell population mimicking a plasma cell neoplasm. Clinically, they can be quite deceptive and often require detailed histopathological examination to exclude malignancy. Examples include cutaneous plasmacytosis and angioendotheliomatosis.
- Cutaneous manifestations of paraproteinemias: These are more common and include skin disorders that occur as a consequence of the presence of abnormal paraproteins produced by neoplastic plasma cells as well as associated dermatopathological conditions.

Skin manifestations as a direct result of plasma cell neoplasms are rare, but cutaneous reactions secondary to paraproteinemia are more frequently encountered. Therefore, a high index of suspicion is needed when encountering unusual or resistant skin conditions, particularly in individuals with known plasma cell disorders or other risk factors. See Table 4.1.

R. Gniadecki (✉)
Division of Dermatology, University of Alberta, Edmonton, AB, Canada
e-mail: r.gniadecki@ualberta.ca

M. Taparia
Division of Hematology, University of Alberta Hospital, Edmonton, AB, Canada

J. Deschenes
Department of Pathology and Laboratory Medicine, Cross Cancer Institute, Edmonton, AB, Canada
e-mail: Jean.Deschenes@albertaprecisionlabs.ca

J. Hardin
Division of Dermatology, University of Calgary, Calgary, AB, Canada
e-mail: Jori.hardin@albertahealthservices.ca

E. Mahe
Department of Pathology & Laboratory Medicine, and Hematology & Hematological Malignancies, University of Calgary, Calgary, AB, Canada
e-mail: etienne.mahe@albertaprecisionlabs.ca

R. Gniadecki et al. (eds.), *Diseases of Blood and Skin*, https://doi.org/10.1007/978-3-031-65292-9_4

Table 4.1 Plasma cell disorders and paraproteinemias as well as their benign simulators (plasma cell-rich reactive lesions) involving the skin

Plasma cell neoplasms
Solitary cutaneous plasmacytoma
Extramedullary cutaneous multiple myeloma
Plasma cell neoplasms with associated paraneoplastic syndrome: POEMS, TEMPI, AESOP
Paraproteinemias-induced skin lesions
MGUS
Cold agglutinin disease
Heavy chain diseases
Plasma cell-rich reactive cutaneous lesions
Cutaneous plasmacytosis
Angioplasmacellular pseudolymphoma (pediatric)
Pretibial lymphoplasmacytic plaque
Pseudolymphomatous angiokeratoma of children
IgG4-related disease (Chap. 15)
Cutaneous Castleman disease (Chap. 15)
Cutaneous plasma cell granuloma
Zoon balanitis
Syphilis
Lyme disease (*Borrelia* sp.)
Immunodeficiency-related lymphoproliferative disease (plasma cell variant) (Chap. 10)

4.1 Cutaneous Plasmacytoma

4.1.1 Practice Essentials

- Cutaneous plasmacytoma is an umbrella term describing the proliferation of plasma cells in the skin.
- Plasmacytomas are found in two main variants: as an extramedullary spread of the underlying multiple myeloma (extramedullary cutaneous multiple myeloma, ECMM) and a solitary cutaneous plasmacytoma (SCP), which is a proliferation of plasma cells in the skin without evidence of systemic disease.
- Clinical manifestations are firm, erythematous nodules which develop in any region of the skin. Multiple lesions indicate ECMM.
- Prognosis is poor in ECMM but favorable in SCP in the absence of other risk factors (monoclonal gammopathy, abnormal serum free light chain ratio, bone marrow plasmacytosis).

4.1.2 Clinical Manifestations

SCP without evidence of multiple myeloma is an exceedingly rare entity, documented only in isolated case reports [1, 2]. Clinically, SCP presents as a non-tender, red-to-purple nodule or plaque that is usually non-ulcerated (Fig. 4.1). The lesions can manifest across a broad age range and appear on any part of the skin. Since the clinical features are not specific, the diagnosis is generally confirmed through biopsy. It is important to note that the presence of multiple lesions strongly suggests systemic multiple myeloma rather than SCP [3, 4]. The prognosis for SCP is typically excellent, provided there are no signs of systemic disease. In clinical practice, it might be difficult, if not impossible, to differentiate SCP from plasma-cell-rich primary cutaneous marginal zone lymphoma (pcMZL/LPD). It is even possible that some of the reported cases of SCP represented in fact MZL. Fortunately, both diseases

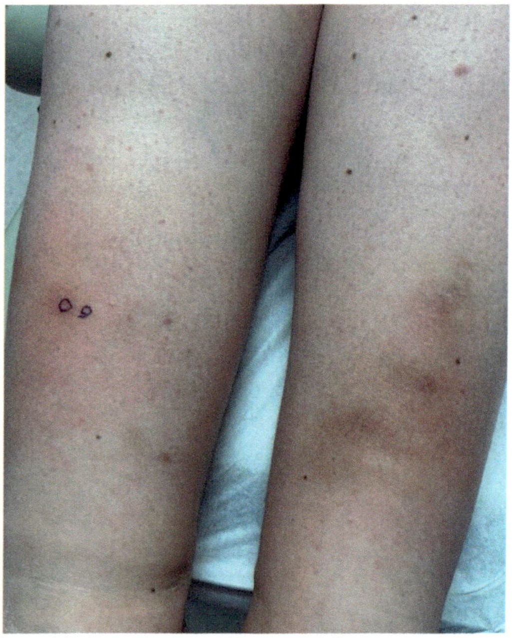

Fig. 4.1 Pretibial lymphoplasmacytic plaque. The biopsy showed a dense infiltration of monotypic plasma cells IgG4/κ. There was no sign of systemic malignancy or IgG4 disease

have a benign course, and the prognosis and therapy for all practical reasons are the same.

ECMM represents a distinct clinical scenario. It usually emerges in patients already diagnosed with multiple myeloma (or osseous plasmacytoma) and may result from hematogenous spread. Most commonly, these cutaneous lesions occur as a continuous extension to the overlying skin from an adjacent bone lesion [5]. Some rare instances have been reported where ECMM was triggered by invasive procedures such as bone marrow aspiration [6]. Among extramedullary manifestations of multiple myeloma, skin involvement is most common, accounting for over 40% of all extramedullary presentations in newly diagnosed cases [5, 7]. Clinically, ECMM lesions closely resemble those of SCP and can manifest as either single or multiple nodules or plaques.

In the differential diagnosis, one should consider Waldenström macroglobulinemia/lymphoplasmacytic lymphoma (WM/LPL), which can also produce skin changes and accompanying paraproteinemia. In these cases, the cutaneous lymphoplasmacytic infiltrate often manifests as violaceous plaques and nodules, frequently on the face. These lesions may display a remarkable symmetry, potentially resembling other dermatological conditions like rosacea or lupus erythematosus [8]. The confusion with plasma cell neoplasms may occasionally arise at the time of histopathological examination, if the lymphoid component of the lesions is not appreciated. The prognosis for patients with ECMM is notably less favorable compared to those with multiple myeloma but without extramedullary involvement.

4.1.3 Diagnosis and Staging

4.1.3.1 Skin Biopsy

The histological appearance is similar to myeloma with diffuse mature, immature, or plasmablastic plasma cells. Malignant cells stain positively with CD138, CD38, MUM1 and CD79a, but are generally negative for CD19, PAX5, and CD45, with variable expression of CD20, CD56, Cyclin D1 and CD117 [9]. It is not possible to differentiate between SCP and ECMM based on skin biopsy.

4.1.3.2 Diagnostic Approach

Cutaneous plasmacytomas are very rare and systemic disease should be ruled out in all patients. Unfortunately, there are no specific studies on cutaneous plasmacytomas, and the recommendations suggested below are based on the data gathered from bone plasmacytomas, which have a worse prognosis and higher risk of progressing to multiple myeloma compared to plasmacytoma in soft tissues [10].

Blood cell counts and blood chemistry, including LDH, calcium, immunoglobulins, serum free light chain ratio, and serum protein electrophoresis, should be ordered in all patients. The presence of a monoclonal protein and/or abnormal serum free chain ratio (outside the normal range of 0.26–1.65) are indicative of a worse prognosis and may herald progression to multiple myeloma [11, 12].

All patients should receive a bone marrow aspiration and a biopsy to rule out plasma cell neoplasms using sensitive immunohistochemistry and flow cytometry (assessing κ and λ light chains expression among plasma cells) [10]. Patients with bone plasmacytomas who have bone marrow plasmacytosis have a higher risk of progression to MM [13, 14].

For imaging studies, PET/CT seems to be the procedure of choice because most plasmacytomas have a high uptake of FDG [12]. MRI imaging of the bones increases sensitivity to detect myeloma bone lesions [10].

4.1.4 Differential Diagnosis

Distinguishing between SCP and ECMM primarily relies on comprehensive bone marrow, blood tests, and imaging studies. However, when systemic involvement is absent, SCP can pose a diagnostic challenge, being easily confounded with other skin conditions that feature abundant plasma cells.

For example, plasma cell-rich primary cutaneous marginal zone lymphoma also contains significant numbers of monotypic plasma cells that tend to cluster at the periphery of the lesions, and can at times overrun the B lymphoid cells (see Chap. 10). Lymphoplasmacytic lymphoma (most commonly Waldenström macroglobulinemia, LPL/WM) may present similar challenges at the morphological level. In cases with ambiguous morphological or phenotypic results, demonstration of the MYD88 p.L265P mutation may assist in the differential diagnosis and will favor LPL/WM over marginal zone lymphoma or plasma cell neoplasm. Furthermore, in instances where SCP exhibits plasmablastic morphology, it can be histopathologically indistinguishable from cutaneous involvement by plasmablastic lymphoma—a subtype of aggressive, large B-cell lymphoma frequently associated with HIV infection and typically EBV positive [7]. Among patients with immunosuppression, there may be the development of immunodeficiency-related plasma cell lymphoproliferations (Chap. 10).

Contrary to SCP, plasma cell-rich reactive lesions with features mimicking malignancy have a polytypic but often florid population of cytologically reactive plasma cells with limited nuclear atypia, expressing both κ and λ light chains. These plasma cells are often accompanied by a variety of other lymphoid cells and histiocytes. The so-called "cutaneous plasmacytosis" predominantly affects Asian males and often presents as a diffuse eruption of pigmented plaques on the trunk and head [15]. In children, angioplasmacellular pseudolymphoma, which includes pretibial lymphoplasmacytic plaque and acral pseudolymphomatous angiokeratoma of children (APACHE), is most common [16]. These lesions appear as benign, grouped papules or plaques, usually located on distal extremities, and similar manifestations have been described in adults as well [17, 18].

In the context of IgG4-related disease, the skin may show polytypic plasma cell-rich infiltrates that bear resemblance to class-switched primary cutaneous marginal zone lymphoma (pcMZL/LPD). Castleman disease features a dermal infiltrate of polyclonal plasma cells that are usually accompanied by well-developed secondary lymphoid structures [19]. Lastly, cutaneous plasma cell granuloma is characterized by well-circumscribed, brownish, dermal nodules containing a polytypic plasma cell-rich infiltrate along with other inflammatory cells [20, 21].

4.1.5 Treatment

SCP is commonly managed through surgical excision or radiotherapy [10]. When radiotherapy is the chosen modality, the recommended dosing is generally within the 40–50 Gy range, following guidance from studies on bone plasmacytomas. Importantly, it is advised that at least a 2 cm margin of adjacent, unaffected skin be included within the radiation field to ensure comprehensive treatment and to minimize the risk of local recurrence. In cases where SCP lesions recur, a combined approach of surgery followed by adjuvant radiotherapy may offer an effective treatment strategy.

4.2 Plasma Cell Neoplasms with Associated Paraneoplastic Syndrome: POEMS, TEMPI, AESOP

4.2.1 Practice Essentials

- POEMS, AESOP, and TEMPI syndromes are recognized in WHO classification as specific paraneoplastic syndromes associated with plasma cell neoplasms.
- Patients have monoclonal paraproteinemia (usually λ type).
- Skin signs include skin thickening, scleroderma-like changes, and telangiectasias.
- Therapy relies on the treatment of the underlying plasma cell disease.

4.2.2 Clinical Manifestations

4.2.2.1 POEMS Syndrome

POEMS syndrome is a paraneoplastic syndrome associated with an underlying monoclonal plasma cell disorder, often of the λ light chain variety. The acronym POEMS stands for Polyneuropathy, Organomegaly, Endocrinopathy, Monoclonal protein, and Skin changes. Additional frequently observed features that are not encapsulated in the acronym include edema, ascites, pleural effusions, osteosclerotic bone lesions, Castleman disease, and thrombocytosis [22].

Skin changes seen in POEMS syndrome are quite varied and can include hyperpigmentation, eruptive hemangiomas, hypertrichosis, acrocyanosis, leukonychia, sclerodermoid changes, finger clubbing, and facial flushing (Table 4.2; Fig. 4.4). The diagnostic criteria for POEMS syndrome are elaborated in the medical literature and clinical guidelines, and feature a specific combination of these characteristics (see Table 4.3).

The disease tends to have a chronic course, with a median survival of approximately 14 years. Certain features, such as fingernail clubbing, effusions, edema, ascites, and respiratory symptoms, have been identified as predictors for shorter overall survival [23].

Table 4.2 Frequency of symptoms in POEMS syndrome

Symptom	% Affected
Polyneuropathy	100
Monoclonal plasma cell dyscrasia	100
Organomegaly (hepatomegaly, splenomegaly, or other)	45–85
Lymphadenopathy	26–74
Castleman disease	11–25
Endocrinopathy	67–84
Papilloedema	29–64
Extravascular volume overload	29–87
Bone lesions	27–97
Thrombocytosis	54–88
Skin changes	68–89
Hyperpigmentation	46–93
Acrocyanosis	19
Hypertrichosis	26–74
Skin thickening	5–43

Table 4.3 Diagnostic criteria for POEMS syndrome [23]

Major criteria	Minor criteria
Mandatory	Organomegaly
Polyneuropathy	Extravascular volume overload (edema, ascites, pleural effusion)
Monoclonal plasma cell disorder (almost exclusively λ light chain restricted)	Endocrinopathy
Other	Skin changes
Castleman disease[a]	Papilloedema
Osteosclerotic lesions	Thrombocytosis or polycythemia
Elevated serum or plasma VEGF (vascular endothelial growth factor) levels	
Diagnosis: 3 major criteria (including both mandatory criteria) and 1 minor criterion	

[a] Patients with Castleman disease missing one or both of the mandatory criteria above but who still fulfill 3 major and 1 minor criteria are not "classic POEMS" but are rather designated "Castleman disease POEMS" [24]

4.2.2.2 AESOP

AESOP syndrome is an acronym for *Adenopathy and Extensive Skin Patch Overlying a Plasmacytoma* [25–28]. The cardinal features are a slowly enlarging violaceous skin patch or plaque and enlarged regional lymph nodes. Two morphological forms were described: a smooth, shiny macule and the morphea-like variant, with a "peau d'orange" appearance. The lesions are usually found above the ribs, the sternum, or the scalp. AESOP may be the first sign of POEMS syndrome [28]. Biopsy from the cutaneous patch overlying the plasmacytoma shows increased dermal mucin and vascular hyperplasia. In all described cases, the skin lesion was overlying a solitary plasmacytoma of bone. AESOP syndrome, when recognized at an early stage, may lead to the detection of a solitary plasmacytoma of bone, which may be curable.

4.2.2.3 TEMPI Syndrome

The acronym describes the following constellation of symptoms: telangiectasia, elevated erythropoietin and erythrocytosis, monoclonal gammopathy, perinephric fluid collections, and intrapulmonary shunting [29–31]. Like in POEMS syndrome, the gammopathy is λ light

Table 4.4 Diagnostic criteria for TEMPI syndrome [31]

Major criteria	
	Telangiectasia
	Elevated erythropoietin and erythrocytosis
	Monoclonal gammopathy
Minor criteria	
	Perinephric fluid
	Intrapulmonary shunting
Other	
	Venous thrombosis

chain restricted [31]. Males and females aged 35–56 years are affected. Skin manifestations are telangiectases on the upper part of the body: face, neck, and the upper trunk (Table 4.4). Patients with TEMPI syndrome are at risk of cerebral thrombosis and venous thrombosis.

4.2.3 Treatment

The treatment of the underlying paraproteinemia and plasma cell disorder may sometimes provide regression of signs of the disease. POEMS and TEMPI are associated with a worse prognosis.

4.3 Skin Manifestations of Paraproteinemias

4.3.1 Practice Essentials

- Paraproteinemias frequently manifest in the skin.
- Depositions of paraproteins in the skin are rare; most skin manifestations are secondary, reactive dermatoses that are induced by the presence of the paraprotein.
- Skin changes can serve as an important clinical clue to the underlying paraproteinemia.

Skin manifestations are frequently associated with paraproteinemias, often serving as the initial presentation of an underlying plasma cell dyscrasia or hematological condition. The wide array of skin lesions that may occur can either be the result of direct paraprotein deposition in the skin or an indirect effect of the circulating abnormal protein. These manifestations can range from localized infiltrations to generalized skin disorders, and can provide invaluable clues to the diagnosis of the underlying hematologic condition.

The classification presented here draws from a seminal paper from Mayo Clinic [32], with some important modifications. In this original work, skin manifestations of monoclonal gammopathies were divided into four categories:

1. Skin infiltrations due to malignant plasma cells or paraprotein deposition
2. Skin disorders strongly associated with monoclonal gammopathy
3. Skin disorders anecdotally associated with monoclonal gammopathy
4. Cutaneous conditions related to paraproteins but not specific to the diagnosis of monoclonal gammopathy

In our updated classification, we have elected to exclude categories 3 and 4, as they were largely based on anecdotal evidence and did not contribute to a rigorous diagnostic framework. In addition, we have followed the current WHO classification [33] to consider plasma cell skin infiltrations and associated paraneoplastic syndromes in separate chapters, focusing here specifically on the cutaneous manifestations of paraproteinemias.

Moreover, we have refined Category 2 into two distinct subcategories. The first subcategory, which we will refer to as Category 2, includes skin disorders that are so strongly associated with paraproteinemias that their presence in a new patient should trigger further diagnostic workup for an underlying plasma cell disorder; i.e., they are actionable on their own for a diagnostic workup. These conditions are rarely encountered in the absence of underlying paraproteinemia. The second subcategory, Category 3, includes skin disorders that may occur alongside paraproteinemias but can also be observed in patients without any underlying plasma cell pathology. They are not automatically actionable and do not necessarily trigger a diagnostic work up. See Table 4.5.

Table 4.5 Skin manifestations of sparaproteinemias

Category 1. Depositions of paraproteins in the skin	Macroglobulinemia cutis
	Light chain and heavy chain deposition diseases (monoclonal immunoglobulin deposition disease, MIDD)
	Light chain amyloidosis
	Cryoglobulinemic vasculopathies
	Follicular spicules of the nose
	Crystal-storing histiocytosis
Category 2. Skin disorders strongly associated with paraproteinemias	Scleromyxedema
	Scleredema
	Necrobiotic xanthogranuloma
	Normolipemic plane xanthoma
	Schnitzler syndrome
Category 3. Skin disorders comorbid to paraproteinemias	Neutrophilic dermatoses
	Pyoderma gangrenosum
	Sweet's syndrome
	Subcorneal pustular dermatosis
	Erythema elevatum diutinum

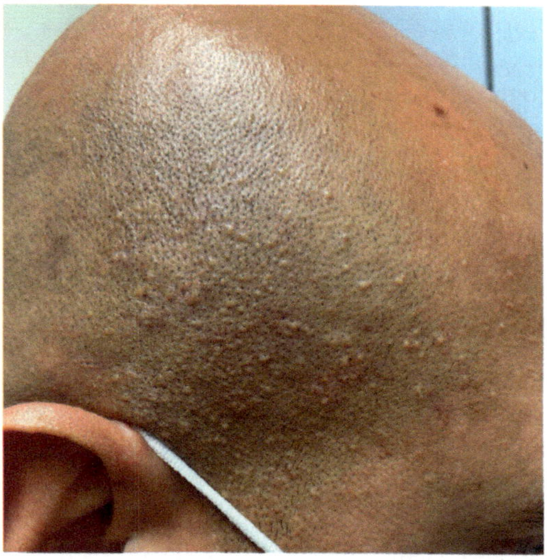

Fig. 4.2 IgM storage papules on the scalp skin in a patient with Waldenström's macroglobulinemia

4.3.2 Clinical Manifestations

4.3.2.1 Category 1: Depositions of Paraproteins in the Skin

Macroglobulinemia Cutis

Macroglobulinemia cutis represents a rare but specific cutaneous manifestation that arises due to the deposition of IgM paraproteins in the skin. This clinical entity is generally observed in patients with Waldenström's macroglobulinemia or, less commonly, in multiple myeloma. Two distinct patterns are recognized: IgM storage papules and immunobullous macroglobulinemia cutis.

IgM storage papules (Fig. 4.2) present as translucent, flesh-colored elevations on the skin, commonly localized to the extensor surfaces of the limbs. These papules harbor periodic acid-Schiff (PAS)-positive deposits that also stain positively for IgM upon direct immunofluorescence examination. Importantly, they are not stained by amyloid stains and do not represent amyloid, distinguishing them from other types of cutaneous deposits [32, 34, 35]. In some cases, the IgM paraproteins exhibit an affinity for plasma membranes, culminating in the development of skin blistering. This condition is referred to as immunobullous macroglobulinemia cutis [36–38]. In these instances, pathological deposition of paraproteins at the dermo-epidermal junction can be readily identified through direct immunofluorescence.

Given the rarity of this condition, management guidelines are sparse. However, there are reports indicating that immunobullous macroglobulinemia cutis can respond favorably to rituximab therapy or a multiagent chemotherapy regimen.

Light Chain and Heavy Chain Deposition Diseases (Monoclonal Immunoglobulin Deposition Disease, MIDD)

MIDD includes light chain deposition disease (LCDD, which is the most common subtype, often involving κ light chain), heavy chain deposition disease (HCDD), or a mixture of both heavy and light chain deposition (LHCDD) [39]. MIDD represents paraprotein disorders complicating some monoclonal plasma cell disorders or B-cell lymphoproliferative disorders, in which abundant and often fragmented monoclonal immunoglobulin light chains or heavy chains are deposited in various tissues either in combination or as pure populations. These pathogenic chain deposits most commonly affect the kidneys, heart, lungs, and peripheral nervous system. Skin involvement in these deposition diseases is exceedingly rare but can exhibit features similar to those seen in light-chain amyloidosis.

The distinguishing factor between LCDD and light chain amyloidosis lies in the conformational state of the deposited paraprotein. In light chain deposition diseases, the paraprotein retains its native conformation, whereas, in amyloidosis, it adopts a fibrillar β-pleated, hydrophobic conformation [40]. The cutaneous manifestations in light chain and heavy chain deposition diseases are typically characterized by skin lesions that closely mimic those seen in light chain amyloidosis on hematoxylin/eosin sections, with immunofluorescence expression of a specific light chain (κ most commonly) but are negative for amyloid stains, such as Congo red, thioflavin T, or amyloid P immunostaining. Additionally, these deposition diseases can lead to cutis laxa, a condition marked by sagging or inelastic skin [40, 41].

Light-Chain (AL) Amyloidosis

Light-chain (AL) amyloidosis represents a severe and often fatal condition resulting from the aberrant processing and deposition of the variable portions of monoclonal light chains. The majority of affected individuals, more than 90%, exhibit an underlying monoclonal gammopathy, most frequently monoclonal gammopathy of undetermined significance (MGUS) or multiple myeloma, and less commonly, Waldenström macroglobulinemia or solitary bone plasmacytoma. In patients with AL amyloidosis, serum and urine protein electrophoresis and immunoelectrophoresis will identify an M spike in virtually all cases. Most commonly, IgG is detected, followed by light chain-only M spikes, and, less commonly, IgA, IgM or IgD. The light chain detected in the abnormal deposits is most commonly of λ type (60–80% of cases) [42].

Cutaneous manifestations are a common feature in AL amyloidosis, occurring in approximately 40% of patients. These skin symptoms often present as perioral and periorbital purpura and ecchymoses, which are notably sensitive to mechanical trauma, such as pinching [43]. Macroglossia, or an enlarged tongue, serves as another hallmark feature. Additionally, patients may manifest waxy papules and plaques, occasionally undergoing sclerodermatous or bullous transformations. These skin changes bear similarities to those seen in macroglobulinemia cutis and LCDD. In areas affected by these skin changes, alopecia can also develop.

The prognosis for untreated AL amyloidosis is dire, with a median survival time ranging from 12 to 18 months. The disease shows a predilection for females, who constitute approximately 75% of patients [43]. Multiorgan involvement is common, potentially leading to a constellation of severe complications that may include nephrotic syndrome, renal failure, congestive heart failure, and peripheral neuropathy. Therefore, early diagnosis and aggressive management are critical to improve outcomes.

Cryoglobulinemic Vasculopathy

Cryoglobulinemic vasculopathy is a complex condition seen in patients with plasma cell disorders and immunosecretory lymphomas, notably those with type I (monoclonal) and type II (mixed, monoclonal, and polyclonal) cryoglobulinemias. The condition arises due to the deposition of abnormal monoclonal immunoglobulins, predominantly IgM, but also IgG and IgA, in the microvasculature. These abnormal proteins have the property of precipitating at low temperatures, leading to microvascular occlusion not just in the skin, but also in other tissues. The prevalence of this condition varies, affecting about 5% of patients with multiple myeloma and up to 37% of those with Waldenström macroglobulinemia [32]. Clinically, the cutaneous manifestations are diverse and often severe, encompassing purpura, ulcerations, and necrosis, commonly seen on the lower legs or face. Other skin-related symptoms may include cold urticaria, Raynaud's phenomenon, livedo reticularis, and inflammatory macules and papules (Fig. 4.3). Intriguingly, patients may also present with papular, purple lesions mimicking Kaposi's sarcoma due to vascular occlusion and endothelial cell hyperproliferation, also known as reactive angioendotheliomatosis, a rare nonspecific vascular reactive lesions observed in patients with a variety of systemic conditions, including cryoglobulinemia [40, 44].

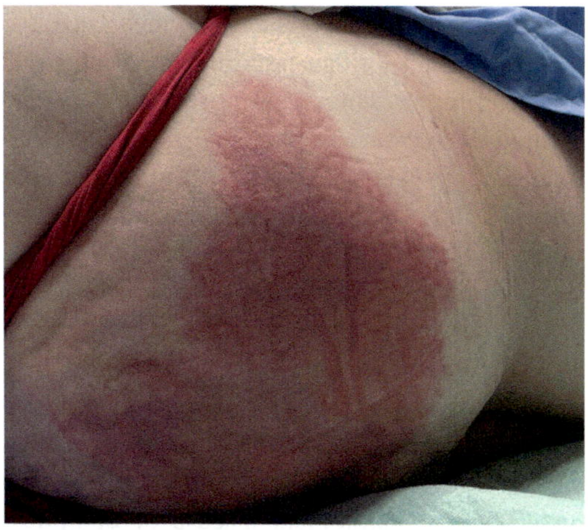

Fig. 4.3 Cryoglobulinemic vasculopathy presenting as a painful area of erythema in a patient with Waldenström macroglobulinemia

In addition to cutaneous features, systemic manifestations are not uncommon and include neuropathy, nephropathy, and less frequently, gastrointestinal disturbances [45]. Hyperviscosity syndrome may occur in some cases, with manifestations ranging from neurologic symptoms such as headache and confusion to ocular issues like blurred vision and visual loss, as well as rhino-otological symptoms including epistaxis and hearing loss. In severe instances, it can culminate in multiorgan failure, necessitating immediate treatment.

An extreme and life-threatening form of the condition is known as cryocrystalglobulinemia. In this variant, the paraprotein actually crystallizes within the vessels, leading to catastrophic vasculopathy affecting various organs, including the kidneys (resulting in renal failure), central nervous system (causing neurologic symptoms), liver, and lungs. The cutaneous manifestations in these cases are particularly severe, featuring necrotic ulcers, hemorrhagic blisters, and gangrene [40].

Diagnosis is typically confirmed through direct serum cryoglobulin measurements and is further supported by characteristic clinical and histopathological findings. Skin biopsies show vasculitic changes, often leucocytoclastic, inflammatory or non-inflammatory purpura, intravascular hyaline material that is PAS positive and post-inflammatory sequelae [46].

Follicular Spicules of the Nose

Follicular spicules of the nose present as horn-like, filiform spicules originating from the follicular ostia, primarily on the nose. These spicules are not just a cosmetic concern but are often a harbinger of underlying gammopathy, most frequently cryoglobulinemia [47, 48]. It is noteworthy that this condition has not been described in the absence of a coexisting paraproteinemia, underlining its diagnostic significance.

Histologically, these spicules are composed of columns of homogeneous, eosinophilic, horny material protruding from dilated, and/or distorted follicular openings [49]. Additional findings may include small vessel thrombotic vasculopathy and vasculitis. The presence of paraprotein, often IgG λ, within these spicules and in the infundibular epidermis has been confirmed by several studies [47, 49–51].

It is essential to differentiate these spicules from other skin conditions with similar presentations. For example, spicules resulting from an infestation of Demodex mites show different histopathological features, where the spicules consist of dead mites surrounded by eosinophilic material [52]. Lesions in folliculotropic mycosis fungoides, another condition affecting the face, may exhibit a "spiculate" appearance. However, the underlying histopathology, often showing follicular mucinosis, is distinctly different from that of follicular spicules associated with paraproteinemia. Trichodysplasia spinulosa, caused by polyomavirus in immunosuppressed individuals, may also present with similar spicules but typically has a more severe presentation, including papules that can extend beyond the nose to the cheeks.

Given the high likelihood of an associated underlying gammopathy, follicular spicules of the nose should prompt further evaluation to rule out paraproteinemia and other related disorders.

Crystal-Storing Histiocytosis

Crystal-storing histiocytosis is an exceedingly rare condition characterized by the accumulation of crystallized paraprotein within the lysosomes of histiocytes across various organs, including the skin [40, 53]. Predominantly, this condition is associated with κ paraproteins.

Clinically, the most consistent sign of the disease is facial swelling. Beyond that, the manifestations are markedly heterogeneous, ranging from indurated, pigmented patches and plaques to sometimes ulcerative lesions. These cutaneous presentations are nonspecific, and the definitive diagnosis typically hinges on skin biopsy findings.

Histopathologically, the biopsy reveals an abundance of histiocytes that are positive for CD68 and CD163, with their cytoplasm densely packed with crystalline inclusions. These inclusions appear eosinophilic and refractile under light microscopy. These crystals are immunostained with κ or λ light chain antibodies.

4.3.2.2 Category 2 Skin Disorders Strongly Associated with Paraproteinemias

Scleromyxedema

Scleromyxedema is a rare but severe dermatological condition closely associated with monoclonal gammopathies. Skin lesions are caused by the accumulation of mucin (heavily glycosylated proteins made by fibroblasts) following fibroblast proliferation. In the absence of thyroid disease, scleromyxedema almost invariably develops in patients with monoclonal gammopathies, either associated with MGUS, multiple myeloma, or plasmacytomas [54, 55]. In the vast majority of cases, over 80%, patients with scleromyxedema have IgG and λ paraproteinemia [56].

Clinically, the disease manifests as a generalized eruption of firm, waxy, and slightly translucent papules, primarily affecting the face, ears, and dorsal hands. The skin changes are sclerodermatous in nature, but notably lack significant epidermal alterations or inflammation. Histological analysis typically reveals increased fibroblast numbers and fibrosis, along with widely separated collagen fibers due to mucin deposits in the dermis that stain positive with alcian blue and colloidal iron (see Fig. 18.3; Chap. 18).

The condition often extends beyond the skin, leading to a range of extracutaneous manifestations that contribute to the disease's morbidity. Such manifestations include dysphagia, hoarseness, and aspiration due to laryngeal involvement; myopathy, either proximal or generalized; polyarthritis; various central nervous system symptoms such as encephalopathy, seizures, vertigo, and psychosis; sicca syndrome; cardiac issues such as arrhythmias or myocardial infarctions; and lung involvement leading to dyspnea. Carpal tunnel syndrome with median neuropathy is also frequently reported [57].

The course of scleromyxedema is often progressive, and mortality rates are significant, ranging from 15% to 50% [56, 58]. The leading causes of death are usually the progression of the underlying hematological disease or complications related to central nervous system involvement. As for therapeutic options, intravenous immunoglobulin has shown promising results, providing a rapid response in at least 50% of patients, and thus may be considered a first-line treatment. Other treatment modalities include melphalan, systemic corticosteroids, thalidomide, and plasmapheresis.

Scleredema (Formerly Scleredema Adultorum)

Scleredema is another rare dermatological condition characterized by skin thickening and woody induration, often accompanied by non-pitting edema. Unlike scleromyxedema, which is most frequently associated with IgG λ paraproteins, scleredema can develop in the context of IgG2-κ, IgG3-κ, or IgA-κ paraproteins [59, 60].

Clinically, the disorder typically starts on the face and neck and may spread to the scalp and upper trunk, while usually sparing the hands and feet. It manifests in three primary clinical variants: the classical type triggered by a febrile illness, diabetes-associated scleredema, and paraneoplastic scleredema, which is particularly relevant in the context of paraproteinemias and accounts for about 25% of all cases. Paraneoplastic scleredema is often linked with monoclonal gammopathies or B-cell lymphomas (see Fig. 18.4; Chap. 18).

Histologically, scleredema is characterized by dermal and subcutaneous thickening, attributed to increased glycosaminoglycans that separate the collagen fibers. Unlike scleromyxedema, there is no deposition of mucin proteins in scleredema.

Internal organ involvement is less frequent but can occur, particularly affecting the heart, joints, and eyes [61, 62]. Additionally, scleredema can be a skin manifestation of POEMS syndrome.

Unlike the classical variant, paraneoplastic scleredema does not tend to resolve spontaneously and presents a therapeutic challenge. Various treatment options have been tried with varying degrees of success, including PUVA (psoralen plus ultraviolet A), electron beam radiation, intravenous immunoglobulins, broadband ultraviolet A (UVA1) phototherapy, and extracorporeal photopheresis. These therapies have been beneficial in isolated cases [63–67], but no universal standard of care exists, making the management of scleredema complex and often individualized.

Necrobiotic Xanthogranuloma and Normolipemic Plane Xanthoma

Necrobiotic xanthogranuloma and diffuse normolipemic xanthoma are paraneoplastic skin conditions, most often associated with monoclonal gammopathies. Both of these conditions occur without concomitant hyperlipidemia, making them distinct from more common forms of xanthomas [68].

In the vast majority (80–90%) of cases of both necrobiotic xanthogranuloma and normolipemic plane xanthoma, an underlying monoclonal gammopathy is present. IgG paraproteinemias are the most commonly associated gammopathies, specifically MGUS in approximately 50% and multiple myeloma in around 40% of cases. The rest may be linked to Waldenström macroglobulinemia, chronic myelomonocytic leukemia, chronic lymphocytic leukemia, or non-Hodgkin lymphoma. Notably, xanthomas often serve as the initial clinical indicator of these underlying hematological disorders.

Clinically, normolipemic xanthomas may mimic their hyperlipidemic counterparts, presenting as yellowish, soft plaques or nodules. Necrobiotic xanthogranulomas, on the other hand, manifest predominantly as firm nodules, papules, or plaques in the periorbital area (Fig. 4.4). These lesions may also show signs of ulceration, crusting, or telangiectasia. While less common, lesions can also appear on the upper extremities and trunk. Exceptionally, these lesions can involve extracutaneous sites like the oral mucosa, eyes, bones, liver, or lungs [68, 69].

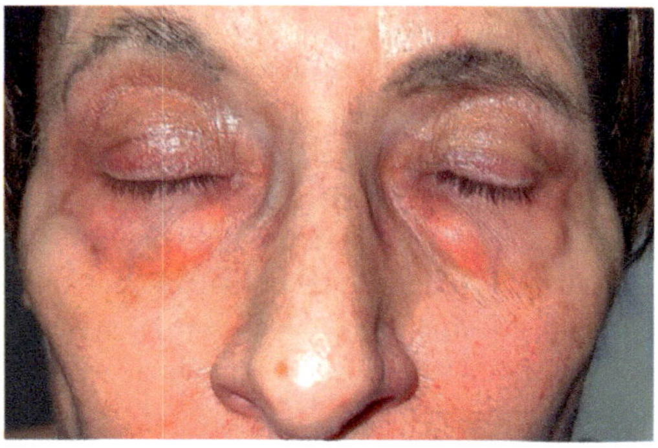

Fig. 4.4 Necrobiotic xanthogranuloma involving bilateral eyelids in a patient with POEMS syndrome

Histopathologically, normolipemic xanthomas share features with the hyperlipidemic variant, such as lipid-laden histiocytes. Necrobiotic xanthogranuloma, however, shows granulomatous inflammation consisting of lymphocytes, foreign body-like giant cells, Touton giant cells, and areas of collagen necrobiosis.

Differentiating between these paraneoplastic conditions and other xanthomas relies on clinical and histopathological evaluations. The distinction between normolipemic and hyperlipidemic xanthomas can be challenging due to overlapping features and the occasional presence of hyperlipidemia in patients with gammopathies. Certain markers like low levels of complement C4 and C1 inhibitor have been suggested to indicate a paraneoplastic origin.

Regarding treatment, options are limited and often focus on managing the underlying hematologic disease. Surgical excision of the skin lesions may offer symptomatic relief. Some isolated cases have responded to systemic corticosteroids or intravenous immunoglobulin.

Schnitzler Syndrome

Schnitzler syndrome is an autoinflammatory condition closely associated with monoclonal paraproteinemia, most often of the IgM type, although IgG has been reported less frequently. The syndrome typically presents in adults aged 40 to 60 years and is characterized by a recurrent, often burning, urticarial rash accompanied by systemic manifestations such as fever, arthralgia, myalgia, and hepatosplenomegaly (Fig. 4.5). Laboratory findings usually reveal leukocytosis and elevated levels of erythrocyte sedimentation rate (ESR) and C-reactive protein (CRP).

Given the symptomatology and lab findings, the differential diagnosis for Schnitzler syndrome is broad, and it includes conditions such as chronic idiopathic urticaria, urticarial vasculitis, systemic adult-onset Still's disease, and other rare autoinflammatory disorders like Muckle-Wells syndrome and mevalonate kinase deficiency (hyper-IgD syndrome). Accurate diagnosis is crucial as the management strategies for these conditions vary significantly. The proposed diagnostic criteria for Schnitzler syndrome are detailed in Table 4.6.

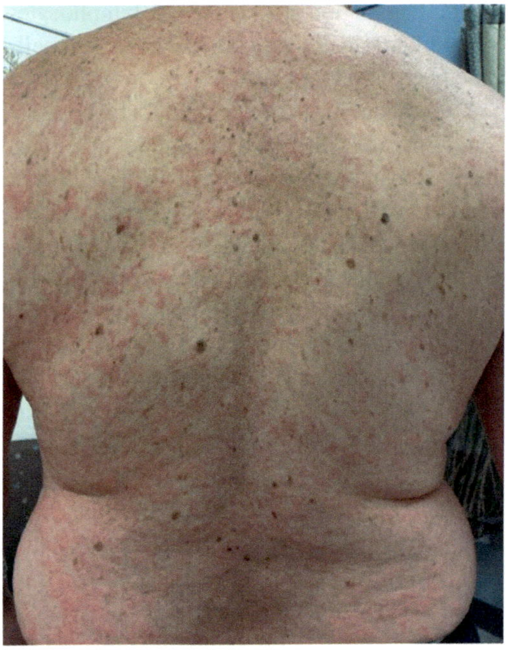

Fig. 4.5 Schnitzler syndrome. Persistent urticarial eruption in a patient with MGUS

Table 4.6 Diagnostic criteria for Schnitzler syndrome [70]

Major criteria	Minor criteria
Chronic urticarial rash	Recurrent fever
Monoclonal IgM or IgG	Bone abnormalities (assessed by scintigraphy, magnetic resonance, or elevation in alkaline phosphatase)
	Neutrophilic dermal infiltrate on skin biopsy
	Leukocytosis and/or elevated CRP
Definite diagnosis: 2 major criteria and 2 minor criteria (if IgM) or 3 minor criteria (if IgG gammopathy)	
Probable diagnosis: 2 major criteria and 1 minor criterion (if IgM) or 2 minor criteria (if IgG)	

Treatment of Schnitzler syndrome is imperative, not only to control symptoms but also to prevent the potentially severe long-term complication of AA amyloidosis, a condition resulting from the deposition of serum amyloid A (SAA) protein. For mild cases, treatment may involve colchicine, nonsteroidal anti-inflammatory drugs, or hydroxychloroquine. However, for patients who do not respond to these treatments or are severely affected, targeted therapies like IL-1 receptor antagonists, including anakinra or canakinumab, are often considered. In selected cases, the anti-IL-6 antibody, tocilizumab, has also proven to be effective.

Due to the potential for severe complications, patients with Schnitzler syndrome should be closely monitored. Monitoring should include periodic measurements of SAA protein levels and quantification of the monoclonal paraprotein to assess treatment efficacy and the need for modification of therapeutic approaches.

4.3.2.3 Category 3. Skin Disorders Comorbid to Paraproteinemias

Pyoderma Gangrenosum (PG)

PG is a neutrophilic, ulcerative disease. There are six different clinical forms, the most common being ulcerative PG, manifesting with one or several painful, non-healing ulcers. Other types are vesiculobullous PG (blisters leaving superficial erosions), pustular PG where the patients develop sterile pustules on the skin, most commonly on the upper extremities, upper trunk and the head, vegetative (granulomatous), peristomal, and perioperative. Patients may report systemic symptoms such as fever and joint pain. Besides its classic association with inflammatory bowel disease and arthritic syndromes (such as rheumatoid arthritis), PG is associated with monoclonal gammopathies and different hematological malignancies, the most common being myelodysplastic syndrome and myeloid leukemias. PG in patients with paraproteinemia is usually of the classic, ulcerative type and affects middle-aged to elderly patients (median age 50–60 years), more commonly males. In most patients, PG precedes the diagnosis of paraproteinemia [71]. IgA gammopathy is the most common type in patients with comorbid PG [72]. PG in patients with leukemias is usually of the vesiculobullous type.

Ulcerative PG has numerous differential diagnoses and is a diagnosis of exclusion since skin pathology is rather unspecific. The diagnosis is made clinically in patients who present with a rapidly progressive, painful, necrotic ulcer(s) with irregular, violaceous, and undermined border, in whom other causes of cutaneous ulceration have been excluded (namely infection) (see Chap. 18; Fig. 18.4). Minor diagnostic criteria are the history of pathergy (development of pustule or ulcer after skin trauma), presence of a systemic disease associated with PG, biopsy showing neutrophilic skin infiltrate in an absence of infection, and response to systemic corticosteroids in medium to high doses. PG, in the context of paraproteinemia, is resistant to treatment. The therapy comprises a combination of systemic corticosteroid, intravenous immunoglobulins, and, if not contraindicated by the underlying hematological condition, immunosuppressives (cyclosporin A, mycophenolate mofetil, anti-TNF α agents).

Sweet's Syndrome

Sweet's syndrome is a relatively common, reactive, neutrophilic dermatosis, the incidence of which is increased in patients with plasma cell disorders. Patients present with an acute onset fever, neutrophilia, and tender, red to violaceous edematous papules or plaques, most commonly symmetrically distributed on the extremities, head, and neck. The lesions give an impression of translucency because of severe dermal edema (see Chap. 18; Fig. 18.1). Biopsy shows dense dermal neutrophilic infiltrate.

Besides this classic manifestation, Sweet's syndrome may present as a subacute, relapsing disease with minimal (or absent) systemic symptoms and peripheral neutrophilia. There are also intermediate forms between Sweet's syndrome and PG where skin lesions are more pustular, bullous, ulcerative, or located in subcutaneous fat (subcutaneous Sweet's syndrome).

Most cases are idiopathic, but approximately 20% of cases occur in the setting of an underlying hematologic malignancy. The most common associations are myelodysplastic syndrome and myeloid leukemias and only a minority are found in patients with plasma cell disorders with paraproteinemias [73, 74].

The pattern of paraproteinemia associated with Sweet's syndrome has not been investigated but case reports often describe IgG λ or IgA. p-ANCA are often positive in paraproteinemia-associated Sweet's syndrome, but its relevance is unclear [75].

First-line treatments are high-potency topical or systemic corticosteroids. Dapsone, potassium iodide, and colchicine may also be effective.

Subcorneal Pustular Dermatosis (SPD)

SPD is a superficial, blistering skin disease characterized by superficial vesicles and flaccid blisters filled with yellow pus. Hypopyon is a characteristic feature: the neutrophils in the blister fluid settle gravitationally to the inferior portion of the blister, leaving clear fluid in the superior portion. The lesions have a predilection for the flexural areas (axillae, groin), but are also commonly found on the trunk and proximal extremities.

SPD may be idiopathic but is also frequently associated with various diseases, such as various hematological malignancies (CLL, lymphomas), solid tumors, or inflammatory diseases (*Mycoplasma pneumoniae* infection, autoimmune disorders). A minority is associated with paraproteinemias, most commonly IgA type or IgG cryoglobulinemias [73, 76, 77].

Dapsone is the treatment of choice for SPD.

Erythema Elevatum Diutinum (EED)

EED is a chronic fibrosing neutrophilic vasculitis with granuloma formation. EED typically presents as symmetric, brownish-red nodules and plaques, most frequently seen on the extensor surfaces such as the backs of the hands, fingers, elbows, knees, and ankles. Over time, these lesions may become firmer and take on a more yellowish or brown hue due to fibrosis. EED is associated with a variety of systemic diseases, but hematologic abnormalities and especially IgA gammopathy are most commonly observed [78]. This relationship has raised the suspicion that EED may have an immune-complex mediated pathogenesis. In addition to IgA gammopathy, associations with other conditions like HIV, rheumatoid arthritis, and inflammatory bowel disease have also been reported.

EED responds to dapsone (first-line therapy). Alternatively, sulfapyridine, colchicine, or systemic corticosteroids can be considered.

Acquired Cutis Laxa

Acquired cutis laxa is a striking skin disorder when the cutaneous connective tissue loses elasticity due to the damage of elastic fibers (Fig. 4.6). The skin appears sagging and wrinkled. Cutis laxa may appear focally or involve the entire skin. Cutis laxa was described as a comorbidity to MGUS, myeloma, and heavy chain deposition disease [40, 41, 79]. It is unclear whether paraproteins are deposited in the skin, causing elastic tissue damage, or whether elastic tissue pathology is indirect due to inflammatory reaction.

Cutis laxa should be differentiated from mycosis fungoides with granulomatous slack skin (Chap. 7).

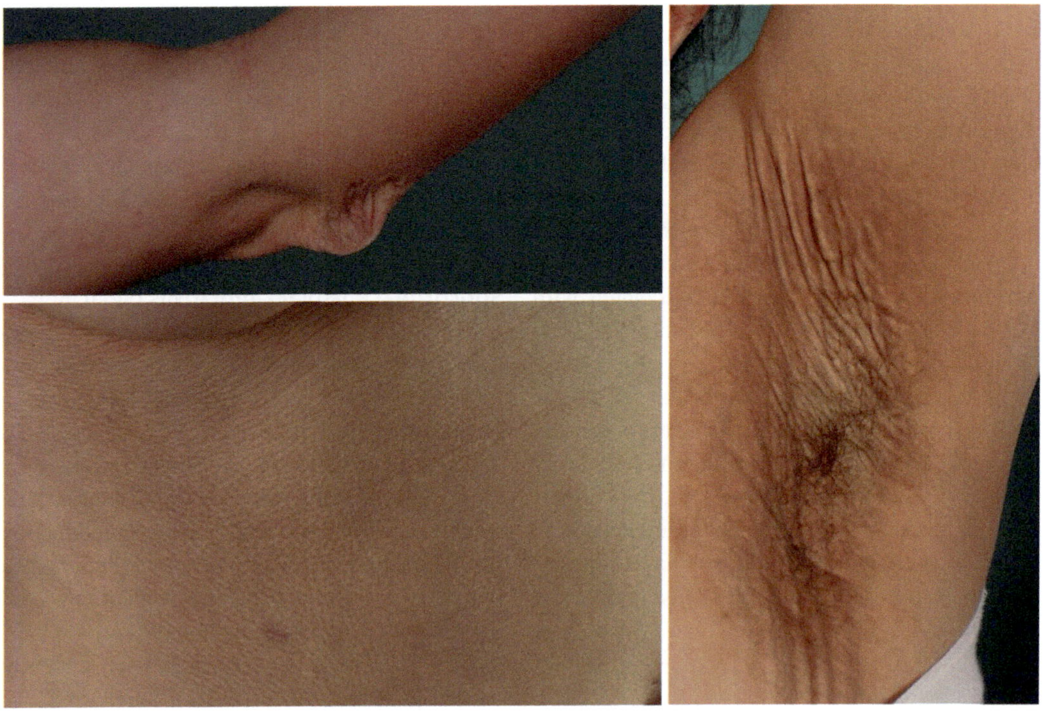

Fig. 4.6 Cutis laxa in a female patient with MGUS. Note sagging and wrinkling of the skin in the axillae and over the elbows, and wrinkling of the skin on the abdomen

References

1. Tüting T, Bork K. Primary plasmacytoma of the skin. J Am Acad Dermatol. 1996;34:386–90.
2. Koletsa T, Patsatsi A, Kostopoulos I, Kartsios C, Korantzis I, Sotiriadis D. A case of a primary cutaneous plasmacytoma presenting in adolescence. Am J Dermatopathol. 2012;34:537–40.
3. Shah A, Klimo P, Worth A. Multiple myeloma first observed as multiple cutaneous plasmacytomas. Arch Dermatol. 1982;118:922–4.
4. Patterson JW, Parsons JM, White RM, Fitzpatrick JE, Kohout-Dutz E. Cutaneous involvement of multiple myeloma and extramedullary plasmacytoma. J Am Acad Dermatol. 1988;19:879–90.
5. Requena L, Kutzner H, Palmedo G, Calonje E, Requena C, Pérez G, et al. Cutaneous involvement in multiple myeloma: a clinicopathologic, immunohistochemical, and cytogenetic study of 8 cases. Arch Dermatol. 2003;139:475–86.
6. Bladé J, Beksac M, Caers J, Jurczyszyn A, von Lilienfeld-Toal M, Moreau P, et al. Extramedullary disease in multiple myeloma: a systematic literature review. Blood Cancer J. 2022;12:45.
7. Walsh NM, Kutzner H, Requena L, Cerroni L. Plasmacytic cutaneous pathology: a review. J Cutan Pathol. 2019;46:698–708.
8. Stien S, Durot E, Durlach A, Beylot-Barry M, Adamski H, Beltraminelli H, et al. Cutaneous involvement in Waldenström's Macroglobulinaemia. Acta Derm Venereol. 2020;100:adv00225.
9. Torlakovic E, Torlakovic G, Nguyen PL, Brunning RD, Delabie J. The value of anti-pax-5 immunostaining in routinely fixed and paraffin-embedded sections: a novel pan pre-B and B-cell marker. Am J Surg Pathol. 2002;26:1343–50.
10. Caers J, Paiva B, Zamagni E, Leleu X, Bladé J, Kristinsson SY, et al. Diagnosis, treatment, and response assessment in solitary plasmacytoma: updated recommendations from a European Expert Panel. J Hematol Oncol. 2018;11:10.
11. Wilder RB, Ha CS, Cox JD, Weber D, Delasalle K, Alexanian R. Persistence of myeloma protein for more than one year after radiotherapy is an adverse prognostic factor in solitary plasmacytoma of bone. Cancer. 2002;94:1532–7.
12. Fouquet G, Guidez S, Herbaux C, Van de Wyngaert Z, Bonnet S, Beauvais D, et al. Impact of initial FDG-PET/CT and serum-free light chain on transformation of conventionally defined solitary plasmacytoma to multiple myeloma. Clin Cancer Res. 2014;20:3254–60.
13. Hill QA, Rawstron AC, de Tute RM, Owen RG. Outcome prediction in plasmacytoma of bone: a risk model utilizing bone marrow flow cytometry and light-chain analysis. Blood. 2014;124:1296–9.
14. Paiva B, Chandia M, Vidriales M-B, Colado E, Caballero-Velázquez T, Escalante F, et al. Multiparameter flow cytometry for staging of solitary bone plasmacytoma: new criteria for risk of progression to myeloma. Blood. 2014;124:1300–3.
15. Gutierrez RA, Jacobson R, Dawson A, Haemel A, North J. Cutaneous and systemic plasmacytosis with concurrent lymphoid hyperplasia. J Cutan Pathol. 2023;50:379–82.
16. Fernandez-Flores A, Suarez Peñaranda JM, De Toro G, Alvarez Cuesta CC, Fernández-Figueras MT, Kempf W, et al. Expression of peripheral node addressins by plasmacytic plaque of children, APACHE, TRAPP, and primary cutaneous angioplasmacellular hyperplasia. Appl Immunohistochem Mol Morphol. 2018;26:411–9.
17. Okada M, Funayama M, Tanita M, Kudoh K, Aiba S, Tagami H. Acral angiokeratoma-like pseudolymphoma: one adolescent and two adults. J Am Acad Dermatol. 2001;45:S209–11.
18. Mitteldorf C, Palmedo G, Kutzner H, Kauer F, Prestin M, Schuster C, et al. Diagnostic approach in lymphoplasmacytic plaque. J Eur Acad Dermatol Venereol. 2015;29:2206–15.
19. Zapata-Salazar NA, Gómez-Flores M, Ocampo-Candiani J, Chavez-Alvarez S. Cutaneous manifestations of castleman disease: histopathological characteristics and review of literature. Am J Dermatopathol. 2021;43:926–31.
20. Chen Y-F, Chao C-M, Liu H-N. Cutaneous plasma cell granuloma: report of a case with novel histologic and immunohistochemical findings. Int J Dermatol. 2009;48:409–11.
21. El Shabrawi-Caelen L, Kerl K, Cerroni L, Soyer HP, Kerl H. Cutaneous inflammatory pseudotumor—a spectrum of various diseases? J Cutan Pathol. 2004;31:605–11.
22. Li J, Zhou D-B. New advances in the diagnosis and treatment of POEMS syndrome. Br J Haematol. 2013;161:303–15.
23. Dispenzieri A. POEMS syndrome: 2011 update on diagnosis, risk-stratification, and management. Am J Hematol. 2011;86:591–601.
24. Dispenzieri A. POEMS syndrome: 2021 update on diagnosis, risk-stratification, and management. Am J Hematol. 2021;96:872–88.
25. Lipsker D, Rondeau M, Massard G, Grosshans E. The AESOP (adenopathy and extensive skin patch overlying a plasmacytoma) syndrome: report of 4 cases of a new syndrome revealing POEMS (polyneuropathy, organomegaly, endocrinopathy, monoclonal protein, and skin changes) syndrome at a curable stage. Medicine. 2003;82:51–9.
26. Dagrosa AT, Cowdrey MCE, LeBlanc RE, Lansigan F, Kaur P, Carter JB. Adenopathy and extensive skin patch overlying a plasmacytoma with unusual histologic findings in a patient with polyneuropathy, organomegaly, endocrinopathy, monoclonal protein and skin changes syndrome and Castleman disease. J Cutan Pathol. 2019;46:784–9.
27. Sanchez EG, Ramos C, Ratnarajah K, Bravo FP, Del Solar MA, Le M, et al. Adenopathy and

extensive skin patch overlying plasmacytoma syndrome-the clue to early diagnosis of polyneuropathy, organomegaly, endocrinopathy, monoclonal gammopathy, and skin changes: a case series and literature review. SAGE Open Med Case Rep. 2022;10:2050313X221091602.
28. Rongioletti F, Failla MC, Atzori L, Ferreli C. Skin manifestations of POEMS and AESOP syndrome in the same patient revealing plasma cell dyscrasia. J Cutan Pathol. 2016;43:1167–71.
29. Sykes DB, Schroyens W, O'Connell C. The TEMPI syndrome—a novel multisystem disease. N Engl J Med. 2011;365:475–7.
30. Xu J, Liu W, Fan F, Zhang B, Zhao F, Hu Y, et al. TEMPI syndrome: update on clinical features, management, and pathogenesis. Front Endocrinol. 2022;13:886961.
31. Sykes DB, O'Connell C, Schroyens W. The TEMPI syndrome. Blood. 2020;135:1199–203.
32. Daoud MS, Lust JA, Kyle RA, Pittelkow MR. Monoclonal gammopathies and associated skin disorders. J Am Acad Dermatol. 1999;40:507–35; quiz 536–8.
33. Alaggio R, Amador C, Anagnostopoulos I, Attygalle AD, Araujo IBO, Berti E, et al. The 5th edition of the World Health Organization classification of haematolymphoid tumours: lymphoid neoplasms. Leukemia. 2022;36:1720–48.
34. Rongioletti F, Patterson JW, Rebora A. The histological and pathogenetic spectrum of cutaneous disease in monoclonal gammopathies. J Cutan Pathol. 2008;35:705–21.
35. Camp BJ, Magro CM. Cutaneous macroglobulinosis: a case series. J Cutan Pathol. 2012;39:962–70.
36. Chattopadhyay M, Rytina E, Dada M, Bhogal BS, Groves R, Handfield-Jones S. Immunobullous dermatosis associated with Waldenström macroglobulinaemia treated with rituximab. Clin Exp Dermatol. 2013;38:866–9.
37. Whittaker SJ, Bhogal BS, Black MM. Acquired immunobullous disease: a cutaneous manifestation of IgM macroglobulinaemia. Br J Dermatol. 1996;135:283–6.
38. West NY, Fitzpatrick JE, David-Bajar KM, Bennion SD. Waldenström macroglobulinemia-induced bullous dermatosis. Arch Dermatol. 1998;134:1127–31.
39. Dalmia S, Asgari E, Hwang K, Aljama M. Monoclonal immunoglobulin deposition disease—a review of current and emerging data. Blood. 2023;142:6757.
40. Alegría-Landa V, Cerroni L, Kutzner H, Requena L. Paraprotein deposits in the skin. J Am Acad Dermatol. 2017;77:1145–58.
41. Majithia RA, George L, Thomas M, Fouzia NA. Acquired cutis laxa associated with light and heavy chain deposition disease. Indian Dermatol Online J. 2018;9:44–6.
42. Merlini G. AL amyloidosis: from molecular mechanisms to targeted therapies. Hematology Am Soc Hematol Educ Program. 2017;2017:1–12.
43. Andrei M, Wang JC. Cutaneous light chain amyloidosis with multiple myeloma: a concise review. Hematol Oncol Stem Cell Ther. 2019;12:71–81.
44. Aguayo-Leiva I, Vano-Galván S, Salguero I, Carrillo-Gijón R, Vallés A, Herrera P, et al. Reactive angioendotheliomatosis in a patient with myelodysplastic syndrome presenting as a cellulitis-like plaque. Eur J Dermatol. 2009;19:182–3.
45. Ramos-Casals M, Stone JH, Cid MC, Bosch X. The cryoglobulinaemias. Lancet. 2012;379:348–60.
46. Cohen SJ, Pittelkow MR, Su WP. Cutaneous manifestations of cryoglobulinemia: clinical and histopathologic study of seventy-two patients. J Am Acad Dermatol. 1991;25:21–7.
47. Requena L, Sarasa JL, Ortiz Masllorens F, Martín L, Piqué E, Olivares M, et al. Follicular spicules of the nose: a peculiar cutaneous manifestation of multiple myeloma with cryoglobulinemia. J Am Acad Dermatol. 1995;32:834–9.
48. Satta R, Casu G, Dore F, Longinotti M, Cottoni F. Follicular spicules and multiple ulcers: cutaneous manifestations of multiple myeloma. J Am Acad Dermatol. 2003;49:736–40.
49. Tomasini C, Michelerio A, Brazzelli V. Eruptive ulcerative follicular spicules heralding progression of smoldering multiple myeloma. J Cutan Pathol. 2019;46:844–51.
50. Bork K, Böckers M, Pfeifle J. Pathogenesis of paraneoplastic follicular hyperkeratotic spicules in multiple myeloma. Follicular and epidermal accumulation of IgG dysprotein and cryoglobulin. Arch Dermatol. 1990;126:509–13.
51. Braun RP, Skaria AM, Saurat J-H, Borradori L. Multiple hyperkeratotic spicules and myeloma. Dermatology. 2002;205:210–2.
52. Zahr AA. Facial spinulate demodicosis. Clin Cosmet Investig Dermatol. 2021;14:1211–4.
53. Kanagal-Shamanna R, Xu-Monette ZY, Miranda RN, Dogan A, Zou D, Luthra R, et al. Crystal-storing histiocytosis: a clinicopathological study of 13 cases. Histopathology. 2016;68:482–91.
54. Cokonis Georgakis C-D, Falasca G, Georgakis A, Heymann WR. Scleromyxedema. Clin Dermatol. 2006;24:493–7.
55. Heymann WR. Scleromyxedema. J Am Acad Dermatol. 2007;57:890–1.
56. Dinneen AM, Dicken CH. Scleromyxedema. J Am Acad Dermatol. 1995;33:37–43.
57. Frayha RA. Papular mucinosis, destructive arthropathy, median neuropathy, and sicca complex. Clin Rheumatol. 1983;2:277–84.
58. Rongioletti F, Merlo G, Cinotti E, Fausti V, Cozzani E, Cribier B, et al. Scleromyxedema: a multicenter study of characteristics, comorbidities, course, and therapy in 30 patients. J Am Acad Dermatol. 2013;69:66–72.
59. Beers WH, Ince A, Moore TL. Scleredema adultorum of Buschke: a case report and review of the literature. Semin Arthritis Rheum. 2006;35:355–9.
60. Angeli-Besson C, Koeppel MC, Jacquet P, Andrac L, Sayag J. Electron-beam therapy in scleredema adulto-

rum with associated monoclonal hypergammaglobulinaemia. Br J Dermatol. 1994;130:394–7.
61. Rimon D, Lurie M, Storch S, Halon D, Eisenkraft S, Laor A, et al. Cardiomyopathy and multiple myeloma. Complications of scleredema adultorum. Arch Intern Med. 1988;148:551–3.
62. Curtis AC, Shulak BM. Scleredema adultorum. Not always a benign self-limited disease. Arch Dermatol. 1965;92:526–41.
63. Hager CM, Sobhi HA, Hunzelmann N, Wickenhauser C, Scharenberg R, Krieg T, et al. Bath-PUVA therapy in three patients with scleredema adultorum. J Am Acad Dermatol. 1998;38:240–2.
64. Aichelburg MC, Loewe R, Schicher N, Sator P-G, Karlhofer FM, Stingl G, et al. Successful treatment of poststreptococcal scleredema adultorum Buschke with intravenous immunoglobulins. Arch Dermatol. 2012;148:1126–8.
65. Kroft EBM, Berkhof NJG, van de Kerkhof PCM, Gerritsen RMJP, de Jong EMGJ. Ultraviolet A phototherapy for sclerotic skin diseases: a systematic review. J Am Acad Dermatol. 2008;59:1017–30.
66. Stables GI, Taylor PC, Highet AS. Scleredema associated with paraproteinaemia treated by extracorporeal photopheresis. Br J Dermatol. 2000;142:781–3.
67. Hong KR, Hong JY, Chung EH, Lee SH, Lee SW, Kim JE. Monoclonal gammopathy-associated scleredema adultorum of buschke in a patient with diabetes mellitus successfully treated with intravenous immunoglobulin and narrow-band ultraviolet B phototherapy: a case report. Ann Dermatol. 2021;33:586–8.
68. Szalat R, Arnulf B, Karlin L, Rybojad M, Asli B, Malphettes M, et al. Pathogenesis and treatment of xanthomatosis associated with monoclonal gammopathy. Blood. 2011;118:3777–84.
69. Spicknall KE, Mehregan DA. Necrobiotic xanthogranuloma. Int J Dermatol. 2009;48:1–10.
70. Simon A, Asli B, Braun-Falco M, De Koning H, Fermand J-P, Grattan C, et al. Schnitzler's syndrome: diagnosis, treatment, and follow-up. Allergy. 2013;68:562–8.
71. Montagnon CM, Fracica EA, Patel AA, Camilleri MJ, Murad MH, Dingli D, et al. Pyoderma gangrenosum in hematologic malignancies: a systematic review. J Am Acad Dermatol. 2020;82:1346–59.
72. Powell FC, Schroeter AL, Su WP, Perry HO. Pyoderma gangrenosum and monoclonal gammopathy. Arch Dermatol. 1983;119:468–72.
73. Prat L, Bouaziz J-D, Wallach D, Vignon-Pennamen M-D, Bagot M. Neutrophilic dermatoses as systemic diseases. Clin Dermatol. 2014;32:376–88.
74. Bourke JF, Keohane S, Long CC, Kemmett D, Davies M, Zaki I, et al. Sweet's syndrome and malignancy in the U.K. Br J Dermatol. 1997;137:609–13.
75. Bayle P, Laplanche G, Gorguet B, Oksman F, Boulinguez S, Bazex J. Neutrophilic dermatosis: a case of overlapping syndrome with monoclonal antineutrophil cytoplasmic autoantibody activity. Dermatology. 1994;189:69–71.
76. Takata M, Inaoki M, Shodo M, Hirone T, Kaya H. Subcorneal pustular dermatosis associated with IgA myeloma and intraepidermal IgA deposits. Dermatology. 1994;189(Suppl 1):111–4.
77. Kasha EE Jr, Epinette WW. Subcorneal pustular dermatosis (Sneddon-Wilkinson disease) in association with a monoclonal IgA gammopathy: a report and review of the literature. J Am Acad Dermatol. 1988;19:854–8.
78. Yiannias JA, el-Azhary RA, Gibson LE. Erythema elevatum diutinum: a clinical and histopathologic study of 13 patients. J Am Acad Dermatol. 1992;26:38–44.
79. Maruani A, Arbeille B, Machet M-C, Barbet C, Laure B, Martin L, et al. Ultrastructural demonstration of a relationship between acquired cutis laxa and monoclonal gammopathy. Acta Derm Venereol. 2010;90:406–8.

5 Primary Cutaneous Lymphomas: Classification

Robert Gniadecki, Minakshi Taparia, Jean Deschenes, Jori Hardin, and Etienne Mahe

Primary cutaneous lymphomas constitute a unique subset of mature lymphoproliferative disorders with an initial clinical presentation restricted to the skin. This heterogeneous group encompasses both T-cell and B-cell lymphomas, each exhibiting varied clinical manifestations (Table 5.1).

Contrary to the prevailing belief that primary cutaneous lymphomas arise from lymphocytes already residing in the skin [2], recent experimental evidence suggests a different point of origin. It has been postulated that the initial malignant transformation occurs extracutaneously, perhaps in locations such as the thymus or bone marrow [3–7]. Following this initial transformation, mutated lymphoid precursors generate skin-homing lymphocytes that eventually colonize the skin, leading to the formation of clinically noticeable skin lesions.

From a clinical standpoint, a diagnosis of primary cutaneous lymphoma is established when skin lesions manifest before any signs of systemic involvement. Generally, a time gap of at least 6 months exists between the appearance of cutaneous lesions and clinically detectable systemic disease. However, many low-grade primary cutaneous lymphomas may never disseminate to other tissues or do so only infrequently. This distinction underscores the notion that even if the disease's origin may be extracutaneous, its primary manifestation is invariably in the skin.

It is important to note that while the nosology of primary cutaneous lymphomas may draw upon histopathological similarities to nodal lymphomas, these are fundamentally separate clinicopathological entities. Often, primary cutaneous lymphomas have a significantly better prognosis compared to their histologically similar nodal counterparts, which is reflected in differing therapeutic approaches. Consequently, precise differentiation between primary cutaneous lymphomas and secondary lymphomatous skin infiltrates is imperative for accurate patient prognostication

R. Gniadecki (✉)
Division of Dermatology, University of Alberta, Edmonton, AB, Canada
e-mail: gniadeck@ualberta.ca

M. Taparia
Division of Hematology, University of Alberta Hospital, Edmonton, AB, Canada

J. Deschenes
Department of Pathology and Laboratory Medicine, Cross Cancer Institute, Edmonton, AB, Canada
e-mail: Jean.Deschenes@albertaprecisionlabs.ca

J. Hardin
Division of Dermatology, University of Calgary, Calgary, AB, Canada
e-mail: Jori.hardin@albertahealthservices.ca

E. Mahe
Department of Pathology & Laboratory Medicine, and Hematology & Hematological Malignancies, University of Calgary, Calgary, AB, Canada
e-mail: etienne.mahe@albertaprecisionlabs.ca

R. Gniadecki et al. (eds.), *Diseases of Blood and Skin*, https://doi.org/10.1007/978-3-031-65292-9_5

Table 5.1 WHO classification of primary cutaneous lymphomas [1]

Primary cutaneous T-cell lymphomas	Primary cutaneous B-cell lymphomas
Mycosis fungoides	Primary cutaneous marginal zone lymphoma
Primary cutaneous CD4-positive small or medium T-cell lymphoproliferative disorder	Primary cutaneous follicle center lymphoma
Primary cutaneous CD30-positive T-cell lymphoproliferative disorder: Lymphomatoid papulosis	Primary cutaneous diffuse large B-cell lymphoma, leg type
Primary cutaneous CD30-positive T-cell lymphoproliferative disorder: Primary cutaneous anaplastic large cell lymphoma	EBV-positive mucocutaneous ulcer
Subcutaneous panniculitis-like T-cell lymphoma	NK/T-cell lymphomas
Primary cutaneous γδ T-cell lymphoma	Cutaneous NK/T-cell lymphoma, nasal type
Primary cutaneous CD8-positive aggressive epidermotropic cytotoxic T-cell lymphoma	EBV-positive T- and NK-cell lymphoid proliferations and lymphomas of childhood
Primary cutaneous peripheral T-cell lymphoma, NOS	Severe mosquito bite allergy
Primary cutaneous acral CD8-positive lymphoproliferative disorder	Hydroa vacciniforme lymphoproliferative disorder

and management. Failure to make this distinction can lead to inappropriate and unnecessarily aggressive treatment strategies.

References

1. Alaggio R, Amador C, Anagnostopoulos I, Attygalle AD, Araujo IBO, Berti E, et al. The 5th edition of the World Health Organization classification of haematolymphoid tumours: lymphoid neoplasms. Leukemia. 2022;36:1720–48.
2. Clark RA. Resident memory T cells in human health and disease. Sci Transl Med. 2015;7:269rv1.
3. Iyer A, Hennessey D, O'Keefe S, Patterson J, Wang W, Wong GK-S, et al. Branched evolution and genomic intratumor heterogeneity in the pathogenesis of cutaneous T-cell lymphoma. Blood Adv. 2020;4:2489–500.
4. Iyer A, Hennessey D, O'Keefe S, Patterson J, Wang W, Wong GK-S, et al. Skin colonization by circulating neoplastic clones in cutaneous T-cell lymphoma. Blood. 2019;134:1517–27.
5. Iyer A, Hennessey D, O'Keefe S, Patterson J, Wang W, Salopek T, et al. Clonotypic heterogeneity in cutaneous T-cell lymphoma (mycosis fungoides) revealed by comprehensive whole-exome sequencing. Blood Adv. 2019;3:1175–84.
6. Iyer A, Hennessey D, Gniadecki R. Clonotype pattern in T-cell lymphomas map the cell of origin to immature lymphoid precursors. Blood Adv. 2022;6:2334–45.
7. Harro CM, Sprenger KB, Chaurio RA, Powers JJ, Innamarato P, Anadon CM, et al. Sézary syndrome originates from heavily mutated hematopoietic progenitors. Blood Adv. 2023;7:5586–602.

Primary Cutaneous T-Cell Lymphoid Neoplasms

6

Robert Gniadecki, Minakshi Taparia, Jean Deschenes, Jori Hardin, and Etienne Mahe

6.1 Practice Essentials

- Primary cutaneous T-cell lymphoid neoplasms (CTCL) comprise a heterogeneous group of neoplasms ranging from aggressive lymphoma to clinically benign lymphoproliferative disorders.
- The most common disease is mycosis fungoides (MF), followed by small-medium $CD4^{+}$ lymphoproliferative disorder.
- The accurate diagnosis of CTCL depends on clinicopathological correlation.

R. Gniadecki (✉)
Division of Dermatology, University of Alberta, Edmonton, AB, Canada
e-mail: gniadeck@ualberta.ca

M. Taparia
Division of Hematology, University of Alberta Hospital, Edmonton, AB, Canada

J. Deschenes
Department of Pathology and Laboratory Medicine, Cross Cancer Institute, Edmonton, AB, Canada
e-mail: Jean.Deschenes@albertaprecisionlabs.ca

J. Hardin
Division of Dermatology, University of Calgary, Calgary, AB, Canada
e-mail: Jori.hardin@albertahealthservices.ca

E. Mahe
Department of Pathology & Laboratory Medicine, and Hematology & Hematological Malignancies, University of Calgary, Calgary, AB, Canada
e-mail: etienne.mahe@albertaprecisionlabs.ca

6.2 Classification of Primary Cutaneous T-Cell Lymphoid Neoplasms (CTCL)

Primary cutaneous T-cell neoplasms make up the majority of primary cutaneous lymphomas, accounting for about three-quarters of all cases [1]. The classification and nomenclature of these neoplasms are primarily based on clinicopathological patterns, with key associated histopathological and phenotypic features. The entities in this group can broadly be divided into two main categories. The largest group represents bona fide malignancies that exhibit all the hallmarks of cancer, i.e., fulfilling the criteria of a lymphoma. Lymphomas are considered a subset of lymphoproliferative disorders (LPD), but the term lymphoproliferative disorder also encompasses primary cutaneous lymphoproliferative diseases that display some histopathological or molecular features of cancer but have a clinically benign or very indolent clinical course. These entities with borderline and indolent clinical behavior, which are not clear-cut lymphomas, are hence simply called "lymphoproliferative disorders" for lack of a better term. For example, primary cutaneous anaplastic large cell lymphoma (pcALCL), which shows indolent behavior, is considered part of the spectrum of CD30-positive lymphoproliferative disorders; yet, this category also includes lymphomatoid papulosis, a clinical benign process that shows some overlapping features with the related lymphoma.

R. Gniadecki et al. (eds.), *Diseases of Blood and Skin*, https://doi.org/10.1007/978-3-031-65292-9_6

Another key concept is that the majority of primary cutaneous T-cell lymphoid neoplasms represent distinct clinicopathological entities that should be distinguished from their nodal counterparts, even if they share similar names. Overall, the prognosis of primary cutaneous T-cell lymphomas is generally better than that of nodal T-cell lymphomas. Only a few primary cutaneous T-cell lymphomas exhibit aggressive behavior with early systemic dissemination, including entities like primary cutaneous γδ T-cell lymphoma (pcGDTCL), and primary cutaneous CD8+ aggressive epidermotropic cytotoxic T-cell lymphoma (pcCD8-AECTCL).

Here is a proposed classification of primary cutaneous T-cell lymphoid neoplasms, based on the updated 2018 WHO-EORTC classification of primary cutaneous lymphomas, the 2022 International Consensus Classification of Mature Lymphoid Neoplasms (ICC, 2022), and WHO-HAEM 5th edition (2022), corresponding relative frequency and average disease-specific survival [2–5].

Disease	Frequency[a]	Five-year disease-specific survival[a]
Mature T-cell neoplasms		
Mycosis fungoides (MF)		Average 85%, stage I MF >90%, stage ≥IIB <50%
Classic type (Alibert-Bazin)	30%	
Folliculotropic MF (fMF)	5%	
Granulomatous slack skin disease		
Pagetoid reticulosis		
Granulomatous MF[b]	5%	
Gamma-delta (γδ) MF[b]		
Interstitial MF[b]		
Sézary syndrome (SS)	2%	35%
Primary cutaneous CD8+ aggressive epidermotropic cytotoxic T-cell lymphoma (pcCD8-AECTCL)	<1%	0–20%
Primary cutaneous γδT-cell lymphoma (pcGDTCL)	<1%	0–10%
Subcutaneous panniculitis-like T-cell lymphoma (pcSPTCL)	1%	95%
Primary CD30+ lymphoproliferative disorders		
Lymphomatoid papulosis	10%	100%
Primary cutaneous anaplastic large-cell lymphoma (pcALCL)	2%	95%
Benign CD30+ intravascular lymphoproliferative disease	<1%	100%
Primary cutaneous CD4+ small/medium T-cell lymphoproliferative disorder	40%	100%
Primary cutaneous acral CD8+ T-cell lymphoproliferative disorder	<1%	100%
Primary cutaneous peripheral T-cell lymphoma, NOS	2%	15%
NK/T cells neoplasms		
Extranodal NK-/T-cell lymphoma	<1%	0–15%
EBV-positive T- and NK-cell lymphoid proliferations and lymphomas of childhood	<1	Data not available
(Systemic) chronic active EBV disease		
Hydroa vacciniforme lymphoproliferative disorder		
Severe mosquito bite allergy		
Systemic EBV-positive T-cell lymphoma of childhood		

[a]Based on Refs. [5, 6] and unpublished data from lymphoma registries from the University of Copenhagen, Denmark and the University of Alberta/University of Calgary, Canada

[b]Not included in the updated 2018 WHO-EORTC classification of primary cutaneous lymphomas, or in the upcoming 5th edition of the WHO-HAEM5 (2022)

References

1. Hristov AC, Tejasvi T, Wilcox RA. Cutaneous T-cell lymphomas: 2021 update on diagnosis, risk-stratification, and management. Am J Hematol. 2021;96:1313–28.
2. Campo E, Jaffe ES, Cook JR, Quintanilla-Martinez L, Swerdlow SH, Anderson KC, et al. The International Consensus Classification of Mature Lymphoid Neoplasms: a report from the Clinical Advisory Committee. Blood. 2022;140:1229–53.
3. Falini B, Martino G, Lazzi S. A comparison of the International Consensus and 5th World Health Organization classifications of mature B-cell lymphomas. Leukemia. 2023;37:18–34.
4. Campo E, Jaffe ES, Cook JR, et al. The International Consensus Classification of Mature Lymphoid Neoplasms: a report from the Clinical Advisory Committee. Blood. 2022;140(11):1229–53.
5. Willemze R, Cerroni L, Kempf W, Berti E, Facchetti F, Swerdlow SH, et al. The 2018 update of the WHO-EORTC classification for primary cutaneous lymphomas. Blood. 2019;133:1703–14.
6. Scarisbrick JJ, Prince HM, Vermeer MH, Quaglino P, Horwitz S, Porcu P, et al. Cutaneous lymphoma international consortium study of outcome in advanced stages of mycosis fungoides and sézary syndrome: effect of specific prognostic markers on survival and development of a prognostic model. J Clin Oncol. 2015;33:3766–73.

Mycosis Fungoides and Sézary Syndrome

7

Robert Gniadecki, Minakshi Taparia, Jean Deschenes, Jori Hardin, and Etienne Mahe

7.1 Mycosis Fungoides

7.1.1 Practice Essentials

- Mycosis fungoides is the most common type of primary cutaneous T-cell lymphoma.
- Early-stage, typical MF (Alibert-Bazin) presents with patches and plaques on sun-protected areas of the skin and has an excellent prognosis with a low risk of stage progression.
- Early-stage MF may clinically and histopathologically mimic a number of other inflammatory or neoplastic diseases and diagnosis is made by clinicopathological correlation.
- Some histological subtypes (folliculotropic MF, granulomatous MF, γδMF, interstitial MF) may have a more aggressive course.
- Development of tumors, large cell transformation, and extracutaneous involvement negatively affect prognosis.
- Therapy is individual, dependent on the stage and prognosis of the disease, and comprises skin-directed therapies (e.g., topical corticosteroids, phototherapy, radiotherapy, mechlorethamine), targeted therapies (HDACi, rexinoids, mogamulizumab, brentuximab), single agent and combination chemotherapies, and allogeneic bone marrow transplant.

7.1.2 Clinical Presentation

Mycosis fungoides (MF) stands as the most common type of primary cutaneous T-cell lymphoma (CTCL). Its clinical presentation can be highly diverse, often resembling various benign inflammatory skin conditions as well as systemic T-cell lymphomas with secondary skin infiltration.

R. Gniadecki (✉)
Division of Dermatology, University of Alberta, Edmonton, AB, Canada
e-mail: r.gniadecki@ualberta.ca

M. Taparia
Division of Hematology, University of Alberta Hospital, Edmonton, AB, Canada
e-mail: mtaparia@ualberta.ca

J. Deschenes
Department of Pathology and Laboratory Medicine, Cross Cancer Institute, Edmonton, AB, Canada
e-mail: Jean.Deschenes@albertaprecisionlabs.ca

J. Hardin
Division of Dermatology, University of Calgary, Calgary, AB, Canada
e-mail: Jori.hardin@albertahealthservices.ca

E. Mahe
Department of Pathology & Laboratory Medicine, and Hematology & Hematological Malignancies, University of Calgary, Calgary, AB, Canada
e-mail: etienne.mahe@albertaprecisionlabs.ca

R. Gniadecki et al. (eds.), *Diseases of Blood and Skin*, https://doi.org/10.1007/978-3-031-65292-9_7

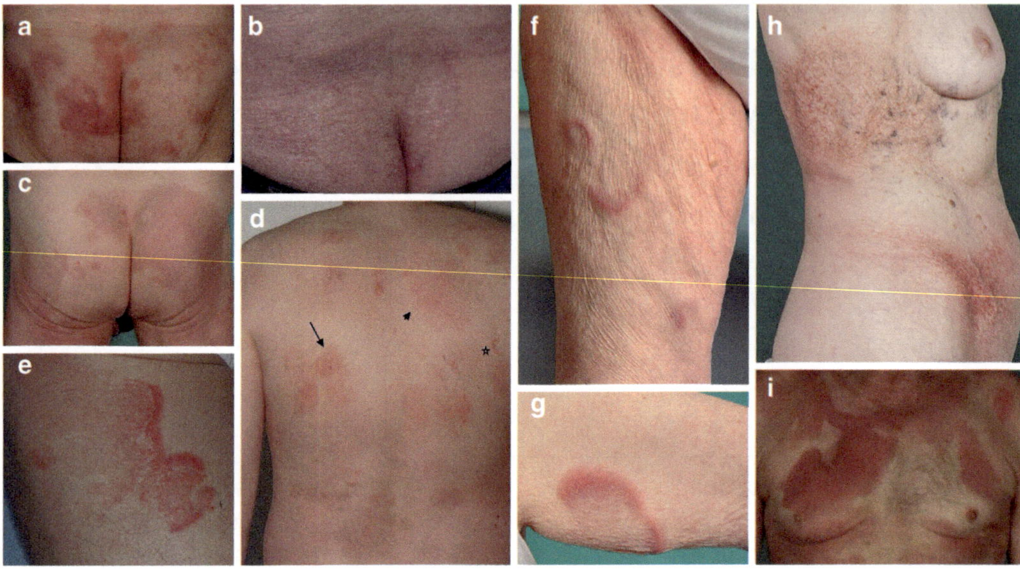

Fig. 7.1 Early mycosis fungoides (MF), Alibert-Bazin type. (**a–e**) The initial lesions reported by patients manifest as scaly, flat patches, frequently observed on the buttocks, upper legs, and lower back. Notice the morphologic heterogeneity of the lesions: well-demarcated patches (**d**, arrow), eczematous, poorly demarcated areas of erythema (redness) (**d**, arrowhead), and arcuate lesions (**d**, star), along with asymmetry in color and shape (**e**). (**f, g**) Rapidly growing lesions often adopt arcuate, reniform shapes. (**h, i**) Further progression of the lesions to large plaques (**h**—large, atrophic plaques historically termed large-plaque parapsoriasis) or thicker, infiltrated plaques exhibiting variability in shape and color (**i**)

In its classic presentation, known as Alibert-Bazin type,[1] MF initially appears as erythematous, scaly patches and plaques (Fig. 7.1). These skin lesions tend to emerge on sun-protected areas of the lower trunk, buttocks, and thighs. The size of these lesions can vary, ranging from approximately 10 mm to larger patches spanning 20–30 cm. Moreover, there can be asymmetry in the shape of the lesions. Within the same patient, the morphology of these lesions may differ, ranging from well-demarcated, scaly plaques with a psoriasiform appearance to horseshoe- or reniform-shaped annular plaques.

MF typically affects males in the age range of 50–60 years, although it can develop at any age, including in children. In about two-thirds of patients, MF remains in this early stage for years or even decades, and it doesn't significantly impact life expectancy. However, for approximately one-third of patients, the disease progresses to the tumor stage, which is associated with a substantially reduced 5-year overall survival rate of approximately 50% [1–3] (Fig. 7.2). The exact cause of death in MF is not fully understood, but most patients who pass away do not exhibit signs of disease dissemination. Death is more likely attributed to factors such as immunosuppression, cachexia (muscle wasting and weight loss), and secondary infections [4]. Additionally, MF is linked to several comorbidities, including cardiovascular disease, thromboembolism, pulmonary disease, and secondary cancers, which can also contribute to increased mortality [5, 6].

7.1.2.1 Clinical Variants

MF exhibits numerous clinical variants, with many distinct clinical-pathological presentations compared to the classic Alibert-Bazin type, which stand out because they involve a preferred histological compartment (e.g., folliculotropic

[1]The eponym commemorates two French dermatologists, Jean-Louis Alibert (1768–1837) and Pierre-Antoine-Ernest Bazin (1807–1878) who were the first to describe MF and its typical clinical evolution.

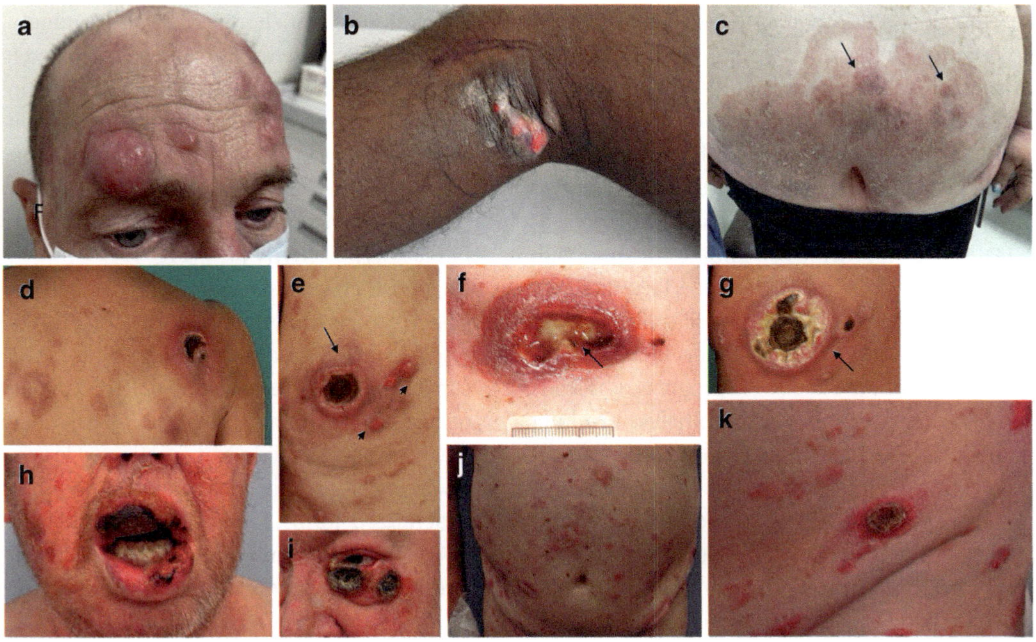

Fig. 7.2 Advanced (tumor stage) mycosis fungoides (MF). Tumors may manifest clinically as exophytic, dome-shaped nodules emerging on previously unaffected skin (**a**) or within pre-existing plaques (**b, c** [arrows]). (**d–g**) Some tumors exhibit early necrosis and ulceration. Observe the annular shape of the tumor (arrows), resembling the configuration of early MF plaques, and the emergence of smaller tumors in the proximity of the larger lesion (arrowheads in **e**). (**h–k**) Widespread lesions comprising plaques and tumors in a patient with advanced MF. The development of tumors in the oral mucosa or conjunctiva (**h, i**) represents an unfavorable prognostic sign

or mucosal MF), display a peculiar distribution (e.g., palmoplantar or intertriginous MF, unilesional MF), are accompanied by pigmentary changes (e.g., hypo- or hyperpigmented MF) or show remarkable clinical features that simulate other dermatoses (e.g., ichthyosiform MF, pigmented purpura-like MF, bullous MF). Most of these variants, while they may represent diagnostic challenges, lack significant prognostic implications and their natural history does not differ significantly from classic MF. However, some are specifically recognized in the WHO-EORTC (2018) classification and more recent WHO and ICC classifications because of their distinctive clinical features, natural history and/or prognosis. See Table 7.1.

- **Folliculotropic MF.** Among the clinical subtypes of MF, folliculotropic MF (fMF) stands out as particularly important due to its distinct

Table 7.1 Clinical variants of MF [7]

Bullous/vesicular mycosis fungoides
Erythodermic mycosis fungoides
Follicular mucinosis
Folliculotropic mycosis fungoides[a]
Granulomatous slack skin[a]
Hyperpigmented mycosis fungoides
Hypopigmented mycosis fungoides
Icthyosiform mycosis fungoides
Intertriginous mycosis fungoides
Mucosal mycosis fungoides
Pagetoid reticulosis[a]
Palmoplantar/acral mycosis fungoides
Pigmented purpura-like mycosis fungoides
Poikilodermatous mycosis fungoides
Pustular mycosis fungoides
Spiky mycosis fungoides
Unilesional mycosis fungoides
Vegetating/papillomatous mycosis fungoides
Verrucous/hyperkeratotic mycosis fungoides

[a]Specific variant recognized in the WHO-EORTC 2018 classification

clinical and histopathological features and its relative frequency, representing approximately 10% of all cases of MF, which makes it the most common non-classic variant of MF [3, 8]. fMF is defined by histopathological characteristics and has distinct clinical features. Unlike the classic Alibert-Bazin presentation of MF, fMF often initiates in areas with large hair follicles, such as the face or scalp. The initial lesions in fMF are typically papules that can enlarge, forming thick plaques and tumors. As the disease progresses, it leads to the destruction of hair follicles, resulting in localized hair loss. One notable clinical manifestation of fMF is the accumulation of mucin within affected hair follicles, a condition referred to as "follicular mucinosis." Clinically, this presents as milia-like follicular white papules. When squeezed, these papules produce a white, mucinous discharge.

Over time, fMF tends to involve various skin areas, often affecting the back, axillae, genital areas, and thighs. The WHO-HAEMR 5th edition recognizes a distinction should be made between the early and advanced stages of fMF, as the latter shows a worse clinical course [9]. Lesions in fMF are typically thicker than those seen in classic MF, and tumors may develop early in the disease course. This aggressive nature is one reason why fMF is often resistant to therapy and carries a worse prognosis [3, 8]. However, once fMF reaches the tumor stage, the prognosis is similar to classic MF [10]. Additionally, it is important to emphasize that folliculotropism or follicular mucinosis can sometimes be incidental findings in biopsies from classic MF and should not be the sole criteria for diagnosing fMF. A characteristic clinical pattern of lesions is essential for an accurate diagnosis of fMF (Fig. 7.3).

- **Granulomatous slack skin disease** is a rare manifestation of MF characterized by pendulous, lax skin folds caused by elastolysis [11]. This form of MF is typically resistant to therapy and has a worse prognosis compared to Alibert-Bazin MF. However, limited data are available due to the rarity of the disease. It is worth noting that shorter survival in granulomatous slack skin disease may be attributed to a higher association with secondary lymphomas [12]. Some evidence suggest that granulomatous slack skin disease and granulomatous MF (gMF) are two manifestations of a continuum, fundamentally different by the degree of elastolytic activity [13] (Fig. 7.4).
- **Pagetoid reticulosis** (Woringer-Kolopp disease) is a clinically indolent form of MF that often presents as an enlarging single, scaly, superficial, well-demarcated patch, typically on the feet. In some cases, the disease may manifest with multiple or disseminated lesions involving other skin areas, referred to as the generalized form (Ketron-Goodman disease) [14]). While the unilesional form is well-recognized as an indolent, localized MF-like lesion, the status of Ketron-Goodman disease remains debated [15]. Pagetoid reticulosis should be differentiated from the palmoplantar MF, and, at times, this is only possible by histopathological features (Fig. 7.5).
- **Gamma-delta MF** (γδMF) is histopathologically defined by the immunohistochemical expression of γδTCR chains by the malignant cells. Gene rearrangement studies showing γ chain rearrangement and/or β chain rearrangement have no diagnostic importance in this definition, except to show the presence of monoclonal T cells. Clinically, it may exhibit subtle deviations from the Alibert-Bazin MF presentation. Initial lesions in γδMF can appear anywhere on the skin and often manifest as violaceous papules or nodules, or diffuse erythematous areas. Palpation may reveal deep infiltration into the subcutis. The distinction between γδMF and primary cutaneous γδ T-cell lymphoma (pcGDTCL) is somewhat controversial and primarily based on histopathological characteristics [16]. Although some authors claim that γδMF has a similar prognosis to classic MF, all our patients with γδMF had progressive disease, were quickly relapsing after therapy, and developed systemic metastases (Figs. 7.6 and 7.7).
- **Granulomatous MF (gMF)** is histopathologically defined by the presence of a granulo-

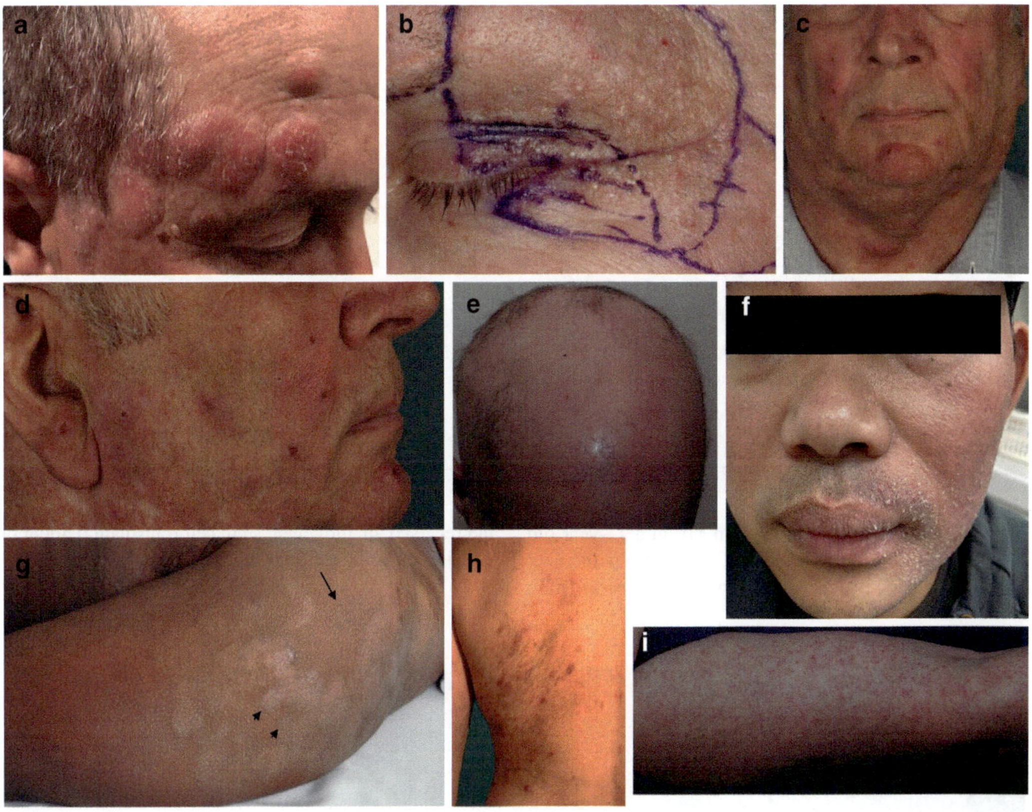

Fig. 7.3 Folliculotropic mycosis fungoides (fMF). (**a**) In contrast to Alibert-Bazin MF lesions developing on sun-protected areas of the trunk and proximal lower extremities, fMF's initial presentation often involves plaques and tumors on the face and scalp. (**b**) Milia-like lesions result from follicular mucinosis. (**d–f**) Atypical fMF presentations include acneiform (folliculitic) lesions on the face, total alopecia with subtle signs of hair follicle involvement (perifollicular redness with minimal infiltration [**e**]), or deep, asymmetric infiltration of the cheek (**f**). (**g–i**) fMF on the trunk and limbs. (**g**) Plaques (arrowheads) and follicular accentuation resembling goosebumps (arrows) caused by follicular infiltration by malignant cells. (**h**) Lesions resembling folliculitis on the trunk. (**i**) fMF manifesting as keratosis pilaris-like lesions on the arms

matous inflammatory infiltrate. In comparison to classic MF, gMF typically has a worse prognosis, and stage progression and extracutaneous dissemination may occur early in the disease course. gMF may clinically resemble γδMF. Up to 35% of patients develop early organ metastasis within 2 years of the initial presentation (lung > liver > spleen >CNS) [17] (Fig. 7.8).

- **Interstitial MF** often clinically resembles classic MF and is defined by distinctive histopathological features [18]. The malignant infiltrate in interstitial MF is typically restricted to the dermis, and it often exhibits a $CD8^+$ phenotype with expression of cytotoxic markers. Clinical presentations of interstitial MF may be atypical, with early lesions occurring in unusual areas of the body, such as the arms or lower legs (Fig. 7.9).
- **MF with large cell transformation (LCT)** is characterized by the presence of >25% large cells in the biopsy. LCT is a rare event that negatively influences survival and elevates the risk of extracutaneous dissemination. LCT may manifest at any stage of MF, although it is most commonly observed in stage IIB or higher and is usually detected 5–10 years after diagnosis [19]. Clinical indicators of LCT

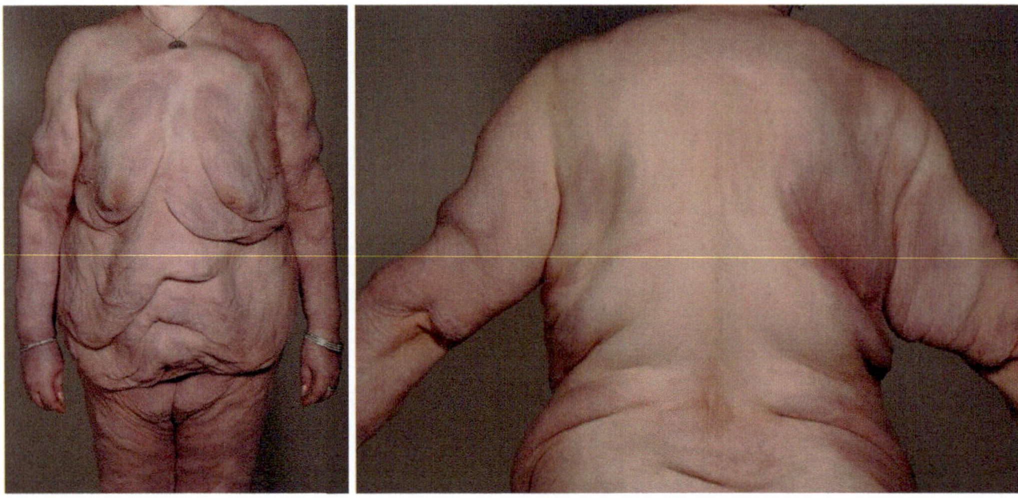

Fig. 7.4 Granulomatous slack skin MF in a 27-year-old female patient. After 15 years of a relatively indolent course, the patient developed large cell transformation and received an allogeneic stem cell transplant. Patient of Dr. Lisa Vaakeva, Helsinki, Finland

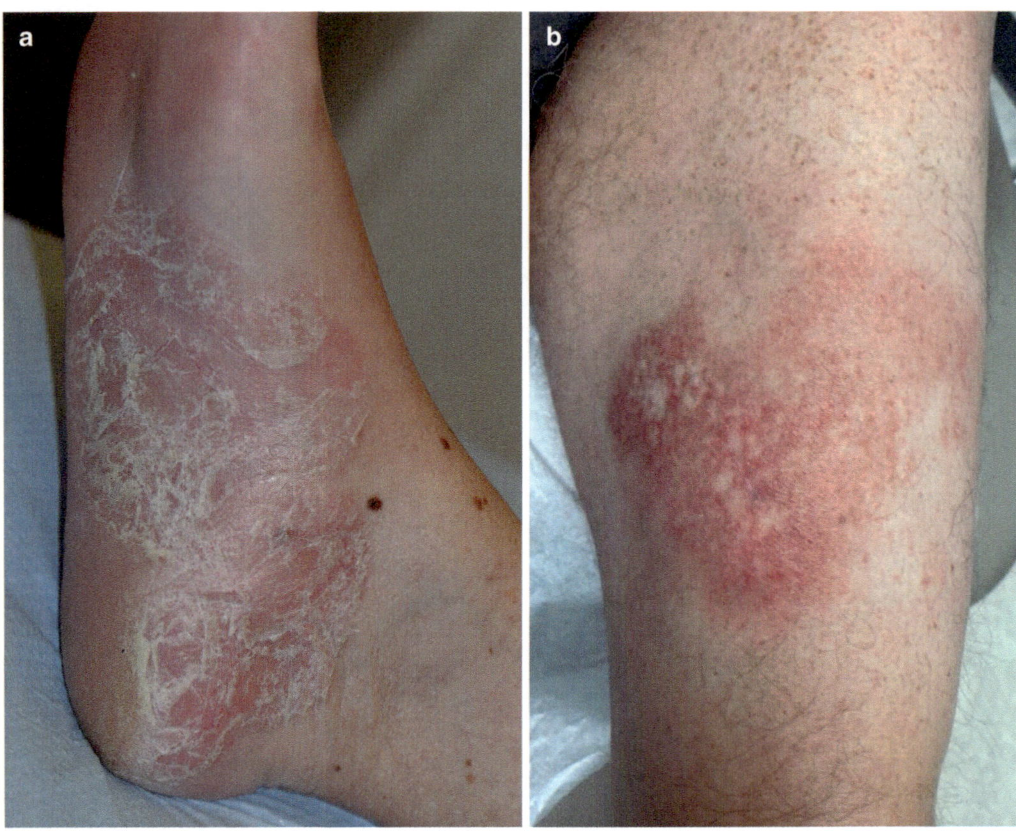

Fig. 7.5 Pagetoid reticulosis presenting on the foot (Woringer-Kolopp disease) (**a**) and on the lower leg as a superficial, slightly scaly patch (**b**)

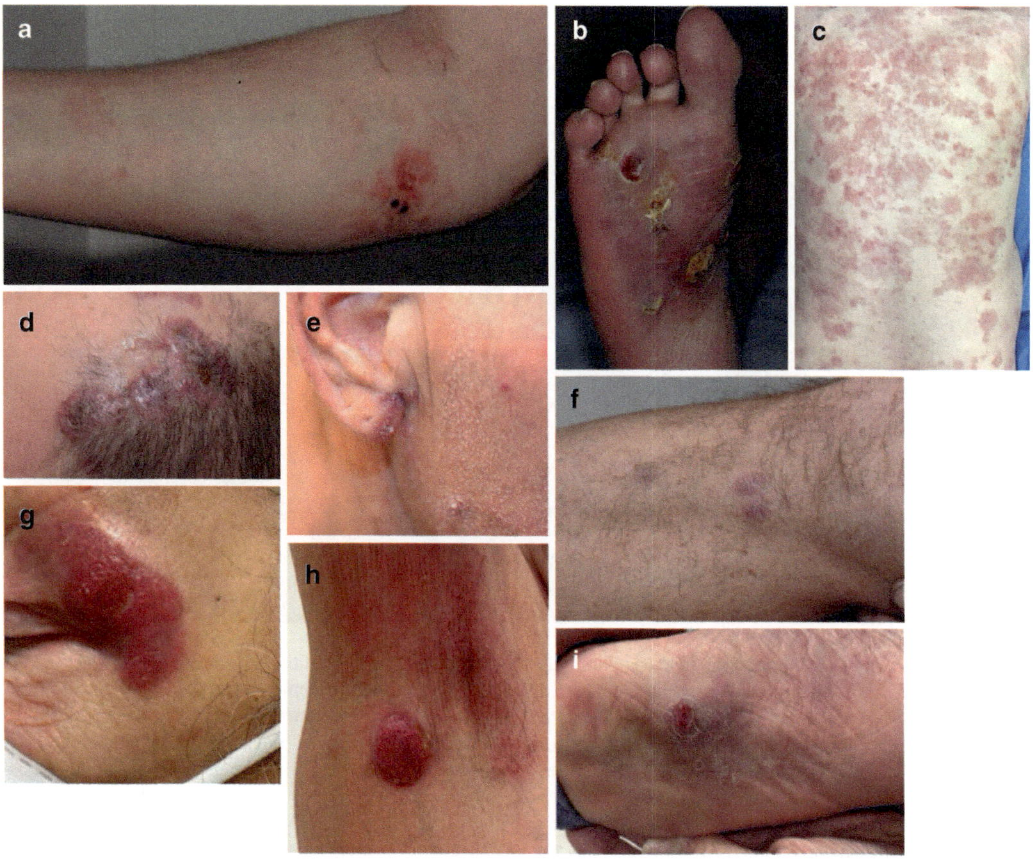

Fig. 7.6 Clinical presentations of gamma-delta mycosis fungoides (γδMF). (**a**) Superficial patches and plaques observed in atypical areas of early involvement for Alibert-Bazin MF (forearms in this instance). Noteworthy is the inclination toward ulceration in the early lesions, a feature not commonly associated with classic MF. (**b**) Initial plantar involvement. (**c**) Early, extensive skin participation characterized by patches and plaques. (**d–f**) Ulcerated plaques on the scalp and earlobe, accompanied by superficial plaques and patches on distal extremities, clinically reminiscent of fMF. (**g–i**) γδMF presentation initially as an ulcerated plaque on the eyelid, progressing over the subsequent 2 years to widespread disease with thick plaques and tumors on the trunk, distal extremities, and the soles (**h, i**)

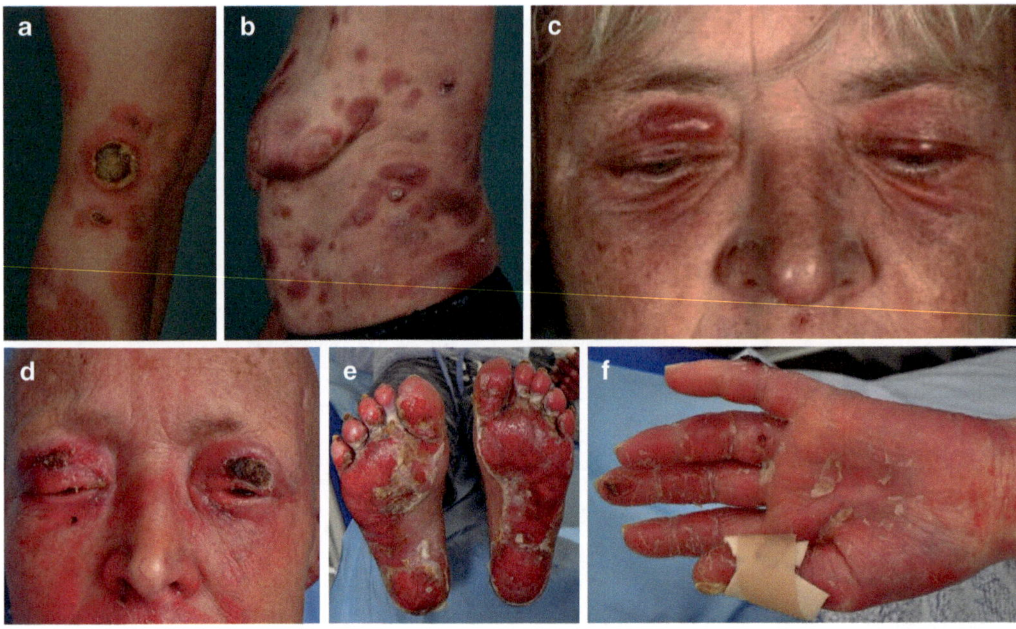

Fig. 7.7 Evolution of gamma-delta mycosis fungoides (γδMF) in a previously healthy, 58-year-old woman. The initial presentation featured a swiftly expanding, ulcerated tumor on the leg, surrounded by superficial patches and plaques (**a**). Biopsy results revealed an epidermotropic, atypical T-cell infiltrate $CD4^+$ $CD3^+$ $CD8^-$ $CD7^-$ $betaF1^+$ with TCRγ and TCRβ monoclonality, leading to the diagnosis of MF, subsequently managed with radiotherapy. Nine months later, a relapse occurred, manifesting as plaque and tumor involvement on the skin of the trunk and face (**b, c**). A biopsy of these lesions identified $\beta F1^-$ $CD4^-$ $CD8^-$ triple-negative, epidermotropic lymphoma, exhibiting identical TCR rearrangements as observed in the initial biopsy. Despite intensive systemic therapy, the patient progressed to an advanced stage, developing resistant lesions on the palms, soles, and eyelids (**d–f**). Notably, our experience with γδMF patients underscores potential discrepancies in biopsy results from different sites, necessitating serial biopsies for an accurate diagnosis

encompass the rapid development of tumors, the appearance of atypical-looking tumors, palpable and deeply infiltrating plaques, or panniculitic lesions. Intriguingly, LCT may also be an incidental finding encountered in routine biopsies of skin lesions. In such instances, additional biopsies may be necessary to ascertain whether LCT is also present in other lesions. Strikingly, nearly 50% of MF-LCT patients may present with extracutaneous dissemination, predominantly involving the lymph nodes, which is a foreboding sign associated with substantial mortality (5-year survival of <10% in patients with extracutaneous dissemination versus >30%) [20, 21]. In some series, even isolated LCT has been deemed a negative prognostic sign [19]. However, widespread LCT suggests an even more aggressive disease. While it has been proposed that $CD30^+$ LCT carries a more favorable prognosis than the $CD30^-$ phenotype, other case series have not demonstrated any prognostic significance of CD30 expression [20, 21] (Fig. 7.10).

- **Metastatic MF** is a rare event characterized by the progression of MF to the stage of organ metastases (M1, IVB), with a prevalence of only 0.1–0.5% in clinical practice [1]. Some patients exhibit organ metastases as a result of a sequential stage progression (e.g., from stage I to IIB to IVA or from stage III to IVA to IVB). However, organ metastases can also arise unpredictably. Risk factors for systemic dissemination encompass gMF,

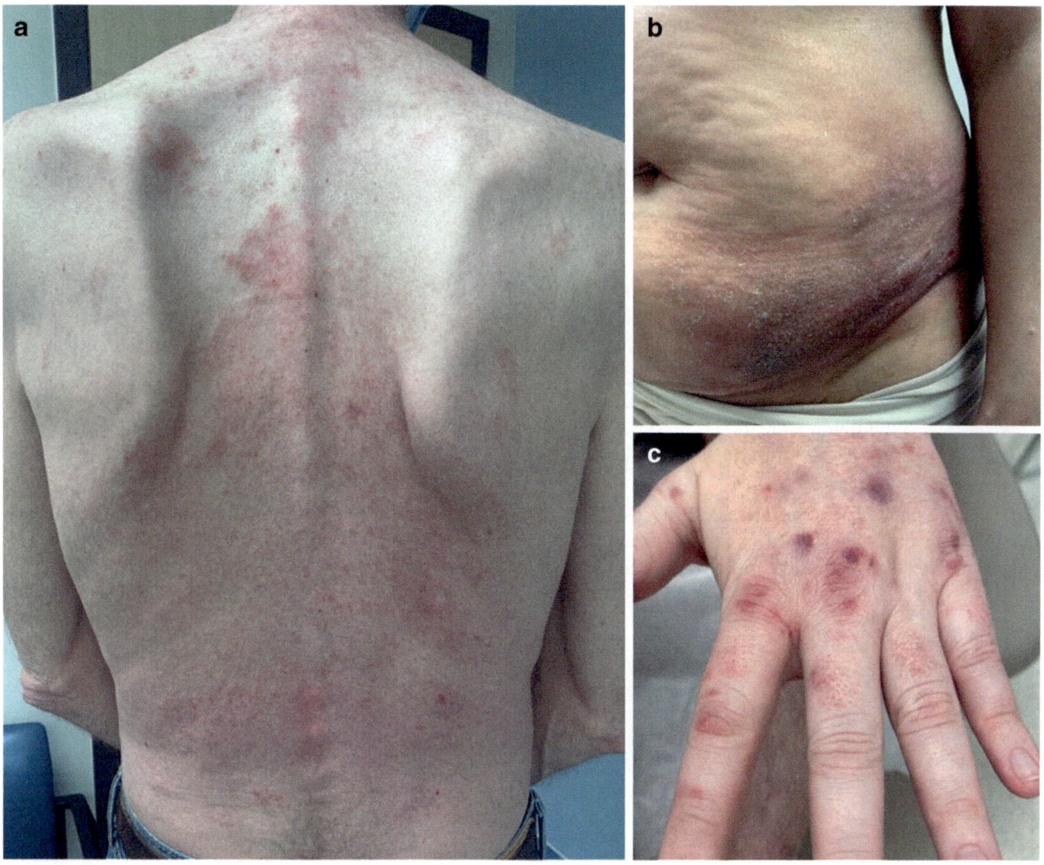

Fig. 7.8 Granulomatous mycosis fungoides (gMF). The cutaneous presentations of gMF may bear semblance to those observed in Alibert-Bazin MF; yet in certain individuals, the lesion distribution pattern diverges from the conventional. (**a**) Slender, diffuse papules and patches observed on the back. (**b**) An infiltrated, indistinctly demarcated plaque situated on the abdomen, and (**c**) a manifestation of papular and nodular lesions on the dorsal hands

the γδ phenotype, large-cell transformation, or concurrent immunosuppression (e.g., due to calcineurin inhibitors or biologics such as TNF α- or IL4/13 inhibitors). Notably, parenchymatous organs may be involved without prior lymph node or peripheral blood involvement. The pattern of organ involvement is variable, but early metastases have been observed in the brain, lungs, liver, and kidneys. Given the unpredictability and low risk of early metastasis detection, most centers do not recommend routine imaging for this purpose, and detection primarily relies on clinical symptoms and signs related to the target organ (Fig. 7.11).

7.1.3 Diagnostic Workup

7.1.3.1 Lesional Skin Biopsy

The interpretation of the skin biopsy for MF is often challenging as it may not definitively yield the diagnosis due to histological similarities with benign lymphocytic infiltrates. At times, the degree of atypia can be quite subtle, and the histological manifestations may exhibit heterogeneity, necessitating multiple biopsies for an accurate diagnosis [22]. Histological clues that aid in the early diagnosis of MF include the presence of epidermotropism of lymphocytes without accompanying spongiosis, the existence of Pautrier microabscesses (well-demarcated lymphocytic

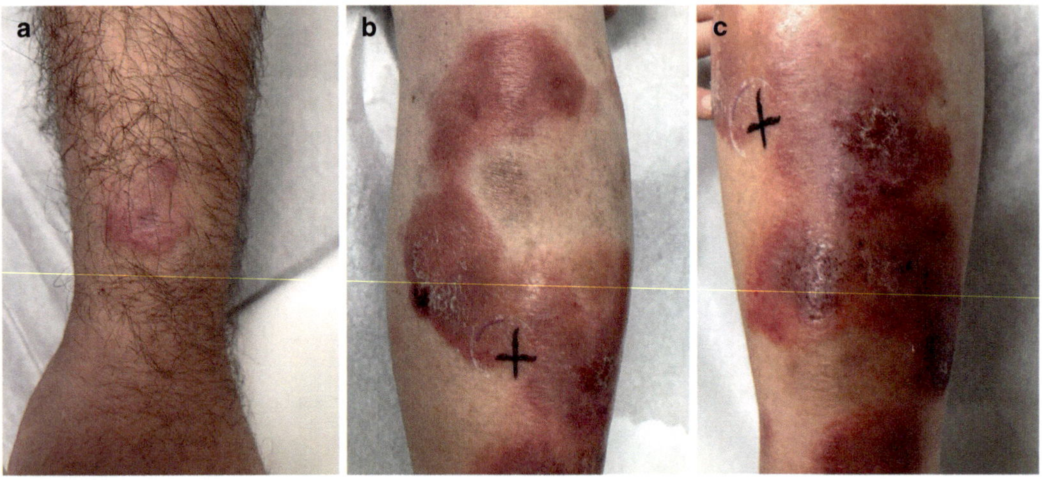

Fig. 7.9 Atypical lesions in interstitial mycosis fungoides (MF). In the initial stages of the disease, a slender plaque manifested on the forearm (**a**). Subsequent to a span of 10 months, the pathology advanced, culminating in the development of substantial, ulcerated plaques on the lower extremities (**b, c**)

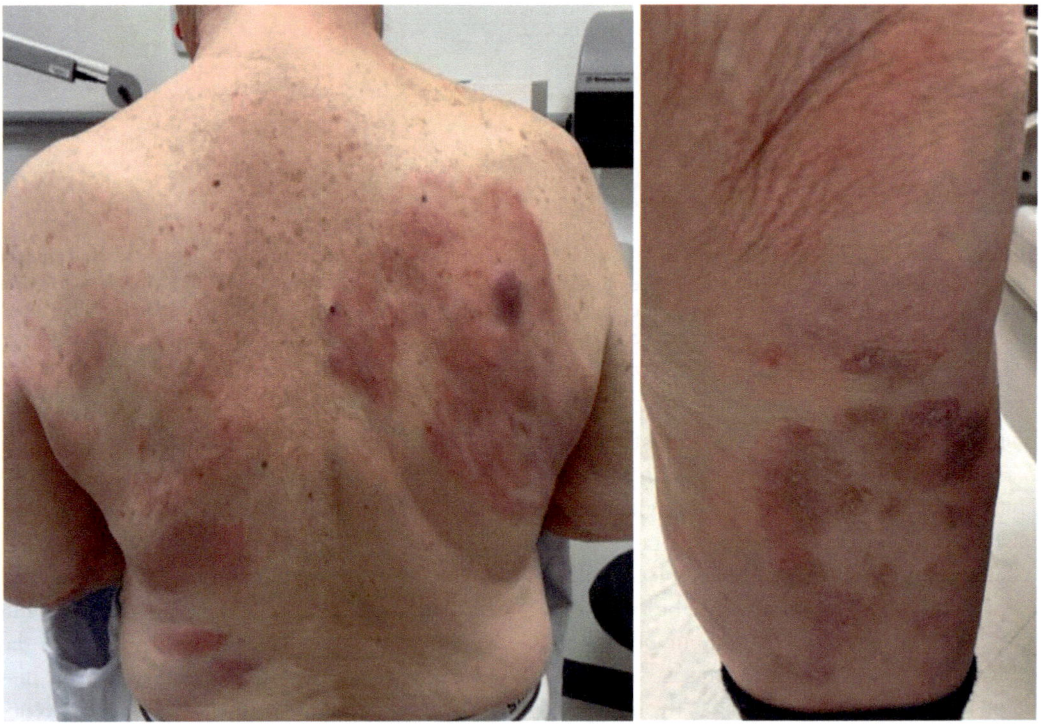

Fig. 7.10 Mycosis fungoides (MF) with large cell transformation. A 69-year-old male patient with a 7-year history of stage IB mycosis fungoides exhibited disease exacerbation, marked by the emergence of a notably large plaque with central necrosis on the right back (**a**) and additional plaques on the lower extremities (**b**). The biopsy revealed the presence of 30% large cells, identified through immunohistochemical markers $CD4^{+}$ $CD4^{+}$ $CD8^{-}$ $CD30^{+}$

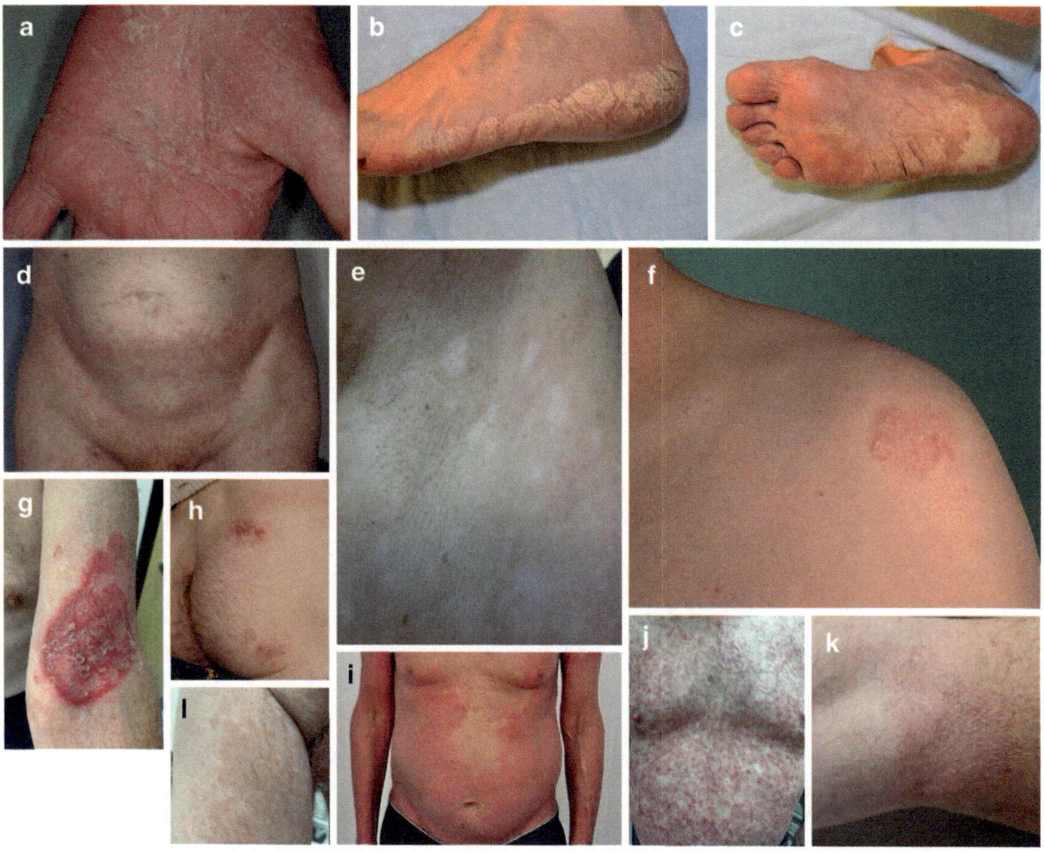

Fig. 7.11 Special manifestations of mycosis fungoides (MF). (**a–c**) Palmar and plantar MF resembling psoriasis or hyperkeratotic eczema. (**d**) Lichenoid MF. (**e**) Hypopigmented MF resembling vitiligo. (**f, g**) Unilesional MF. (**h**) Eczematous MF resembling nummular dermatitis. (**i, j**) Psoriasiform lesions of MF with relative symmetry of distribution and well-demarcated borders. (**k**) Poikilodermatous MF presenting with very thin, atrophic patches with a wrinkled surface reminiscent of cigarette paper. (**l**) Intertriginous MF resembling erythrasma

conglomerates in the epidermis), a linear arrangement ("tagging" or "string of pearls") of lymphocytes along the basal membrane, hyperchromasia and nucleomegaly of lymphocytes within the epidermis compared to the dermis, and infiltration of lymphocytes between dermal collagen fibers.

Immunohistochemistry provides additional diagnostic clues (Table 7.2). Typically, it reveals a mature phenotype, characterized by $CD3^+$ $CD4^+$ expression, with a partial or complete loss of CD7. Unfortunately, loss of CD7 is not uncommon in reactive T-cell populations and may be viewed as sensitive but not specific for the diagnosis of MF, unless it is extensive and marked (less than 10% of tumor cells). Loss of CD2 or CD5 is more specific

Table 7.2 Prognostic significance of MF immunophenotypes

Feature	Prognostic significance
Large cell transformation	Unfavorable prognosis, maybe worse in CD30 negative cases
$CD3^+$, $CD4^-$, $CD8^{+/-}$	Same as $CD4^+$ unless it indicates γδ phenotype (requires additional IHC to prove it)
$CD3^+$ $CD4^+$ $CD8^+$	Worse if accompanied by granulomatous features
$δF1^-$	Indicating γδMF with a worse prognosis
$CD4^-$ $CD8^-$ (double negative)	Hallmark of γδMF, worse prognosis
$CD3^+$ $CD4^+$ TIA-1/ granzyme B^+	Expression of cytotoxic markers may appear in the tumor stage of $CD4^+$ and is associated with an aggressive course

Table 7.3 Comparison of major clinical types of MF

	Clinical features	Typical phenotype observed in lesional cells	Other useful IHC markers	TCR protein defined by IHC	Prognosis
Classic MF (Alibert-Bazin)	Patches and plaques on non-sun-exposed areas (lower back, buttocks and upper thighs) evolving over years to eventually form tumors	$CD3^+$ $CD4^+$ $CD8^-$	Rarely cytotoxic, T-cell follicular helper markers (T_{FH})	TCRαβ	Low-grade, good prognosis in early stages
fMF	Plaques and nodules involving the face and scalp as well as other areas. Areas of hair loss (alopecia). Follicular mucinosis	$CD3^+$ $CD4^+$ $CD8^-$	Similar to classic MF	TCRαβ	More aggressive than classic MF, shorter time to tumor progression
Granulomatous slack skin disease	Pendulous skin folds	$CD3^+$ $CD4^+$ $CD8^-$	Similar to classic MF	TCRαβ	Therapy-resistant, association with other lymphomas
Pagetoid reticulosis	Scaly, well-demarcated patch on the extremity (localized form, Woringer-Kolopp) or multiple scaly patches (disseminated form)	$CD3^+$ $CD4^-$ $CD8^+$	Cytotoxic proteins very rare	TCRαβ	Indolent
γδMF	Nodules, plaques and tumors, distribution often deviate from that of classic MF	$CD3^{+/-}$ $CD4^-$ $CD8^{+/-}$	Cytotoxic proteins common (TIA-1, granzyme B)	TCRγδ	Probably more aggressive than classic MF
gMF	Nodules and plaques on the extremities and the distribution of lesions often deviate from that of classic MF	$CD3^+$ $CD4^+$ $CD8^-$	Similar to classic MF	TCRαβ	More aggressive than classic MF, early metastases
Interstitial MF [18]	Like Alibert-Bazin MF	$CD3^+$ $CD4^-$ $CD8^+$	Cytotoxic proteins common (TIA-1, granzyme B)	TCRαβ	Prognosis like in classic Alibert-Bazin MF

but of lower sensitivity. T-cell antigen loss has more diagnostic significance when it is extensive and/or sharply limited to an intra-epidermal population, as distinguished from dermal populations. CD30 is typically negative or only stains individual cells, while PD-1 staining can vary (Table 7.3).

Occasionally, MF may exhibit a $CD3^+$ $CD8^+$ phenotype, necessitating a differential diagnosis with aggressive epidermotropic $CD8^+$ lymphoma, Pagetoid reticulosis, acral $CD8^+$ lymphoproliferative disease, or even lymphomatoid papulosis (LyP). In very rare instances, MF may display a double-negative phenotype ($CD4^-$ $CD8^-$), which should raise the possibility of γδMF. In such cases, staining with a -δ chain-specific antibody becomes essential to establish the correct diagnosis. It is worth noting that positivity for βF1 (classic TCRαβ) is not always sufficient to rule out γδMF, as a subset of lymphomas may express both markers (βF1 and δF1) [23, 24].

Transformed MF can be challenging to differentiate from co-existing LyP or anaplastic large cell lymphoma (ALCL) that express the CD30 marker (see below). Occasionally, gMF with a large admixture of histiocytes may also resemble LCT-MF. In most cases, the clinical appearance of the lesions can assist in differentiating between these conditions. It is important to note that comorbid LyP or pcALCL does not typically impact patients' prognosis.

7.1.3.2 Molecular Studies

MF is a hypermutated lymphoma characterized by the presence of at least 50 major oncogenes with nonsynonymous somatic mutations. However, the specific constellation of mutations in MF varies widely among patients, rendering tumor genotyping impractical for clinical use.

For nearly three decades, detection of clonal rearrangements of the T-cell receptor genes has been a valuable tool for demonstrating clonality in MF. While the finding of a specifically rearranged TCR gene, which usually implies an underlying monoclonal T-cell population, cannot establish the diagnosis by itself, the confirmation of TCR monoclonality is useful and counts as a valuable additional criterion to reach more diagnostic certainty. TCR rearrangement testing can currently be performed on formalin-fixed, paraffin-embedded tissue using PCR-based methods. Both TCRγ and TCRβ genes are tested, but TCRγ, although more sensitive, is often seen in benign reactive infiltrates of the skin. Therefore, TCRγ is often supplemented by testing the TCRβ gene, which offers higher genetic variability and functional expression in mature T lymphocytes. In most cases, TCRβ testing provides excellent sensitivity and specificity, but false positive TCR results may be observed in normal elderly patients or patients with systemic diseases that affect their immune milieu (e.g., MDS, CLL [25, 26]) as well benign dermatoses such as lupus erythematosus or lichen planus [27], and some of these benign clonal populations have been detected repeatedly over time, with the exact same clonal population. However, the findings of the exact same clonal population (amplicon product) in two separate samples is a strong and specific indicator for a diagnosis of MF in the right clinical-pathological setting [28].

Next-generation sequencing (NGS) has been proposed as an alternative to standard PCR-based testing and may offer increased sensitivity and specificity in identifying clonality, but as it becomes more widely used, limitations similar to those observed with PCR may be uncovered when it comes to detecting clonal populations of uncertain significance in non-neoplastic cutaneous infiltrates [29, 30].

It's important to note that while MF and other cutaneous T-cell lymphomas may exhibit oligoclonality rather than strict monoclonality, this does not diminish the validity of TCR gene rearrangement testing for a specific lesion, where the given clone will translate in a positive TCR testing result. Occasionally, transient clones may be observed in skin and blood samples. These clones are typically absent upon retesting with new samples, although subsequent testing may reveal new transient clones with different sequences. The origin of these transient clones is unclear, but they may represent public clonotypes—normally expanded clones of the CDR3 sequence (the one used for amplification by PCR) and shared among different individuals [31, 32].

7.1.3.3 Flow Cytometry

Flow cytometry of the skin, while not routinely used in the diagnosis of MF, can be valuable, especially in cases with unusual marker expression patterns. This technique involves obtaining single-cell suspensions from fresh skin biopsies, and this is the most technically challenging part of the process. For that reason, it may be especially suited to larger skin tumors, which may be generously harvested. The harvested cells are then analyzed using multicolor flow cytometry, using similar markers to those used for blood mononuclear cells. Flow cytometry of skin samples can be particularly useful for enumerating CD30-positive neoplastic cells, which can aid in qualifying patients for targeted therapies. In cases where MF exhibits atypical surface markers, flow cytometry can help establish the phenotype more accurately, including the coexpression of CD4 and CD8 antigens on the same cell. However, it is worth noting that established protocols for flow cytometry of skin lymphocytes are currently lacking.

Flow cytometry of peripheral blood is rapidly gaining importance and is highly valuable for assessing peripheral blood involvement. It plays a crucial role in diagnosing conditions like Sézary syndrome (SS) and aids in disease staging. The optimal combination of surface marker stainings for peripheral blood flow cytometry is not firmly established, but many laboratories typically use antibodies against CD3, CD4, CD8, CD7, and

CD26. The presence of $CD3^+$ $CD4^+$ cells and the absence of CD7 or CD26 ($CD7^-/CD26^-$) are suggestive of peripheral blood involvement. Both CD7 and CD26 markers are used because leukemic MF cells may occasionally express one or the other. Additionally, the proportion of $CD4^+$ $CD26^-/CD7^-$ cells increases with age, so patient age should be considered when interpreting the results. While various markers like KIR3DL2 and TOX have been proposed for better identification of circulating malignant cells, they have not yet been widely adopted in clinical practice.

Flow cytometry can also be useful for assessing MF involvement in lymph nodes, especially when combined with TCR monoclonality assays. Suitable materials for analysis include fresh tissue from excised lymph nodes or core needle biopsy samples obtained from pathologically enlarged lymph nodes.

7.1.4 Imaging and Staging

Clinical staging of MF is primarily based on clinical features and the presence of extracutaneous involvement in various compartments (Table 7.4).

Stage IA. Patients with typical clinical presentation and expected histopathology ($CD3^+$ $CD4^+$) typically do not require additional imaging. Life expectancy in this stage is similar to that of a matched healthy population. However, this recommendation may not apply to patients with aberrant or high-risk histopathological features, such as the γδ phenotype or gMF, who are at risk of early extracutaneous dissemination despite minimal skin involvement.

Stage IB. For patients in this stage, it is generally recommended to rule out systemic involvement through imaging. This typically involves CT scanning of the chest and abdomen or PET/

Table 7.4 Staging of mycosis fungoides (MF)

TNMB		TNMB classification and staging of mycosis fungoides and Sézary syndrome[a,b]
Skin	T1	Limited patches,[c] papules, and/or plaques[d] covering <10% of the skin surface
	T2	Patches, papules,[c] and/or plaques[c] covering ≥10% of the skin surface
	T2a	Patch only
	T2b	Plaque ± patch
	T3	One or more tumors[e] (≥1 cm in diameter)
	T4	Confluence of erythema ≥80% body surface area
Node	N0	No abnormal lymph nodes; biopsy not required
	N1	Abnormal lymph nodes; histopathology Dutch Gr 1 or NCI LN 0-2
	N2	Abnormal lymph nodes; histopathology Dutch Gr 2 or NCI LN 3
	N3	Abnormal lymph nodes; histopathology Dutch Gr 3-4 or NCI LN 4
	NX	Abnormal lymph nodes; no histologic confirmation
Visceral	M0	No visceral organ involvement
	M1	Visceral involvement (must have pathology confirmation and organ involved should be specified)
	MX	Abnormal visceral site; no histologic confirmation
Blood	B0	Absence of significant blood involvement: ≤5% of peripheral blood lymphocytes or <250/mcL are atypical (Sézary) cells or <15% $CD4^+/CD26^-$ or $CD4^+/CD7^-$ cells of total lymphocytes
	B1	Low blood tumor burden: >5% of peripheral blood lymphocytes are atypical (Sézary) cells or >15% $CD4^+CD26^-$ or $CD4^+CD7^-$ of total lymphocytes but do not meet the criteria of B0 or B2
	B2	High blood tumor burden: ≥1000/mcL Sézary cells[b] determined by cytopathology or ≥1000 $CD4^+CD26^-$ or $CD4^+CD7^-$ cells/μL or other abnormal subset of T lymphocytes by flow cytometry with clone in blood same as that in skin. Other criteria for documenting high blood tumor burden in $CD4^+$ MF/SS include $CD4^+$; $CD7^-$ cells ≥40% and $CD4^+CD26^-$ cells ≥30%

(continued)

Table 7.4 (continued)

TNMB	TNMB classification and staging of mycosis fungoides and Sézary syndrome[a,b]
[a]Adapted from Olsen E, Vonderheid E, Pimpinelli N, et al. Blood 2007;110:1713-1722 and Olsen E, Whittaker S, Kim Y, et al. J Clin Oncol 2011;29;2598–2607	
[b]Sézary syndrome is defined by B2 blood involvement and a clonal rearrangement of *TCR* in the blood (clones should be relevant to clone in the shin)	
[c]Patch = Any size skin lesion without significant elevation or induration. Presence/absence of hypo- or hyperpigmentation, scale, crusting, and/or poikiloderma should he noted	
[d]Plaque = Any size skin lesion that is elevated or indurated. Presence or absence of scale, crusting, and/or poikiloderma should be noted. Histologic features such as folliculotropism or LCT (≥25% large cells), CD30[+] or CD30[−], and clinical features such as ulceration are important to document	
[e]Tumor = at least one ≥1 cm diameter solid or nodular lesion with evidence of depth and/or vertical growth. Note total number of lesions, total volume of lesions, largest size lesion, and region of body involved. Also note if histologic evidence of LCT has occurred. Phenotyping for CD30 is encouraged	

Clinical Staging of MF and SS[f]				
Clinical stage[g]	T (Skin)	N (Node)	M (Visceral)	B (blood involvement)
IA (limited skin involvement)	T1 (patches, papules, and/or plaques covering <10% body surface area [BSA])	N0	M0	B0 or B1
IB (skin only disease)	T2 (patches, papules, and/or plaques covering ≥10% BSA)	N0	M0	B0 or B1
IIA	T1–2	N1–2	M0	B0 or B1
IIB (tumor stage disease)	T3 (one or more tumors [≥1 cm in diameter])	N0–2	M0	B0 or B1
IIIA (erythrodermic disease)	T4 (confluence of erythema ≥80% BSA)	N0–2	M0	B0
IIIB (erythrodermic disease)	T4 (confluence of erythema ≥80% BSA)	N0–2	M0	B1
IVA_1	T1–4	N0–2	M0	B2
IVA_2	T1–4	N3	M0	B0 or B1 or B2
IVB	T1–4	N0–3	M1	B0 or B1 or B2
	Large-cell transformation (LCT)[h]			
[f]Olsen E, Vonderheid E, Pimpinelli N, et al. Blood 2007;110:1713–1722				
[g]Folliculotropism is a histologic feature that can occur irrespective of stage. Histologic evidence of folliculotropic MF is associated with higher risk of disease progression. In selected cases or inadequate response, consider primary treatment for stage IIB (tumor stage disease)				
[h]LCT is a histologic feature that can occur irrespective of clinical stage. LCT often but not always corresponds to a more aggressive growth rate requiring systemic therapies				
Version 2.2020 © National Comprehensive Cancer Network, Inc. 2020. All rights reserved				
The NCCN Guidelines® and this illustration may not be reproduced in any form without the express written permission of NCCN				

CT imaging. While the superiority of PET/CT over standard CT scans has not been firmly established, some studies have advocated for PET scans to detect nodal involvement [33]. It is worth noting that patients with widespread cutaneous disease may have enlarged lymph nodes due to skin inflammation, which may not necessarily indicate malignant involvement. Dermatopathic lymph nodes often show low to moderate uptake of fluorodeoxyglucose (FDG) on PET scans, unlike neoplastic lymph nodes, which avidly accumulate FDG. Hypermetabolic lymph nodes are more appropriate for further invasive diagnosis via biopsy.

- Biopsy of slightly enlarged lymph nodes: The utility of biopsying slightly enlarged lymph nodes that are not hypermetabolic is debatable. In some cases, patients with IA/IB disease may be upstaged to IIA due to lymph node involvement. However, the treatment and long-term prognosis for patients in stage IIA do not substantially differ from those in stage IB, so this upstaging may not have significant clinical significance.
- Bone marrow biopsy: Bone marrow biopsy is generally not clinically useful for staging. Studies have shown that even in early stages, the bone marrow may show molecular signs of lymphomatous involvement [34]. However, the presence of TCR monoclonality in the bone marrow is not strongly correlated with clinical outcomes. In fact, most patients, even in advanced stages, do not show microscopic or molecular bone marrow involvement.
- Additional considerations: Imaging, blood flow cytometry, and lymph node biopsies may help detect comorbid conditions that can accompany MF. Some retrospective studies have reported an increased incidence of solid tumors, especially lung cancer, in patients with MF [5]. Patients with cutaneous lymphoma, including MF, also have an increased risk of other hematologic neoplasms such as B-cell lymphoma, CLL, or Hodgkin lymphoma. Therefore, a comprehensive diagnostic approach is important for patient management and identifying any additional conditions that may require treatment or monitoring.

7.1.5 Clinicopathological Correlations and Differential Diagnoses

7.1.5.1 MF vs Benign, Inflammatory Skin Disease

One of the most significant challenges in dermatology is distinguishing MF, especially in its early stages, from benign inflammatory skin conditions. As described earlier and summarized in Table 7.1, MF is a versatile imitator, and its skin manifestations can resemble numerous inflammatory skin disorders, including eczematous diseases, psoriasis vulgaris, pityriasis lichenoides or pityriasis rosea, benign follicular mucinosis, alopecia areata, keratosis pilaris, vitiligo, skin infections, erythroderma, and more. Since biopsies may not always provide a clear diagnosis in the early stages of MF, diagnostic errors can occur. Resistance of the disease to topical corticosteroids and systemic anti-inflammatory drugs like methotrexate or the appearance of tumors will eventually guide the clinician toward the correct diagnosis.

It is crucial to keep the possibility of MF in mind when prescribing immunosuppressive therapy. Numerous case reports document the unmasking of cutaneous lymphoma with drugs such as cyclosporine, anti-tumor necrosis factor-α agents, and dupilumab (anti-interleukin 4/13) [35–41]. In some instances, discontinuing immunosuppressive agents may not lead to disease remission, and patients may experience a fulminant, fatal course of MF.

7.1.5.2 MF vs Other Primary Cutaneous T-Cell Lymphomas and Malignancies

The diagnosis of MF relies heavily on precise clinicopathological correlation, and atypical clinical presentations or pathological findings should prompt consideration of other types of cutaneous lymphomas, some of which may have an unfavorable prognosis. Patients with suspected plaque-stage MF, cutaneous pseudolymphoma, leukemia cutis, lupus erythematosus tumidus, uticaria pigmentosa, and tinea corporis should enter the differential diagnostic considerations [42]. Patients who primarily present with a tumor are unlikely to have MF, except for fMF, where facial plaques tend to be thicker than those of Alibert-Bazin MF and may rapidly evolve into tumors. In fact, based on our experience, patients who initially present with solitary tumors or tumors that develop simultaneously with patches or plaques often end up with a diagnosis of γδ cutaneous lymphoma, primary cutaneous anaplastic T-cell lymphoma, gMF, γδMF, or aggressive, epidermotropic $CD8^+$ lymphoma. The differential diagnosis between SS and advanced-stage or erythrodermic MF, a common diagnostic challenge, is discussed below.

7.1.5.3 MF vs Cutaneous Metastasis from Systemic T-Cell Lymphoma

Systemic lymphomas that can metastasize to the skin have been discussed in Chap. 3. Notable mimics of MF include adult T-cell leukemia lymphoma, prolymphocytic leukemia, and systemic anaplastic lymphoma. Typically, when cutaneous lesions occur in these cases, they are accompanied by lymphadenopathy, blood involvement, and systemic symptoms. The primary presentation of systemic lymphoma in the skin is unusual. Therefore, in patients with characteristic MF skin lesions (patches and plaques) but no clinical signs of systemic involvement, the likelihood of secondary skin infiltration is very low and, in practice, negligible. However, in cases with atypical clinical presentations, such as the early development of tumors without a preceding patch and plaque stage, or if the lesions are distributed in atypical locations like distant extremities, a search for systemic lymphoma may be warranted.

7.1.6 Therapy

MF is an intractable malignancy with an indeterminate influence on patient survival and disease progression, barring the possible exception of allogeneic bone marrow transplantation. Treatment strategies are stage-dependent and regularly undergo modifications based on emerging evidence [43, 44]. The primary objective of treatment is palliative, aimed at symptomatology relief rather than a curative outcome. Skin-directed therapies are used first line in early MF, because stage I-IIA MF has a low malignant potential and only a minority of patients progress to tumor stage (IIB) or higher. Use of aggressive chemotherapy in the early stages should be discouraged as they, at best, provide only short-term relief, or at worst, may result in accelerated disease progression [45, 46].

7.1.6.1 Topical Steroids, Topical Mechlorethamine, and Topical Carmustine

Topical corticosteroids, particularly medium and high-potency varieties, serve as a cornerstone in managing MF symptoms and are frequently integrated with other treatment strategies. They offer symptomatic relief, notably in reducing pruritus and plaque inflammation. Although some studies report complete remission in over 60% of stage I patients using high-potency steroids [47, 48], our clinical experience suggests a less remarkable efficacy. The primary adverse effect is skin atrophy, more prominent when applied to regions with thinner skin such as the face and groins. Use of topical corticosteroids on the face should be discouraged as they commonly induce skin atrophy, periorificial dermatitis or rosacea and are not particularly effective in fMF, which is the most common type of MF in the face.

Topical mechlorethamine (chlormethine) is another viable option, especially in the form of a stable, non-aqueous diethylene glycol monoethyl ether gel at 0.02% concentration. The gel achieves roughly 20% complete response and around 50% partial response when applied daily, but the maximal response may take months to develop [49, 50]. Dermatitis is a prevalent adverse event occurring in over half of the patients. This is usually managed by treatment adjustments, such as reducing application frequency and combining with emollients or topical steroids [51]. When mechlorethamine is unavailable, carmustine can serve as an alternative (e.g., 0.4% in petrolatum or in isopropyl alcohol), although its efficacy appears to be inferior. Carmustine can also be used for patients with extensive disease as a total skin treatment [52]. The adverse effects of carmustine are similar to those of topical mechlorethamine. In addition, carmustine can be systemically absorbed when applied to larger areas of the skin, leading to systemic toxicities, such as leukopenia, thrombocytopenia, and anemia [53], necessitating appropriate monitoring. [52]

7.1.6.2 Phototherapy

Phototherapeutic modalities, including narrow-band UVB and psoralen and ultraviolet A (PUVA), constitute the mainstay of early-stage (I-IIA) MF treatment due to its relatively benign malignancy potential. In patients with thin plaques, narrow-band UVB demonstrates substantial effectiveness, achieving clearance in up to 90% of patients after roughly 30 treatment sessions under a standard protocol [54, 55]. The treatment's efficacy is prone to relapses, which can vary broadly from 3 months to 1.5 years post-treatment.

PUVA therapy exhibits particular efficacy in patients with thicker skin plaques and achieves similar therapeutic outcomes to narrow-band UVB [56]. The therapy, often administered 2–3 times weekly, is met with hesitation due to its well-documented carcinogenic effects. However, recent data suggests that maintenance therapy may offer a judicious approach to manage long-term responses [57]. In our clinic we only offer maintenance PUVA treatments for patients who have a history of short remissions (<6 months after completion of phototherapy).

Systemic interferon (e.g., pegylated interferon α 90–180 μg/weekly) increases the response rate to phototherapy [58, 59]. Interferon can be used up front for patients with predicted poor response to phototherapy (thick lesions, folliculotropism, gMF) or may be added at a later point if the treatment response is insufficient. We usually start phototherapy without concomitant interferon, but if the patient does not achieve a good partial response after approximately 15 phototherapy session, we add low-dose interferon and continue the treatment until complete (or almost complete) response, after which the phototherapy is interrupted, and the patient remains on maintenance interferon therapy.

Not uncommonly, in spite of the good response to phototherapy, the patients have one or several resistant lesions. Sometimes, the lesions persist because they cannot be sufficiently exposed to ultraviolet radiation, e.g., the lesions hidden in the skin folds (such as genital MF) or lesions in the terminal hair-bearing areas, such as the scalp. Those resistant lesions can be treated with field radiotherapy or other skin-directed therapies, such as topical mechlorethamine, imiquimod, photodynamic therapy (discussed below), or even topical corticosteroids.

High-dose UVA therapy and extracorporeal photopheresis have occasionally been used for MF; however, their efficacy is lower than that of narrow-band UVB or PUVA [60–62].

7.1.6.3 Radiation Therapy

MF is highly radiosensitive, making radiation therapy a cornerstone across all disease stages. Photon radiation to single MF lesions using kilovolt or orthovolt rays yields nearly 100% complete response rates within the dose range of 10–30 Gy. Lesions should be irradiated with a margin of at least 15–20 mm of healthy skin to preempt peripheral relapses. Radiotherapy is used to treat resistant plaques that do not respond to other skin-directed therapies and to manage skin tumors. Multiple lesions can be managed in a single radiotherapy session and cyclical treatments allow for the management of patients even with a relative number of tumors.

Acute adverse events, such as ulceration and radiodermatitis, are usually manageable with appropriate dressings, emollients, and topical corticosteroids. Long-term adverse effects are dose-dependent and include skin pigmentation, skin atrophy, fibrosis, telangiectasias, hair loss, and, in extreme cases, skin cancer.

Chronic ulcerations may develop even at lower cumulative doses and sometimes need skin grafting to accelerate healing [63]. Hair loss is always seen after radiotherapy but hair regrowth takes place within 2 months after treatment. Permanent post-radiation alopecia can be seen at any dose, which is especially problematic in lesions localized to the scalp. The estimated risk is 15% after irradiation of 45 Gy [64]. In our experience, virtually all patients who received >50 Gy of cumulative orthovoltage radiation developed permanent radiation alopecia within the radiation field. The risk of skin cancer, especially of basal cell carcinoma, is linearly correlated to the cumulative dose of radiation and has a latency time of approximately 10 years or more. Therefore, the benefit of radiation should be weighed heavily against the risk of latent skin cancers in patients under 50 years of age.

Compared to photon radiation, electron beam therapy offers a different shape of absorption curve in the skin, being more selective to the superficial 10 mm of the tissue and sparing the deeper layers. Of note is that the biological effects of electrons and photons are identical because electrons are converted to photon radiation when interacting with the tissue. Electron beams can be used on larger skin areas with a low risk of systemic side effects. The technique of total skin electron beam (TSEB) has been developed to treat the entire skin surface in patients with advanced disease. The dosing varies, but current data favor the low-dose TSEB of 12–16 Gy in six to eight fractions [65]. The treatment can be repeated as needed. The complete response rate is high (>90%), but most patients relapse within a year. Side-effects of TSEB comprise radiodermatitis, skin ulceration, alopecia (usually transient), xerosis, and loss of nails. Most patients develop a dysfunction of sweat glands, which results in hypohidrosis and may create problems with hyperthermia in warm environments due to the inability to thermoregulate efficiently.

7.1.6.4 Other Skin-Directed Therapies

Bexarotene gel (1%) has shown moderate efficacy in clinical trials (>50% improvement in >60% of early-stage patients with complete responses in 21% of patients) and low-grade local side effects similar to those of other retinoids [66]. However, the drug is not widely available. Other topical retinoids (e.g., tazarotene) have been used, but the efficacy was low. Immunostimulatory substances such as imiquimod or resiquimod have been tried with some success, but their use is limited by severe local irritation. Photodynamic therapy showed some promise, but the rate of complete remission is very low.

7.1.6.5 Systemic Therapies

Pegylated Interferon α

Pegylated interferon α remains an invaluable systemic agent across all MF stages, often used synergistically with skin-directed treatments. It plays a critical role in managing forms of MF that are poorly responsive to phototherapy, such as fMF and gMF. Typically administered subcutaneously at doses ranging from 135 to 180 μg/week, its short-term side effects like fatigue and flu-like symptoms are manageable. Nevertheless, long-term usage demands vigilant monitoring for more severe adverse events like profound depression, anemia, and chronic fatigue [67, 68].

Low-Dose Methotrexate

Low-dose methotrexate (15–25 mg weekly) is another systemic agent, albeit with modest efficacy, evidenced by an overall response rate of approximately 30% [69]. Nevertheless, its safety profile at low doses makes it a candidate for combination therapies.

7.1.6.6 Targeted Therapies

Histone deacetylase inhibitors (HDACIs), such as romidepsin and vorinostat, offer limited efficacy, with overall response rates hovering around 30%. The most common side effects include gastrointestinal issues like nausea, vomiting, and diarrhea, but severe toxicities are uncommon [70]. Despite their modest overall efficacy, some patients have exhibited striking clinical improvements, including regression of pulmonary metastases in cases of gMF treated with vorinostat alone.

Brentuximab vedotin, an antibody-drug conjugate, targets CD30-positive lymphoma cells and has been approved for the treatment of CD30-positive cutaneous T-cell lymphomas. Intriguingly, the correlation between CD30 expression and clinical response is weak, leading many clinicians to employ brentuximab as a second-line therapy in advanced, CD30-negative MF cases (i.e., <10% cells expressing CD30). The overall response rate ranges from 50% to 60%, with complete responses occurring in approximately 15% of cases [71, 72]. The most common toxicity is peripheral neuropathy, which occurs in about 70% of patients. While neuropathy generally resolves within 1–2 years, it may persist in approximately 20% of patients.

Mogamulizumab, a humanized antibody targeting CCR4, was initially developed for adult T-cell leukemia-lymphoma (ATLL) but has shown effectiveness in MF. The overall response rate approximates 40%, and a comparative trial against vorinostat revealed superior progression-free survival with mogamulizumab. Serious adverse events are rare and include sepsis, pulmonary embolism, and cellulitis [73, 74]. The response rate depends on the degree of blood involvement, being most effective in patients with B1 or higher. In Sézary's syndrome, the overall response rate is 47% versus 28% in MF stage B0. Importantly, mogamulizumab can delete CCR4-expressing regulatory T-cells, which increases the risk of severe acute GvHD in patients who subsequently receive allogeneic hematopoietic stem cell transplantation (allo-HSCT) [75]. A characteristic dermatologic adverse effect of mogamulizumab is skin rash, which can be difficult to differentiate from relapsing MF [76].

7.1.6.7 Chemotherapy

There is no consensus on the use of single agent chemotherapy, and the choice of the drug is based on expert opinion rather than evidence. Monotherapy with gemcitabine is probably used most widely, due to favorable side effect profile and tolerability in older patients. The short-term efficacy is good (overall response rate of 70% given weekly at 1000–1200 mg/m^2 in a 28-day cycle [77]). The efficacy of liposomal doxorubicin and pentostatin are comparable to gemcitabine (overall response rate 41% and 70%, respectively) but those drugs are rarely used due to a less favorable adverse event profile [78, 79].

Multiagent chemotherapy, such as CHOP [80] or EPOCH [80, 81], is used as a palliative therapy for advanced or metastatic MF. The overall response rates are very high (>80%), but the results are short-lived and the relapses may be more difficult to treat than the disease which was not modified by chemotherapy.

7.1.6.8 Surgery

Surgical excision of tumors is rarely mentioned in treatment recommendations but is a viable option for the difficult to treat patients or to address tumors in locations where radiotherapy will produce unwanted adverse effects (e.g., tumors of the scalp). Surgery has a particular role in the treatment of deep, ulcerated tumors that do not respond well to radiotherapy. Excision can be done with a narrow (e.g., 1 cm) margin and the area can be irradiated with low-dose (e.g., 10 Gy) radiation to eradicate residual lymphoma cells. There are no studies on the efficacy of surgery in MF, but our experience with selected patients has been very encouraging.

7.1.6.9 Allogeneic Hematopoietic Stem Cell Transplant

Allo-HSTC is a potentially curative option for patients with high-risk, progressive MF, who failed skin-directed therapies and recommended first-line systemic treatments. The results are encouraging, especially with the low-intensity conditioning where 2-year overall survival rate was ≅ 80%, decreasing to 32% after 7 years. The post-transplant relapse can be rescued by donor lymphocyte infusion. Allo-HSCT has the highest chances of success in patients with good performance status, where a related donor is available, and where the patient achieved very good partial or complete remission of the disease pre-transplant [82, 83].

7.1.7 Typical Treatment Scenarios

7.1.7.1 Early-Stage MF (Stage IA-IIA, Alibert-Bazin MF)

As previously emphasized, the prognosis in early-stage MF is generally favorable. The chief objectives of therapeutic intervention are multifaceted—comprising disease control, mitigation of disease burden, and elevation of the patient's overall quality of life. First-line management typically consists of skin-directed therapies, prominently featuring topical corticosteroids, topical chlormethine, and phototherapy. It is important for clinicians to understand that complete lesion clearance may not always be attainable. However, persistently resistant lesions can usually be well-controlled through targeted applications of topical corticosteroids or focal radiotherapy, depending on factors such as lesion dimensions, anatomical location, and associated clinical symptoms.

Skin-directed therapies such as phototherapy are generally administered in a cyclical fashion. This entails interspersing periods of active treatment with intervals colloquially referred to as "treatment holidays," designed to coincide with phases of disease remission. For patients exhibiting a propensity for swift relapses, the institution of maintenance phototherapy regimes may warrant consideration [57, 84]. In instances of disease instability—characterized by the abrupt onset of new plaques or the geographic extension of the disease to previously unaffected bodily regions—the employment of systemic agents like interferon α, or alternative low-toxicity options such as bexarotene or methotrexate, may be judiciously combined with existing skin-directed treatments.

7.1.7.2 Unilesional MF

A distinct subset of early-stage MF is constituted by cases manifesting as a single lesion, commonly termed "unilesional MF." In such instances, our clinical strategy usually leans towards employing targeted radiotherapy with the intent of lesion eradication. Reassuringly, approximately 50% of the patients managed in this manner demonstrate no subsequent recurrence of the disease.

7.1.7.3 Addressing Pruritus

Pruritus frequently represents the most debilitating symptom in early MF, and yet the therapeutic options available for its effective management are notably limited. Narrow-band UVB phototherapy has proven to be the most efficacious modality and ideally should be integrated with topical corticosteroids and intensive cutaneous moisturization to attenuate pruritogenic inflammation and restore skin barrier functionality. While systemic pharmacotherapy, including antihistamines, gabapentinoids, naltrexone, and aprepitant, has shown some promise in small-scale trials and anecdotal case series, these medications seldom provide substantial relief beyond a placebo effect.

7.1.7.4 The Role of Watchful Waiting

In certain cases, a policy of watchful waiting may represent an acceptable strategy, particularly for patients who are not highly motivated to undergo active treatment and whose disease burden remains sufficiently low so as to not significantly impact their quality of life.

7.1.7.5 Management Strategies for High-Risk Early-Stage Mycosis Fungoides Subtypes (gMF, fMF, γδMF)

The therapeutic approach for high-risk subtypes of early-stage MF, including granulomatous MF (gMF), folliculotropic MF (fMF), and gamma-delta MF (γδMF), generally aligns with the strategies employed for the classical Alibert-Bazin type of MF. Nonetheless, patients with these high-risk variants often necessitate a more aggressive treatment regimen, including the earlier implementation of radiotherapy and the judicious use of systemic, non-chemotherapeutic agents. The management of fMF, in particular, presents unique challenges. Lesions are frequently localized on facial regions—most notably the eyebrows—as well as the scalp. Owing to the depth of the dermal infiltrate, these lesions are less responsive to traditional skin-directed therapies. In such cases, interferon α (IFN α) proves to be invaluable in the early treatment stages, significantly reducing both the lesion count and their thickness. For lesions that exhibit resistance to conventional approaches, radiotherapy is efficacious. However, the potential for permanent hair loss in regions such as the scalp and eyebrows can be a difficult issue for patients, often resulting in treatment hesitancy. Should rapid progression and tumor development occur, allogeneic hematopoietic stem cell transplantation (allo-HSCT) should be seriously considered, given the generally poor prognosis in such scenarios.

7.1.7.6 Implications of Large Cell Transformation (LCT)

Large cell transformation serves as a harbinger of an elevated mutational rate and signifies an imminent risk of disease progression. This holds true even when LCT is localized to a single lesion. Emerging evidence suggests that neoplastic cells in MF have the ability to recirculate among various lesions, thereby potentially seeding new cutaneous regions and mediating disease advancement [85]. While robust empirical evidence is currently lacking, our clinical perspective strongly advocates for the early and radical treatment of transformed lesions, preferably utilizing radiotherapy, as this approach may help arrest further stage progression.

7.1.7.7 Management of Tumoral MF (Stage ≥IIB)

The treatment of MF at stage ≥IIB marked by the presence of cutaneous tumors represents a clinical challenge. A notable exception exists for isolated tumors, which can be managed using targeted or spot radiotherapy. For patients manifesting multiple tumors, systemic interferon can yield favorable outcomes in a subset of cases. However, for those demonstrating resistance or inadequate response, alternative debulking strategies may be employed. These can include systemic administration of agents such as brentuximab, mogamulizumab, histone deacetylase (HDAC) inhibitors, or even single-agent chemotherapeutics. Resistant lesions, in particular, may be viable candidates for radiotherapy. Given the rapid relapse observed in untreated patients, ongoing maintenance therapy is typically requisite. Maintenance regimens can range from skin-directed therapies designed to address early lesion development to systemic interventions employing interferon, bexarotene, or low-dose methotrexate. In the context of extensively disseminated disease, efficacious debulking can often be achieved through total skin electron beam (TSEB) therapy, coupled with boost photon irradiation targeting thicker lesions.

Individuals with tumoral MF frequently require additional supportive therapies. *Staphylococcus aureus* colonization is a common complication that has been implicated in exacerbating disease flares and potentially driving tumor progression. Early intervention with anti-staphylococcal antibiotics is therefore strongly advised. Furthermore, necrotic tumors often become anaerobically infected, resulting in malodorous discharge amenable to treatment with metronidazole. Late-stage mucosal necrotic tumors are generally prognostically unfavorable and a significant source of patient distress. Localized radiotherapy remains the most effective treatment option for these challenging cases.

7.1.7.8 Therapeutic Approaches to Metastatic MF

Metastatic MF represents an unmet medical need, and the outlook for affected patients remains grim. Therapeutic planning must be highly individualized, incorporating a multitude of factors, including performance status, age, comorbidities, and metastatic site involvement. Initial interventions frequently involve a combination approach with single-agent therapy—whether targeted biologic, chemotherapeutic, or HDAC inhibitor—followed by multiagent chemotherapy. Radiotherapy may serve a palliative or supportive role in these advanced cases. For patients who have failed to respond to multiagent chemotherapy regimens, allogeneic hematopoietic stem cell transplantation (allo-HSCT) remains the last viable therapeutic option for potentially eliciting a clinical response.

7.2 Sézary Syndrome

7.2.1 Practice Essentials

- SS is a leukemia/lymphoma syndrome manifesting in its typical form with the triad of erythroderma, lymphadenopathy and leukemic blood involvement.
- SS has intermediate malignant potential with a 5-year survival of approximately 50%.
- Diagnosis is made based on clinicopathological correlation. Differential diagnosis with inflammatory erythroderma can be challenging.
- SS is often treatment resistant. First-line therapies include combination multimodality therapy with topical and systemic corticosteroids, extracorporeal photopheresis, oral retinoids, and pegylated interferon α.

7.2.2 Clinical Presentation

SS is categorized as a leukemia/lymphoma syndrome and is specifically a primary cutaneous, mature T-cell neoplasm. Although closely related to MF, both entities are currently considered to represent separate conditions, and although this is the object of an ongoing debate, it is supported by molecular profiling studies [86].

The diagnosis of SS is traditionally established based on the presence of a distinctive triad: erythroderma, lymphadenopathy, and circulating malignant Sézary cells, which are atypical T-cells. The prognostic landscape of SS is generally unfavorable, with a 5-year mortality rate approximating 50% and a median survival time of around 4 years.

The syndrome predominantly afflicts elderly males, with the majority of patients being over 60 years of age.

In its classical manifestation, SS presents rather abruptly as pruritic erythroderma (redness and scaling present over 80% of body surface area), characteristically sparing the skin folds. The affected skin typically exhibits a deep red to purple hue, punctuated by regions of hyperpigmentation. With disease progression, the skin develops pronounced scaling, notably observed on the palmar and plantar surfaces—referred to as palmar and plantar keratoderma. Additionally, alopecia commonly manifests in the erythrodermic regions.

Unique clinical features can further include onychodystrophy and ectropion. A particularly severe presentation is the so-called "leonine facies," characterized by marked infiltration of the facial skin, especially prominent around the ocular, frontal, and oral regions [87].

It is noteworthy that the classical presentation featuring erythroderma and generalized erythroderma constitutes just one stage in the disease continuum [88]. The initial cutaneous involvement in SS can be remarkably heterogeneous, ranging from MF-like patches and plaques to nonspecific, eczematous, pruritic erythema. The latter may manifest with a predilection for the face and flexural regions, mimicking the clinical presentation of atopic dermatitis. As the disease evolves, patients may transition into the classical erythrodermic stage, though a subset never exhibits this hallmark erythrodermic involvement.

When lymphadenopathy is present, it is typically symmetrical and widespread, often involving the inguinal, axillary, or cervical lymph nodes (Fig. 7.12).

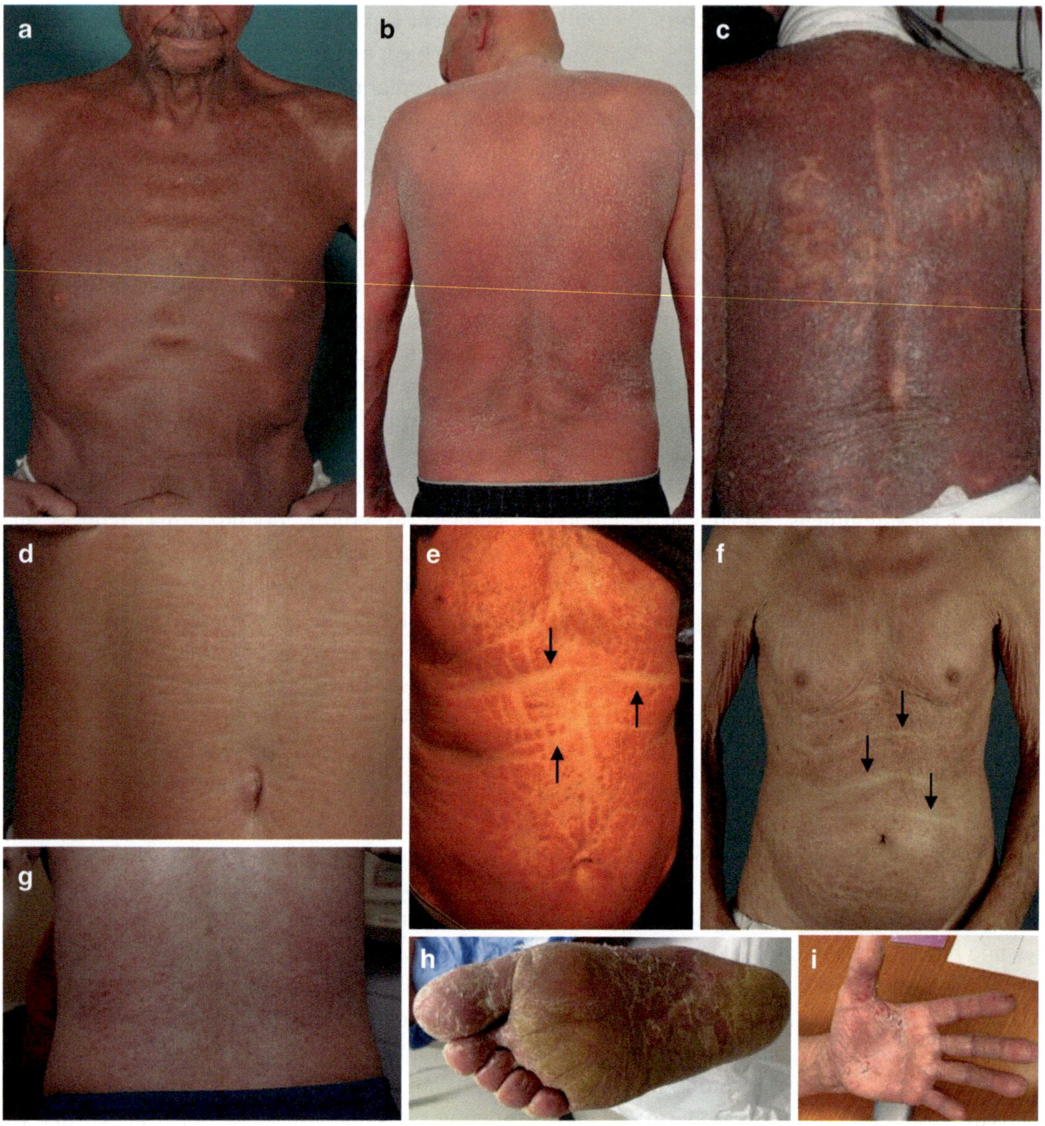

Fig. 7.12 A classic presentation of Sézary syndrome. Most patients exhibit confluent erythroderma (**a, b**). The skin color varies from dark red, purple-red (**a**) to vivid red (**b**). Some patients manifest significant scaling (**b**), and skin lesions may occasionally be more infiltrated with areas of sparing, reminiscent of mycosis fungoides (MF) plaques (**c**). The areas of skin sparing can be observed in skin folds (**d**), which in extreme cases present as papulo-erythroderma with a deck-chair sign (arrows, **e, f**). Erythroderma in a patient in panel (**g**) comprises confluent papular lesions representing folliculotropic infiltration with malignant cells, indistinguishable from folliculotropic MF. There is typically severe involvement of palms and soles with hyperkeratosis and painful skin cracking (**h, i**)

7.2.2.1 Clinical Variants

Mycosis Fungoides-Like SS (MF/SS Overlap)

The relationship between Mycosis Fungoides (MF) and SS remains a subject of ongoing debate. Both conditions share numerous histopathological and molecular similarities. More than 60% of SS patients present with skin lesions characteristic of MF. These MF-like patches and plaques can either manifest initially or develop later, coexisting with erythroderma. As a corollary, one should remember that skin biopsies of patients with SS may or may not be diagnostically specific. Furthermore, the emergence of MF plaques post-successful SS therapy has been observed. From a staging standpoint, there is currently little practical difference between erythrodermic MF with secondary blood involvement (stages ≥ IIIB) and de novo SS; the distinction is often semantic.

Adermopathic SS

Recently described, this variant manifests primarily with blood involvement and minimal to absent skin features [88, 89]. Patients may initially exhibit unexplained lymphadenopathy, lymphocytosis, or nonspecific skin symptoms like itch. Circulating malignant T-cell clones are often discovered incidentally. Over time, some may develop classic erythroderma or MF-like lesions, and the prognosis appears comparable to classic MF.

Atopic Dermatitis-Like SS

This form mimics adult-onset atopic dermatitis (AD), presenting with poorly demarcated erythematous and eczematous regions typically in the head, neck, and flexural areas. These patients may also display other AD features, such as asthma, hay fever, and increased IgE. Biopsy is often inconclusive in the early stages as atypical cells are generally absent. This is not surprising, as it has been well established that patients with SS have a skewed immune response towards T-helper cell type 2 (Th2, overproduction of IL4, IL13, IL31), reminiscent of the pathogenesis of AD. Our experience indicates that systemic immunosuppressive agents, primarily cyclosporine and dupilumab, often trigger this variant. Unlike classic AD, there is no childhood or familial history of the condition, offering a useful differentiating factor (Fig. 7.13).

Smoldering, Nonprogressive SS (Pre-Sézary Syndrome)

Introduced in 1974 by Winkelmann et al., this variant is thought to run a benign course, primarily characterized by erythroderma and minimal, if any, blood involvement [90, 91]. The term "pre-Sézary syndrome" has been coined to signify its putative pre-malignant nature. Blood involvement in pre-SS is minimal, and the condition is highly reminiscent of AD-like SS. In fact, pre-SS manifests itself as an AD-like SS running a protracted, chronic, non-progressive course for years. The use of immunosuppressive drugs, in particular cyclosporine, triggers progression and unmasks SS.

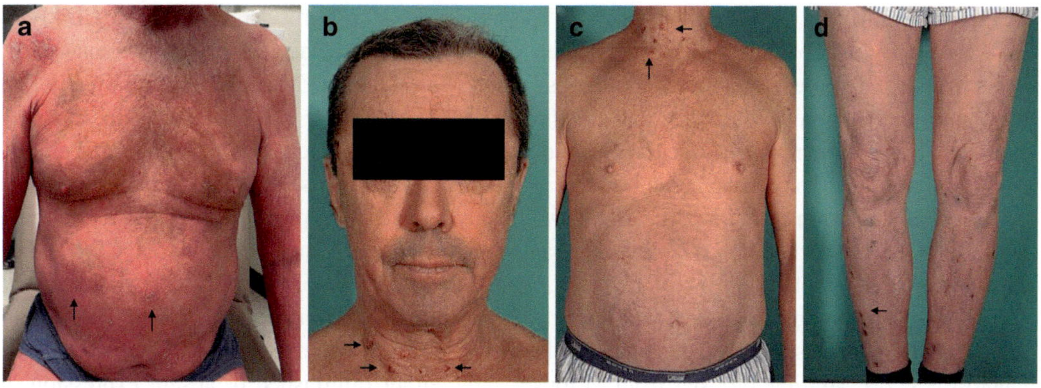

Fig. 7.13 Clinical variants of Sézary syndrome (SS). (**a**) SS/MF overlap with clinically discernible MF plaques on the trunk (arrows). (**b–d**) The atopic dermatitis-like form of SS. This 58-year-old male patient was referred with a 15-year-long history of an itchy, eczematous rash covering the entire skin surface. The initial diagnosis of atopic dermatitis was made based on the biopsy showing spongiotic dermatitis, increased IgE, and a history of asthma and seasonal conjunctivitis. Eventually, the patient developed nodular lesions on the neck and lower extremities (arrows), which were re-biopsied and revealed abnormal T cells. An identical T-cell clone was found in the blood (TCRγ rearrangement)

Erythrodermic Inflammatory Dermatosis

This condition features extensive erythroderma or eczema with T-cell receptor (TCR) clones in the peripheral blood but has not been observed to progress to SS [92]. It's considered a monoclonal T-cell dyscrasia rather than a direct precursor to SS.

7.2.3 Diagnostic Workup

The International Society for Cutaneous Lymphomas proposed that the diagnosis of SS can be made in patients with erythroderma (a necessary criterion) and at least two of the following: Sézary cell count >1000/μL; immunophenotypic T-cell abnormalities in the peripheral blood (CD4/CD8 > 10 or loss of T-cell surface markers, such as CD2, CD3, CD4, CD5, CD7 or CD26); presence of a monoclonal T-cell receptor (TCR) population in the blood; or presence of chromosomally abnormal T-cell clones [93]. However, as described above, many patients with SS may not have erythroderma and in the real world the diagnosis of SS is established based on the clinical-pathological correlations, combining the result of skin histopathology, peripheral blood flow cytometry, lymph node biopsy and molecular studies.

7.2.3.1 Skin Biopsy

The skin biopsy of a patient with SS may often reveal MF-like features. However, the biopsy does not uncommonly present non-specific results, typically showing a perivascular lymphocytic infiltrate. This type of result can be seen in various skin conditions, making the definitive diagnosis of SS problematic on the basis of cutaneous histopathology alone.

Hence, it is paramount to realize that a single biopsy might not be sufficient to conclusively diagnose SS [22]. Multiple biopsies from various sites or repeated biopsies over time may be necessary. This iterative approach aims to capture the variability and evolution of skin manifestations and increases the probability of detecting characteristic histological features of SS.

7.2.3.2 Peripheral Blood Examination

The role of peripheral blood examination in the diagnosis of SS has evolved over time. Traditionally, the identification of circulating Sézary cells in a peripheral blood smear was considered mandatory for diagnosing the condition. However, the limitations inherent to the morphological review of peripheral blood smears, with its relatively low sensitivity and specificity for the identification of Sézary cells, have led to a decline in their use, with some centers even abandoning the technique altogether.

Blood smears can still be beneficial in certain scenarios. For instance, in patients where circulating Sézary cells are plentiful, these cells are often easily identifiable through microscopic examination.

Enumerating $CD4^+$ and $CD8^+$ lymphocyte subsets in the blood is another important diagnostic modality. Typically, an increased CD4/CD8 ratio above a threshold value of 10 is consistent with SS. However, this ratio should not be evaluated in isolation, as it can be artificially elevated due to a reduced number of $CD8^+$ cells. While a drop in $CD8^+$ cells is commonly observed in SS, it is not a specific marker and can occur in various inflammatory and autoimmune diseases. Moreover, CD8 cell count decreases with age [82]. Hence, a more solid confirmation of SS comes from elevated CD4 counts, although this is not always straightforward. Neoplastic CD4 lymphocytes may replace their normal counterparts, affecting the total CD4 cell count minimally.

Flow cytometry has become an increasingly valuable tool for identifying the abnormal phenotype of Sézary cells. Although there is no universally agreed-upon panel of markers, a minimum staining panel generally includes CD7, CD3, CD4, CD8, CD26, and CD45, which can be accommodated by a standard 6-color flow cytometry system [94]. In most instances, Sézary cells show either diminished or absent expression of CD7 and CD26, and sometimes also reduced staining for CD3. Many groups have found this approach lacking specificity since many benign reactive lymphoid populations may feature $CD4^+$ populations with CD7 and/or CD56 loss. Some groups have advocated an approach based on phenotypic aberrations of the $CD4^+$ subset of cells, which appears to be more reliable [95]. The technological expansion of flow cytometry to include T-cell receptor constant β chain-1 (TRBC1) Expression may yet bring improved diagnostic accuracy for the diagnosis of SS [96].

Additional markers, such as $CD158k^+$, $CCR4^+$, KIR3DL2, and $PD\text{-}1^+$, have been identified as potentially useful [97, 98]. However, these are generally not included in routine diagnostic panels and are more commonly utilized in research settings.

7.2.3.3 Molecular Diagnosis (TCR Monoclonality Assays)

Similar to the diagnosis of MF, the T-cell receptor (TCR) gene rearrangement assays play a prominent role in the workup of SS. However, using PCR testing alone to establish a diagnosis of SS is not recommended; molecular data should be included in a multiparameter diagnostic work-up. One can test blood, skin, or a lymph node biopsy, and the diagnosis of SS is supported when the same clonal rearrangement is found in the skin and the blood. The neoplastic clone is identified in the skin in >80% of established SS cases, and the chance of finding a positive clone increases in more advanced diseases [99, 100]. The sensitivity and specificity of TCR assays in relation to isolated blood testing are also believed to be high (both >80%), but those data are relatively old, based on a few patients and exclusively on TCRγ assays. As in mycosis fungoides, the current approach is to examine TCRβ and TCRγ rearrangement to reduce non-specific results, and there are no recent studies that tested this modern approach in relation to blood involvement in SS.

In general, the finding of an isolated cutaneous or peripheral blood clonal rearrangement of the TCRβ gene is more specific than a TCRγ rearrangement. Sometimes the TCRβ clones found in the blood and the skin are not identical. The interpretation of this finding may be difficult and looking at the TCRγ results may be helpful. It has recently been shown that SS may be monoclonal in relation to TCRγ but polyclonal or oligoclonal for TCRβ [31]. Another group of SS patients may show different TCRγ clones in the blood and the skin. One should be cautious and avoid misconstruing as neoplastic a circulating reactive lymphoid population that may show rearrangement of the TCRγ gene, a rare, often age-related, finding, the significance of which remains debated [101]. Another feature of the true neoplastic clone is its stability in time, and the finding of the same clones on repeated testing of new samples supports the diagnosis of T-cell lymphoma.

TCR clonality assays on the pathological lymph nodes reveal the presence of the clone in most cases [102], and the chances of a positive result are higher in histopathologically abnormal lymph nodes.

7.2.3.4 Imaging and Staging

Staging protocols used should closely align with those employed for mycosis fungoides.

PET-CT imaging is highly valuable in SS staging because it can identify pathological lymph nodes based on elevated FDG uptake. This feature allows for the differentiation of pathologically involved nodes from reactive, dermatopathic lymph nodes, a common finding in erythroderma but usually exhibit only moderate levels of FDG uptake [33].

Lymph Node Staging: Although histopathological examination of lymph nodes remains the gold standard for precise staging and excludes dermatopathic changes observed in patients with skin diseases, excisional lymph node biopsies are not always conducted. This hesitancy is generally due to the associated procedural risks and the limited impact such biopsies have on the overall treatment strategy. Recently, ultrasound-guided core needle biopsy has emerged as a viable, less invasive alternative for lymph node staging in SS [103, 104].

Blood Staging: Flow cytometry has the potential to provide the most accurate blood staging by enumerating $CD4^+$ $CD7^-$ (or alternatively $CD4^+$ $CD26^-$) cells. According to established parameters [105], a cell count ranging from 250 to 999 cells/μL is categorized as stable B1, while counts exceeding 1000 cells/μL fall into the B2 category. In scenarios where the CD4/CD8 ratio is elevated but flow cytometry is not available or feasible, the total CD4 cell count can serve as a suitable alternative for blood staging. As mentioned above, the role of flow cytometry continues to evolve, and current guidelines will likely evolve to give this technology an even greater precision and a greater role in disease staging and monitoring.

7.2.4 Clinicopathological Correlations and Differential Diagnoses

The diagnosis of SS may seem straightforward when patients present with the classic diagnostic triad—erythroderma, lymphadenopathy, and blood involvement—along with additional characteristic clinical features such as severe pruritus, alopecia, palmar and plantar keratoderma, sparing of skin in the folds, ectropion, and onychodystrophy. However, such textbook presentations are relatively uncommon, and diagnostic challenges often arise when encountering patients with atypical features or those lacking erythroderma.

The differential diagnosis for erythroderma is covered in Table 7.5 and is crucial for excluding other possible conditions. A common feature across all erythrodermas is the presence of dermatopathic lymph nodes, which are reactive but can mimic lymph node involvement seen in SS. The ratio of CD4 to CD8 cells can also be artificially elevated, often due to a decline in the number of CD8 cells rather than an increase in CD4 cells. Complicating matters, Sézary-like cells have been identified in the blood of patients diagnosed with inflammatory erythroderma. As mentioned before, such patients may also display elevated percentages of $CD4^+$ $CD26^-$ cells or $CD4^+$ $CD7^-$ cells, markers typically indicative of SS.

The diagnosis of SS becomes more probable when the proportion of $CD4^+$ $CD26^-$ cells is greater than 30% and the proportion of $CD4^+$ $CD7^-$ cells surpasses 40%. It's essential to note that the presence of stable TCRβ clones is generally not seen in patients with inflammatory erythroderma. However, false-positive TCRγ clones have been reported in a minority of these patients (less than 5%).

Table 7.5 Differential diagnosis of Sézary syndrome

Cause of acquired erythroderma	Key clinical features differentiating from SS
Idiopathic	Rarely ectropion, onychodystrophy, alopecia, or palmoplantar keratoderma
Atopic dermatitis	History of pediatric AD, very high IgE levels, good response to systemic corticosteroids, rarely ectropion, onychodystrophy, alopecia, or palmoplantar keratoderma.
Psoriasis	Previous history of psoriasis, remnants of plaque psoriasis, absence of alopecia, biopsy usually shows features of psoriasis, psoriatic nail changes
Pityriasis rubra pilaris	Bright red rather than dusky, purple erythroderma in SS, island-like skin sparing, palmoplantar keratoderma with yellow hue
Disseminated eczema of the elderly (Oid-Oid disease, Sulzberger-Garbe eczema)	Exudative lesions, pronounced on lower extremities, rarely ectropion, onychodystrophy, alopecia, or palmoplantar keratoderma
Seborrheic dermatitis	Mostly on face, scalp and the trunk, rarely ectropion, onychodystrophy, alopecia, or palmoplantar keratoderma
Drug reactions	History of drug intake, eosinophilia in the blood and skin biopsy, rarely ectropion, onychodystrophy, alopecia, or palmoplantar keratoderma. Sometimes morphology of papuloerythroderma
Papuloerythroderma of Ofuji	Confluent papules, Asian patients, history of infection or drug intake Deck chair sign
Malignant erythroderma in systemic leukemia and lymphoma	ATLL, T-PLL, angioimmunoblastic lymphoma, other T-cell lymphomas—see Chap. 3

Papuloerythroderma poses a diagnostic challenge due to its resemblance to Sézary

Syndrome. Clinically, papuloerythroderma predominantly manifests on the trunk and extends to the proximal extremities, featuring extensive erythema and confluent flat papules. Characteristically, it spares skin folds on the abdomen, often referred to as the "deckchair sign," due to its similarity to the pattern of sunburn that spares abdominal folds in individuals sunbathing in deck chairs. Primarily affecting Asian patients, papuloerythroderma of Ofuji is typically accompanied by pruritus, peripheral eosinophilia, and elevated IgE levels—features also common in SS, making differentiation between the two conditions exceptionally challenging.

Various etiologies may underlie the papuloerythroderma of Ofuji, including infectious precipitants, drug reactions, or paraneoplastic manifestations. Moreover, skin presentations mimicking papuloerythroderma can occur in other conditions such as bullous pemphigoid, erythrodermic seborrheic dermatitis, hypereosinophilic syndrome, or widespread eczema.

Erythroderma can also develop as an advanced manifestation of mycosis fungoides. In contrast to SS, erythrodermic mycosis fungoides is usually distinguished by the absence of blood involvement and generally carries a more favorable prognosis. However, as previously outlined, when blood involvement is present, the differentiation between erythrodermic mycosis fungoides progressing from stage IIIA to IIIB and SS becomes largely academic. Both conditions share a similar prognosis and management approach, rendering the distinction inconsequential for therapeutic strategy.

7.2.5 Therapy

Unlike early-stage mycosis fungoides (MF), which often responds favorably to skin-directed therapies, SS typically necessitates initial systemic treatment. Established therapeutic agents include extracorporeal photophoresis, oral retinoids, low-dose methotrexate, pegylated interferon α, and HDAC inhibitors, often used in combination. Although topical corticosteroids remain the cornerstone for alleviating erythema and itch, medium doses of systemic prednisone (0.2–0.5 mg/kg) can be employed when topical options prove insufficient. Phototherapy, particularly narrow-band UVB, requires prudent application at reduced dosages, given the photosensitivity and susceptibility to ultraviolet phototherapy burns observed in SS patients.

7.2.5.1 Extracorporeal Photopheresis (ECP)

Increasingly considered as a first-line option—particularly if readily accessible—ECP is an apheresis technique that *ex vivo* sensitizes purified peripheral blood mononuclear cells with 8-methoxypsoralen, followed by ultraviolet A (UVA) irradiation. Standard protocols involve bi-weekly or monthly treatments over two consecutive days. Response predictors include the presence of erythroderma, normal CD8 counts, B1 stage, peripheral eosinophilia, and the absence of significant lymphadenopathy or organ involvement. Notably, ECP has demonstrated efficacy rates of approximately 60% overall and 30% for complete responses [106, 107]. One of ECP's most compelling advantages is its compatibility with other SS treatments.

7.2.5.2 Targeted Therapies

Mogamulizumab appears more efficacious in SS than in MF, achieving an overall response rate of around 50% [74]. Histone deacetylase inhibitors have shown moderate efficacy [108–110]. Meanwhile, low-dose alemtuzumab has been selectively employed for cases with pronounced blood involvement, but its application is restricted due to hematological toxicities and increased infection risks [111].

7.2.5.3 Hematopoietic Stem Cell Transplant

For patients exhibiting rapid disease progression, allogeneic bone marrow transplantation remains a last-resort therapeutic avenue, sharing similar considerations as observed in advanced-stage MF [112].

7.2.5.4 Infectious Complications: A Pervasive Risk

Immunosuppression in SS is multifactorial, often involving reduced B cell and CD8 cell counts, alongside pathological immune polarization from T-helper cell type 1 (Th1) to Th2. The susceptibility to bacterial sepsis—predominantly caused by *Staphylococcus aureus*—renders it the most frequent cause of mortality in SS [113, 114]. Moreover, *S. aureus* colonization not only elevates the risk of lethal sepsis but also fosters lymphoma cell proliferation and exacerbates erythroderma [114, 115]. Thus, rapid initiation of systemic antibiotics is imperative in SS patients showing sudden erythroderma flares [113, 116, 117].

References

1. Agar NS, Wedgeworth E, Crichton S, Mitchell TJ, Cox M, Ferreira S, et al. Survival outcomes and prognostic factors in mycosis fungoides/Sézary syndrome: validation of the revised International Society for Cutaneous Lymphomas/European Organisation for Research and Treatment of Cancer staging proposal. J Clin Oncol. 2010;28:4730–9.
2. Mourad A, Gniadecki R. Overall survival in mycosis fungoides: a systematic review and meta-analysis. J Invest Dermatol. 2020;140:495–497.e5.
3. Scarisbrick JJ, Prince HM, Vermeer MH, Quaglino P, Horwitz S, Porcu P, et al. Cutaneous lymphoma international consortium study of outcome in advanced stages of mycosis fungoides and Sézary syndrome: effect of specific prognostic markers on survival and development of a prognostic model. J Clin Oncol. 2015;33:3766–73.
4. Väkevä L, Lipsanen T, Sintonen H, Ranki A. Morbidity and causes of death in patients with cutaneous T-cell lymphoma in Finland. Acta Derm Venereol. 2017;97:735–8.
5. Lindahl LM, Fenger-Grøn M, Iversen L. Secondary cancers, comorbidities and mortality associated with nitrogen mustard therapy in patients with mycosis fungoides: a 30-year population-based cohort study. Br J Dermatol. 2014;170:699–704.
6. Lindahl LM, Schmidt M, Farkas DK, Sørensen HT, Iversen L. Risk of venous thromboembolism in patients with mycosis fungoides and parapsoriasis: a Danish nationwide population-based cohort study. J Am Acad Dermatol. 2018;78:1077–1083.e4.
7. Virmani P, Myskowski PL, Pulitzer M. Unusual variants of mycosis fungoides. Diagn Histopathol. 2016;22:142–51.
8. Wieser I, Wang C, Alberti-Violetti S, Lyons G, Tran C, Talpur R, et al. Clinical characteristics, risk factors and long-term outcome of 114 patients with folliculotropic mycosis fungoides. Arch Dermatol Res. 2017;309:453–9.
9. Alaggio R, Amador C, Anagnostopoulos I, Attygalle AD, Araujo IBO, Berti E, et al. The 5th edition of the World Health Organization classification of haematolymphoid tumours: lymphoid neoplasms. Leukemia. 2022;36:1720–48.
10. Giberson M, Mourad A, Gniadecki R. Folliculotropism does not affect overall survival in mycosis fungoides: results from a single-center cohort and meta-analysis. Dermatology. 2017;233:320–5.
11. LeBoit PE, Zackheim HS, White CR Jr. Granulomatous variants of cutaneous T-cell lymphoma. The histopathology of granulomatous mycosis fungoides and granulomatous slack skin. Am J Surg Pathol. 1988;12:83–95.
12. Shah A, Safaya A. Granulomatous slack skin disease: a review, in comparison with mycosis fungoides. J Eur Acad Dermatol Venereol. 2012;26:1472–8.
13. Bakr F, Ziaj S, Cardoso J, Wain EM, Theaker J, Whittaker S, et al. Mycosis fungoides and granulomatous slack skin: a single entity with distinct clinical phenotypes. Am J Dermatopathol. 2024;46:14–20.
14. Steffen C. Ketron-Goodman disease, Woringer-Kolopp disease, and pagetoid reticulosis. Am J Dermatopathol. 2005;27:68–85.
15. Larson K, Wick MR. Pagetoid reticulosis: report of two cases and review of the literature. Dermatopathology (Basel). 2016;3:8–12.
16. Ferrier A, Soong L, Alabdulsalam A, Kunimoto B, Zhu X, Deschenes J, et al. Diagnosis of gamma/delta mycosis fungoides requires longitudinal clinical observation. J Am Acad Dermatol. 2021;85:1352–3.
17. Motamedi M, Xiao MZ, Deschenes J, Hardin J, Sterrett R, Street L, et al. Early organ metastasis in granulomatous mycosis fungoides: a systematic review. Dermatology. 2024;240(3):468–73.
18. Reggiani C, Massone C, Fink-Puches R, Cota C, Cerroni L. Interstitial mycosis fungoides: a clinicopathologic study of 21 patients. Am J Surg Pathol. 2016;40:1360–7.
19. O'Donnell M, Zaya R, Correia E, Krishnasamy S, Sahu J, Shi W, et al. Disease characteristics, prognosis, and response to therapy in patients with large-cell transformed mycosis fungoides: a single-center retrospective study. J Am Acad Dermatol. 2022;86:1285–92.
20. Vergier B, de Muret A, Beylot-Barry M, Vaillant L, Ekouevi D, Chene G, et al. Transformation of mycosis fungoides: clinicopathological and prognostic features of 45 cases. French Study Group of Cutaneious Lymphomas. Blood. 2000;95:2212–8.
21. Bontoux C, de Masson A, Thonnart N, Ram-Wolff C, Caraguel F, Batista L, et al. Large-cell transformation is an independent poor prognostic factor

in Sézary syndrome: analysis of 117 cases. Br J Dermatol. 2022;187:815–7.
22. Skov AG, Gniadecki R. Delay in the histopathologic diagnosis of mycosis fungoides. Acta Derm Venereol. 2015;95:472–5.
23. Parekh V, Shim E-H, Knapp CF 3rd, Hughey L, Elmets CA, McKay K. Primary cutaneous T-cell lymphoma with coexpression of T-cell receptors αβ and γδ. Am J Dermatopathol. 2016;38:66–72.
24. Omland SH, Gjerdum LMR, Cerroni L, Gniadecki R. Primary cutaneous γδ T-cell lymphoma positive for both T-cell receptor γ and T-cell receptor β. Pathol Case Rev. 2014;19(4):216–20.
25. Posnett DN, Sinha R, Kabak S, Russo C. Clonal populations of T cells in normal elderly humans: the T cell equivalent to "benign monoclonal gammapathy". J Exp Med. 1994;179:609–18.
26. Epling-Burnette PK, Painter JS, Rollison DE, Ku E, Vendron D, Widen R, et al. Prevalence and clinical association of clonal T-cell expansions in Myelodysplastic Syndrome. Leukemia. 2007;21:659–67.
27. Guitart J, Magro C. Cutaneous T-cell lymphoid dyscrasia: a unifying term for idiopathic chronic dermatoses with persistent T-cell clones. Arch Dermatol. 2007;143:921–32.
28. Thurber SE, Zhang B, Kim YH, Schrijver I, Zehnder J, Kohler S. T-cell clonality analysis in biopsy specimens from two different skin sites shows high specificity in the diagnosis of patients with suggested mycosis fungoides. J Am Acad Dermatol. 2007;57:782–90.
29. Raghavan SS, Wang JY, Gru AA, Marqueling AL, Teng JMC, Brown RA, et al. Next-generation sequencing confirms T-cell clonality in a subset of pediatric pityriasis lichenoides. J Cutan Pathol. 2022;49:252–60.
30. Rea B, Haun P, Emerson R, Vignali M, Farooqi M, Samimi S, et al. Role of high-throughput sequencing in the diagnosis of cutaneous T-cell lymphoma. J Clin Pathol. 2018;71:814–20.
31. Iyer A, Hennessey DC, Gniadecki R. Clonotype pattern in T-cell lymphomas map the cell of origin to immature lymphoid precursors. Blood Adv. 2022;6:2334–45.
32. Iyer A, Hennessey D, O'Keefe S, Patterson J, Wang W, Wong GK-S, et al. Skin colonization by circulating neoplastic clones in cutaneous T-cell lymphoma. Blood. 2019;134:1517–27.
33. Kamstrup MR, Gniadecki R, Friberg L. Integrated positron-emission tomography and computed tomography manifestations of cutaneous T-cell lymphoma. Arch Dermatol. 2012;148:1420–2.
34. Kamstrup MR, Madsen HO, Skovgaard GL, Gniadecki R. Analysis of extracutaneous spread in mycosis fungoides. J Invest Dermatol. 2009;129:2905–7.
35. Park A, Wong L, Lang A, Kraus C, Anderson N, Elsensohn A. Cutaneous T-cell lymphoma following dupilumab use: a systematic review. Int J Dermatol. 2023;62:862–76.
36. Elston DM. Dupilumab and cutaneous T-cell lymphoma. J Am Acad Dermatol. 2020;83:33–4.
37. Poyner EFM, Bacon CM, Osborne W, Frew JA, Weatherhead SC. Dupilumab unmasking cutaneous T-cell lymphoma: report of a fatal case. Clin Exp Dermatol. 2022;47:974–6.
38. Martinez-Escala ME, Posligua AL, Wickless H, Rutherford A, Sable KA, Rubio-Gonzalez B, et al. Progression of undiagnosed cutaneous lymphoma after anti-tumor necrosis factor-alpha therapy. J Am Acad Dermatol. 2018;78:1068–76.
39. Schaefer L, Comfere N, Sokumbi O. Development of cutaneous T-cell lymphoma following biologic treatment: a systematic review. Am J Clin Dermatol. 2023;24:153–64.
40. Pielop JA, Jones D, Duvic M. Transient CD30+ nodal transformation of cutaneous T-cell lymphoma associated with cyclosporine treatment. Int J Dermatol. 2001;40:505–11.
41. Feuerstein JD, Cheifetz AS. Cancer screening in inflammatory bowel disease: a guide to risk management and techniques. Springer; 2019.
42. Jonak C, Tittes J, Brunner PM, Guenova E. Mycosis fungoides and Sézary syndrome. J Dtsch Dermatol Ges. 2021;19:1307–34.
43. Trautinger F, Eder J, Assaf C, Bagot M, Cozzio A, Dummer R, et al. European Organisation for Research and Treatment of Cancer consensus recommendations for the treatment of mycosis fungoides/Sézary syndrome—update 2017. Eur J Cancer. 2017;77:57–74.
44. Mehta-Shah N, Horwitz SM, Ansell S, Ai WZ, Barnes J, Barta SK, et al. NCCN guidelines insights: primary cutaneous lymphomas, version 2.2020. J Natl Compr Canc Netw. 2020;18:522–36.
45. Vermeer MH, Willemze R. Limited effect of chemotherapy in cutaneous lymphoma. Blood. 2015;125:4–5.
46. Hughes CFM, Khot A, McCormack C, Lade S, Westerman DA, Twigger R, et al. Lack of durable disease control with chemotherapy for mycosis fungoides and Sézary syndrome: a comparative study of systemic therapy. Blood. 2015;125:71–81.
47. Zackheim HS, Kashani-Sabet M, Amin S. Topical corticosteroids for mycosis fungoides. Experience in 79 patients. Arch Dermatol. 1998;134:949–54.
48. MacArthur KM, Jariwala N, Kim EJ, Rook AH. Topical carmustine as monotherapy or as multimodality therapy for folliculotropic mycosis fungoides. Acta Derm Venereol. 2017;97:373–4.
49. Lessin SR, Duvic M, Guitart J, Pandya AG, Strober BE, Olsen EA, et al. Topical chemotherapy in cutaneous T-cell lymphoma: positive results of a randomized, controlled, multicenter trial testing the efficacy and safety of a novel mechlorethamine, 0.02%, gel in mycosis fungoides. JAMA Dermatol. 2013;149:25–32.

50. Kim YH, Martinez G, Varghese A, Hoppe RT. Topical nitrogen mustard in the management of mycosis fungoides: update of the Stanford experience. Arch Dermatol. 2003;139:165–73.
51. Alexander-Savino CV, Chung CG, Gilmore ES, Carroll SM, Poligone B. Randomized mechlorethamine/chlormethine induced dermatitis assessment study (MIDAS) establishes benefit of topical triamcinolone 0.1% ointment cotreatment in mycosis fungoides. Dermatol Ther. 2022;12:643–54.
52. Zackheim HS. Topical carmustine (BCNU) in the treatment of mycosis fungoides. Dermatol Ther. 2003;16:299–302.
53. Zackheim HS, Epstein EH Jr, Crain WR. Topical carmustine (BCNU) for cutaneous T cell lymphoma: a 15-year experience in 143 patients. J Am Acad Dermatol. 1990;22:802–10.
54. Brazzelli V, Antoninetti M, Palazzini S, Prestinari F, Borroni G. Narrow-band ultraviolet therapy in early-stage mycosis fungoides: study on 20 patients. Photodermatol Photoimmunol Photomed. 2007;23:229–33.
55. Ponte P, Serrão V, Apetato M. Efficacy of narrow-band UVB vs. PUVA in patients with early-stage mycosis fungoides. J Eur Acad Dermatol Venereol. 2010;24:716–21.
56. Whittaker S, Ortiz P, Dummer R, Ranki A, Hasan B, Meulemans B, et al. Efficacy and safety of bexarotene combined with psoralen-ultraviolet A (PUVA) compared with PUVA treatment alone in stage IB-IIA mycosis fungoides: final results from the EORTC Cutaneous Lymphoma Task Force phase III randomized clinical trial (NCT00056056). Br J Dermatol. 2012;167:678–87.
57. Vieyra-Garcia P, Fink-Puches R, Porkert S, Lang R, Pöchlauer S, Ratzinger G, et al. Evaluation of low-dose, low-frequency oral psoralen-UV-A treatment with or without maintenance on early-stage mycosis fungoides: a randomized clinical trial. JAMA Dermatol. 2019;155:538–47.
58. Rupoli S, Barulli S, Guiducci B, Offidani M, Mozzicafreddo G, Simonacci M, et al. Low dose interferon-alpha2b combined with PUVA is an effective treatment of early stage mycosis fungoides: results of a multicenter study. Cutaneous-T Cell Lymphoma Multicenter Study Group. Haematologica. 1999;84:809–13.
59. Stadler R, Otte HG. Combination therapy of cutaneous T cell lymphoma with interferon alpha-2a and photochemotherapy. Recent Results Cancer Res. 1995;139:391–401.
60. Adışen E, Tektaş V, Erduran F, Erdem Ö, Gürer MA. Ultraviolet A1 phototherapy in the treatment of early mycosis fungoides. Dermatology. 2017;233:192–8.
61. Olek-Hrab K, Silny W, Dańczak-Pazdrowska A, Osmola-Mańkowska A, Sadowska PA, Polańska A, et al. Ultraviolet A1 phototherapy for mycosis fungoides. Clin Exp Dermatol. 2013;38:126–30.
62. Valipour A, Jäger M, Wu P, Schmitt J, Bunch C, Weberschock T. Interventions for mycosis fungoides. Cochrane Database Syst Rev. 2020;7:CD008946.
63. Hunter S, Langemo D, Thompson P, Hanson D, Anderson J. Radiation wounds. Adv Skin Wound Care. 2007;20:438, 440.
64. Shakespeare TP, Dwyer M, Mukherjee R, Yeghiaian-Alvandi R, Gebski V. Estimating risks of radiotherapy complications as part of informed consent: the high degree of variability between radiation oncologists may be related to experience. Int J Radiat Oncol Biol Phys. 2002;54:647–53.
65. Hoppe RT, Harrison C, Tavallaee M, Bashey S, Sundram U, Li S, et al. Low-dose total skin electron beam therapy as an effective modality to reduce disease burden in patients with mycosis fungoides: results of a pooled analysis from 3 phase-II clinical trials. J Am Acad Dermatol. 2015;72:286–92.
66. Breneman D, Duvic M, Kuzel T, Yocum R, Truglia J, Stevens VJ. Phase 1 and 2 trial of bexarotene gel for skin-directed treatment of patients with cutaneous T-cell lymphoma. Arch Dermatol. 2002;138:325–32.
67. Photiou L, van der Weyden C, McCormack C, Miles PH. Systemic treatment options for advanced-stage mycosis fungoides and Sézary syndrome. Curr Oncol Rep. 2018;20:32.
68. Jawed SI, Myskowski PL, Horwitz S, Moskowitz A, Querfeld C. Primary cutaneous T-cell lymphoma (mycosis fungoides and Sézary syndrome): part II. Prognosis, management, and future directions. J Am Acad Dermatol. 2014;70:223.e1–17; quiz 240–2.
69. Zackheim HS, Kashani-Sabet M, McMillan A. Low-dose methotrexate to treat mycosis fungoides: a retrospective study in 69 patients. J Am Acad Dermatol. 2003;49:873–8.
70. Olsen EA, Kim YH, Kuzel TM, Pacheco TR, Foss FM, Parker S, et al. Phase IIb multicenter trial of vorinostat in patients with persistent, progressive, or treatment refractory cutaneous T-cell lymphoma. J Clin Oncol. 2007;25:3109–15.
71. Kim YH, Tavallaee M, Sundram U, Salva KA, Wood GS, Li S, et al. Phase II investigator-initiated study of brentuximab vedotin in mycosis fungoides and Sézary syndrome with variable CD30 expression level: a multi-institution collaborative project. J Clin Oncol. 2015;33:3750–8.
72. Prince HM, Kim YH, Horwitz SM, Dummer R, Scarisbrick J, Quaglino P, et al. Brentuximab vedotin or physician's choice in CD30-positive cutaneous T-cell lymphoma (ALCANZA): an international, open-label, randomised, phase 3, multicentre trial. Lancet. 2017;390:555–66.
73. Duvic M, Pinter-Brown LC, Foss FM, Sokol L, Jorgensen JL, Challagundla P, et al. Phase 1/2 study of mogamulizumab, a defucosylated anti-CCR4 antibody, in previously treated patients with cutaneous T-cell lymphoma. Blood. 2015;125:1883–9.
74. Kim YH, Bagot M, Pinter-Brown L, Rook AH, Porcu P, Horwitz SM, et al. Mogamulizumab ver-

sus vorinostat in previously treated cutaneous T-cell lymphoma (MAVORIC): an international, open-label, randomised, controlled phase 3 trial. Lancet Oncol. 2018;19:1192–204.
75. Fuji S, Inoue Y, Utsunomiya A, Moriuchi Y, Uchimaru K, Choi I, et al. Pretransplantation anti-CCR4 antibody mogamulizumab against adult T-cell leukemia/lymphoma is associated with significantly increased risks of severe and corticosteroid-refractory graft-versus-host disease, nonrelapse mortality, and overall mortality. J Clin Oncol. 2016;34:3426–33.
76. Hirotsu KE, Neal TM, Khodadoust MS, Wang JY, Rieger KE, Strelo J, et al. Clinical characterization of mogamulizumab-associated rash during treatment of mycosis fungoides or Sézary syndrome. JAMA Dermatol. 2021;157:700–7.
77. Zinzani PL, Baliva G, Magagnoli M, Bendandi M, Modugno G, Gherlinzoni F, et al. Gemcitabine treatment in pretreated cutaneous T-cell lymphoma: experience in 44 patients. J Clin Oncol. 2000;18:2603–6.
78. Dummer R, Quaglino P, Becker JC, Hasan B, Karrasch M, Whittaker S, et al. Prospective international multicenter phase II trial of intravenous pegylated liposomal doxorubicin monochemotherapy in patients with stage IIB, IVA, or IVB advanced mycosis fungoides: final results from EORTC 21012. J Clin Oncol. 2012;30:4091–7.
79. Kurzrock R, Pilat S, Duvic M. Pentostatin therapy of T-cell lymphomas with cutaneous manifestations. J Clin Oncol. 1999;17:3117–21.
80. Molin L, Thomsen K, Volden G, Groth O, Hellbe L, Holst R, et al. Combination chemotherapy in the tumour stage of mycosis fungoides with cyclophosphamide, vincristine, vp-16, adriamycin and prednisolone (cop, chop, cavop): a report from the Scandinavian mycosis fungoides study group. Acta Derm Venereol. 1980;60:542–4.
81. Akpek G, Koh HK, Bogen S, O'Hara C, Foss FM. Chemotherapy with etoposide, vincristine, doxorubicin, bolus cyclophosphamide, and oral prednisone in patients with refractory cutaneous T-cell lymphoma. Cancer. 1999;86:1368–76.
82. Iqbal M, Reljic T, Ayala E, Sher T, Murthy H, Roy V, et al. Efficacy of allogeneic hematopoietic cell transplantation in cutaneous T cell lymphoma: results of a systematic review and meta-analysis. Biol Blood Marrow Transplant. 2020;26:76–82.
83. Molina A, Zain J, Arber DA, Angelopolou M, O'Donnell M, Murata-Collins J, et al. Durable clinical, cytogenetic, and molecular remissions after allogeneic hematopoietic cell transplantation for refractory Sezary syndrome and mycosis fungoides. J Clin Oncol. 2005;23:6163–71.
84. Vieyra-Garcia P, Wolf P. Psoralen-ultraviolet A maintenance in mycosis fungoides: the underlying question. Br J Dermatol. 2017;177:336–7.
85. Xiao MZX, Hennessey D, Iyer A, O'Keefe S, Zhang F, Sivanand A, et al. Transcriptomic changes during stage progression of mycosis fungoides. Br J Dermatol. 2022;186:520–31.
86. Vermeer MH, van Doorn R, Dijkman R, Mao X, Whittaker S, van Voorst Vader PC, et al. Novel and highly recurrent chromosomal alterations in Sézary syndrome. Cancer Res. 2008;68:2689–98.
87. Morris L, Tran J, Duvic M. Non-classic signs of Sézary syndrome: a review. Am J Clin Dermatol. 2020;21:383–91.
88. Mangold AR, Thompson AK, Davis MD, Saulite I, Cozzio A, Guenova E, et al. Early clinical manifestations of Sézary syndrome: a multicenter retrospective cohort study. J Am Acad Dermatol. 2017;77:719–27.
89. Thompson AK, Killian JM, Weaver AL, Pittelkow MR, Davis MDP. Sézary syndrome without erythroderma: a review of 16 cases at Mayo Clinic. J Am Acad Dermatol. 2017;76:683–8.
90. Winkelmann RK, Buechner SA, Diaz-Perez JL. Pre-Sézary syndrome. J Am Acad Dermatol. 1984;10:992–9.
91. Buechner SA. Pre-Sézary erythroderma evolving to Sézary syndrome. Arch Dermatol. 1983;119:285.
92. Gniadecki R, Lukowsky A. Monoclonal T-cell dyscrasia of undetermined significance associated with recalcitrant erythroderma. Arch Dermatol. 2005;141:361–7.
93. Vonderheid EC, Bernengo MG, Burg G, Duvic M, Heald P, Laroche L, et al. Update on erythrodermic cutaneous T-cell lymphoma: report of the International Society for Cutaneous Lymphomas. J Am Acad Dermatol. 2002;46:95–106.
94. Illingworth A, Johansson U, Huang S, Horna P, Wang SA, Almeida J, et al. International guidelines for the flow cytometric evaluation of peripheral blood for suspected Sézary syndrome or mycosis fungoides: assay development/optimization, validation, and ongoing quality monitors. Cytometry B Clin Cytom. 2021;100:156–82.
95. Lyapichev KA, Bah I, Huen A, Duvic M, Routbort MJ, Wang W, et al. Determination of immunophenotypic aberrancies provides better assessment of peripheral blood involvement by mycosis fungoides/Sézary syndrome than quantification of CD26− or CD7− CD4+ T-cells. Cytometry B Clin Cytom. 2021;100:183–91.
96. Horna P, Shi M, Olteanu H, Johansson U. Emerging role of T-cell receptor constant β Chain-1 (TRBC1) expression in the flow cytometric diagnosis of T-cell malignancies. Int J Mol Sci. 2021;22:1817.
97. Klemke C-D, Brade J, Weckesser S, Sachse MM, Booken N, Neumaier M, et al. The diagnosis of Sézary syndrome on peripheral blood by flow cytometry requires the use of multiple markers. Br J Dermatol. 2008;159:871–80.
98. Vermeer MH, Moins-Teisserenc H, Bagot M, Quaglino P, Whittaker S. Flow cytometry for the assessment of blood tumour burden in cutaneous T-cell lymphoma: towards a standardized approach. Br J Dermatol. 2022;187:21–8.
99. Ponti R, Quaglino P, Novelli M, Fierro MT, Comessatti A, Peroni A, et al. T-cell receptor gamma gene rearrangement by multiplex polymerase chain

reaction/heteroduplex analysis in patients with cutaneous T-cell lymphoma (mycosis fungoides/Sézary syndrome) and benign inflammatory disease: correlation with clinical, histological and immunophenotypical findings. Br J Dermatol. 2005;153:565–73.
100. López Aventín D, Gallardo F, Colomo L, Moragón E, Vela MC, Duran Jordà X, et al. Diagnostic value of genotypic analysis in primary cutaneous lymphomas using standardized BIOMED-2 polymerase chain reaction protocols: experience in daily clinical practice. Acta Derm Venereol. 2021;101:adv00460.
101. Kandolf-Sekulović L, Cikota B, Dinić M, Škiljević D, Magić Z. T-cell receptor-G gene rearrangement analysis in the diagnosis of patients with Erythroderma / Dijagnostički Značaj Analize Preuređenja Gena Gama Lanca T-Ćelijskog Receptora Kod Pacijenata Sa Eritrodermijom. Serb J Dermatol Venerol. 2009;1:17–26.
102. Fraser-Andrews EA, Mitchell T, Ferreira S, Seed PT, Russell-Jones R, Calonje E, et al. Molecular staging of lymph nodes from 60 patients with mycosis fungoides and Sézary syndrome: correlation with histopathology and outcome suggests prognostic relevance in mycosis fungoides. Br J Dermatol. 2006;155:756–62.
103. Calvani J, de Masson A, de Margerie-Mellon C, de Kerviler É, Ram-Wolff C, Gruber A, et al. Image-guided lymph node core-needle biopsy predicts survival in mycosis fungoides and Sézary syndrome. Br J Dermatol. 2021;185:419–27.
104. Cury-Martins J, Netto SDC, de Castro SCC, Siqueira SAC, Giannotti MA, Zerbini MCN, et al. Image-guided lymph node core needle biopsy in mycosis fungoides/Sézary syndrome: direct comparison to surgical excision. J German Soc Dermatol. 2022;20:1008–10.
105. Scarisbrick JJ, Hodak E, Bagot M, Stranzenbach R, Stadler R, Ortiz-Romero PL, et al. Blood classification and blood response criteria in mycosis fungoides and Sézary syndrome using flow cytometry: recommendations from the EORTC cutaneous lymphoma task force. Eur J Cancer. 2018;93:47–56.
106. Knobler R, Arenberger P, Arun A, Assaf C, Bagot M, Berlin G, et al. European dermatology forum—updated guidelines on the use of extracorporeal photopheresis 2020—part 1. J Eur Acad Dermatol Venereol. 2020;34:2693–716.
107. Alfred A, Taylor PC, Dignan F, El-Ghariani K, Griffin J, Gennery AR, et al. The role of extracorporeal photopheresis in the management of cutaneous T-cell lymphoma, graft-versus-host disease and organ transplant rejection: a consensus statement update from the UK Photopheresis Society. Br J Haematol. 2017;177:287–310.
108. Deschamps O, Ram-Wolff C, Beylot-Barry M, Grange F, Skowron F, Dereure O, et al. Treatment of mycosis fungoides and Sézary syndrome with romidepsin: a series of 32 cases from the French Study Group for Cutaneous Lymphoma. Br J Dermatol. 2019;180:423–4.
109. Reddy SA. Romidepsin for the treatment of relapsed/refractory cutaneous T-cell lymphoma (mycosis fungoides/Sézary syndrome): use in a community setting. Crit Rev Oncol Hematol. 2016;106:99–107.
110. Piekarz RL, Frye R, Turner M, Wright JJ, Allen SL, Kirschbaum MH, et al. Phase II multi-institutional trial of the histone deacetylase inhibitor romidepsin as monotherapy for patients with cutaneous T-cell lymphoma. J Clin Oncol. 2009;27:5410–7.
111. Bernengo MG, Quaglino P, Comessatti A, Ortoncelli M, Novelli M, Lisa F, et al. Low-dose intermittent alemtuzumab in the treatment of Sézary syndrome: clinical and immunologic findings in 14 patients. Haematologica. 2007;92:784–94.
112. Polansky M, Talpur R, Daulat S, Hosing C, Dabaja B, Duvic M. Long-term complete responses to combination therapies and allogeneic stem cell transplants in patients with Sézary syndrome. Clin Lymphoma Myeloma Leuk. 2015;15:e83–93.
113. Talpur R, Bassett R, Duvic M. Prevalence and treatment of Staphylococcus aureus colonization in patients with mycosis fungoides and Sézary syndrome. Br J Dermatol. 2008;159:105–12.
114. Vadivel CK, Willerslev-Olsen A, Namini MRJ, Zeng Z, Yan L, Danielsen M, et al. Staphylococcus aureus induce drug resistance in cancer T cells in Sézary Syndrome. Blood. 2024;143(15):1496–512.
115. Lindahl LM, Willerslev-Olsen A, Gjerdrum LMR, Nielsen PR, Blümel E, Rittig AH, et al. Antibiotics inhibit tumor and disease activity in cutaneous T-cell lymphoma. Blood. 2019;134:1072–83.
116. Lewis DJ, Holder BB, Duvic M. The "Duvic regimen" for erythrodermic flares secondary to Staphylococcus aureus in mycosis fungoides and Sézary syndrome. Int J Dermatol. 2018;57:123–4.
117. Emge DA, Bassett RL, Duvic M, Huen AO. Methicillin-resistant Staphylococcus aureus (MRSA) is an important pathogen in erythrodermic cutaneous T-cell lymphoma (CTCL) patients. Arch Dermatol Res. 2020;312:283–8.

Aggressive Cutaneous T-Cell and NK/T-Cell Lymphomas

8

Robert Gniadecki, Minakshi Taparia,
Jean Deschenes, Jori Hardin, and Etienne Mahe

8.1 Practice Essentials

- Primary cutaneous CD8$^+$ aggressive epidermotropic cytotoxic T-cell lymphoma (pcCD8-AETCL), primary cutaneous γδ T-cell lymphoma (pcGDTCL), NK/T-lymphoma, and cutaneous peripheral T-cell lymphoma (not otherwise specified) comprise the clinical category of "aggressive cutaneous lymphomas."
- Mortality in patients with extracutaneous involvement is high (>90% at 5 years). Patients presenting with skin-only disease seem to have a better prognosis.
- Clinical manifestations are heterogeneous (plaques, tumors, ulcers); the lesions can be solitary or multiple.
- There is no consensus regarding the optimal therapeutic approach. Allogeneic hematopoietic stem cell transplant is a promising option for eligible patients.

Aggressive NK/T-cell lymphomas presenting in the skin encompass three entities that may be considered primary to the skin but also include systemic extranodal NK/T-cell lymphoma, out of the many additional neoplasms that may show an initial skin presentation which represents secondarily cutaneous involvement in the setting of a systemic disease. These other entities will not be addressed here because they are not considered "aggressive" or are extremely rare.

The aggressive, primary cutaneous neoplasms are represented by primary cutaneous CD8$^+$ aggressive epidermotropic cytotoxic T-cell lymphoma (pcCD8-AETCL), primary cutaneous γδ T-cell lymphoma (pcGDTCL), and the poorly characterized, heterogenous category of cutaneous peripheral T-cell lymphoma, not otherwise specified (PTCL-NOS) as outlined in Table 8.1. Among these, pcCD8-AETCL and pcGDTCL are clearly aggressive and formally classified as primary cutaneous. On the other hand, cutaneous PTCL-NOS is a heterogeneous group of lym-

R. Gniadecki (✉)
Division of Dermatology, University of Alberta, Edmonton, AB, Canada
e-mail: gniadeck@ualberta.ca

M. Taparia
Division of Hematology, University of Alberta Hospital, Edmonton, AB, Canada

J. Deschenes
Department of Pathology and Laboratory Medicine, Cross Cancer Institute, Edmonton, AB, Canada
e-mail: Jean.Deschenes@albertaprecisionlabs.ca

J. Hardin
Division of Dermatology, University of Calgary, Calgary, AB, Canada
e-mail: Jori.hardin@albertahealthservices.ca

E. Mahe
Department of Pathology & Laboratory Medicine, and Hematology & Hematological Malignancies, University of Calgary, Calgary, AB, Canada
e-mail: etienne.mahe@albertaprecisionlabs.ca

R. Gniadecki et al. (eds.), *Diseases of Blood and Skin*, https://doi.org/10.1007/978-3-031-65292-9_8

Table 8.1 Comparison of clinical and histopathological features of aggressive cutaneous lymphomas

Disease	Skin lesions	Expressed markers	Absent markers	Molecular
pcCD8-AETCL	Oval and annular eroded, necrotic plaques	CD3, CD8, CD7, TCRβF1, cytotoxic markers (TIA-1, granzyme B, perforin) Ki67 high	CD4, CD30, CD56, TCRδ (δF1), EBER	Monoclonal TCRβ and TCRγ
pcGDTCL	Ulcerated plaques, tumors, panniculitis	CD3, TCRδ, CD56 (most cases), cytotoxic markers (TIA-1, granzyme B, perforin)	TCRβ (βF1), CD5, CD4, CD8 (occasionally positive), EBER, CD30 (occasionally positive)	Usually monoclonal TCRγ and occasionally TCRβ
Extranodal NK/T--lymphoma	Necrotic tumors on the extremities, head and neck	CD2, CD3 (intracytoplasmic), CD56, EBV (EBER$^+$ virtually all cases) Cytotoxic markers (TIA-1, granzyme B, perforin) Variably positive: CD30, CD8, CD5, p53	CD4, TCL1, CD20 (rarely positive), CD123 Mostly negative: TCRβ (βF1), δF1	Small subset contains a monoclonal T cell population
Cutaneous peripheral T-cell lymphoma, NOS	One or several tumors, plaques, ulcers	Variable expression of CD2, CD3, CD4, CD5, CD7, CD8 Subset expresses T_{FH} markers (CXCL13, PD1, CD10, ICOS, BCL6) May rarely express cytotoxic markers (TIA-1, granzyme B, perforin)	Variable loss of T-cell antigens	Monoclonal TCRβ and TCRγ, EBER$^-$

phoid neoplasms with variable clinical aggressiveness, including some lymphomas expressing T-follicular helper (T_{FH}) phenotype [1]. Although they initially manifest in the skin, it is currently unclear that they always represent primary cutaneous entities. Nonetheless, rare cases are described where patients present solely with skin lesions and have a protracted but progressive skin-limited course, without clinically identifiable systemic involvement.

Extranodal NK/T-cell lymphoma (so-called "nasal type" in the ICC 2022) is addressed in more details below and ranks among the aggressive systemic lymphoid neoplasms that may be salient in their skin presentation, or secondarily involve the skin, although they are now considered not to be primary skin lymphomas.

Other systemic entities with variable aggressiveness, variable systemic components, and diverse types of cutaneous involvement, such as NK/T-cell variant of intravascular large cell lymphoma (very rare), angioimmunoblastic T-cell lymphoma, T-cell prolymphocytic leukemia (T-PLL) and adult T-cell leukemia/lymphoma (ATCLL) are considered in more detail in Chap. 3.

Aggressive cutaneous lymphomas are rare, comprising less than 1% of all cutaneous T-cell lymphomas (CTCL). Clinical manifestations vary widely, ranging from isolated skin tumors to multiple plaques or tumors and deep panniculitis-like lesions. These aggressive cutaneous lymphomas are characterized by high-grade tumors with rapid growth and a propensity for extracutaneous dissemination. They are notably refractory to conventional treatments, and the 5-year survival rate is dismal, generally below 10%.

It is worth noting that blastic plasmacytoid dendritic cell neoplasm (BPDCN) was once grouped within aggressive cutaneous lymphomas. However, according to updated classifications, this tumor type is no longer categorized as primary cutaneous, despite the skin being frequently involved, particularly in early disease stages.

Given the heterogeneity of clinical presentations, the diagnosis relies heavily on histopathological findings. Common histological traits across pcCD8-AETCL, pcGDTCL, and NK/T-lymphoma include the expression of cytotoxic markers such as granzyme B or TIA-1. Consequently, some authors group these entities under the umbrella term "aggressive cutaneous cytotoxic lymphomas."

8.2 Primary Cutaneous CD8+ Aggressive Epidermotropic Cytotoxic T-Cell Lymphoma (pcCD8-AECTCL)

8.2.1 Clinical Presentation

Among the aggressive lymphomas, pcCD8-AECTCL stands out as the most distinct in its clinical presentation.

The diagnosis of this rare lymphoma should always be the result of careful clinical-pathological correlation. Though the exact demographics are not well-defined, the majority of affected individuals are adults. Notably, while this disease has been reported in pediatric patients, in the few cases we have encountered, its appearance was linked with underlying immunodeficiency.

Clinically, patients typically present with superficial, eroded plaques, which are often covered with a distinct black necrotic eschar [2] (Fig. 8.1). These plaques can take on annular, reniform, and arcuate patterns reminiscent of mycosis fungoides (MF). However, unlike MF, these plaques are more widespread and can extend to the mucosal regions, including the oral cavity and conjunctiva, as well as the soles and palms. Also, their appearance is usually relatively recent and without long-standing preceding chronicity. The lesions tend to be more painful than itchy. While tumors can arise in advanced disease stages, many patients succumb to the disease before this occurs.

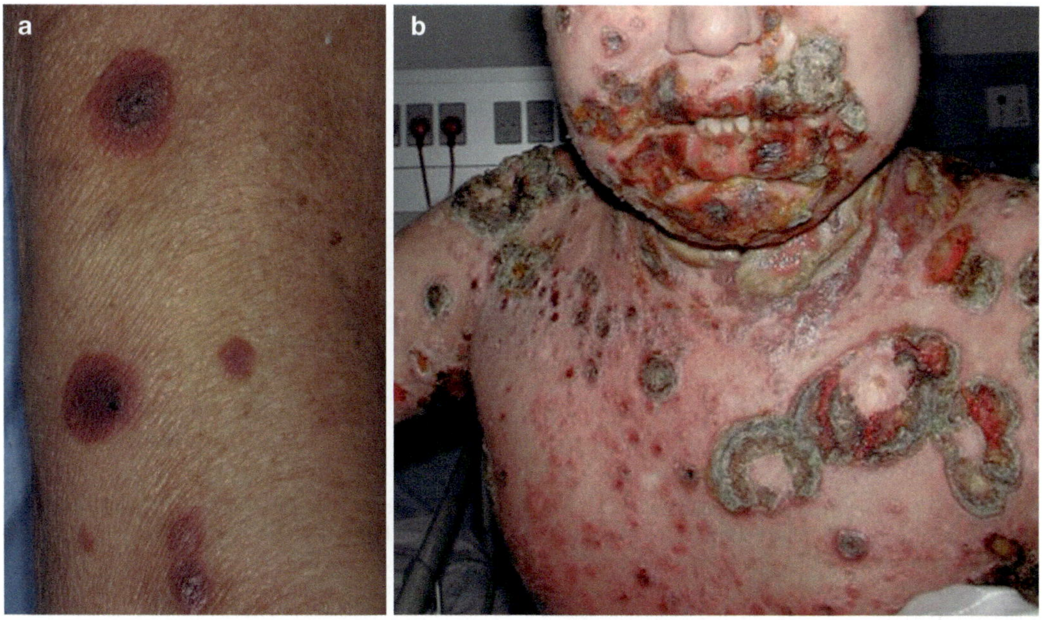

Fig. 8.1 Primary cutaneous CD8+ aggressive epidermotropic cytotoxic T-cell lymphoma (pcCD8-AECTCL). (**a**) Typical lesions in pcCD8-AECTCL are relatively flat, oval, and well-demarcated, with a tendency to develop necrosis in the center. The patient in panel (**b**) is a 14-year-old male with an autosomal recessive hyper IgE syndrome caused by a mutation in the dedicator of cytokinesis 8 gene (DOCK8) who developed very aggressive pcCD8-AECTCL as a complication of immunodeficiency. Note numerous, yet superficial and necrotic, ulcerative lesions. This patient succumbed to the lymphoma despite intensive chemotherapy and allogeneic bone marrow transplant

8.2.2 Skin Biopsy

A skin biopsy will suggest the diagnosis. Histologically, it often reveals a dense lymphocytic infiltrate in the dermis, diffuse or nodular, with frequent angiotropic and angiocentric features. Prominent epidermotropism is a histological hallmark of this entity. It is accompanied by intraepidermal lymphocytic abscesses, epidermal vesiculation, necrosis, and blistering. The immunophenotype reflects cytotoxic T cells ($CD3^+$, $CD8^+$ and TIA-1/granzyme/perforin$^+$), though the expression of other markers can vary; notably, loss of CD2 and/or CD5 is common, and CD30 as well as EBV are both negative [2–4]. The diagnostic features are summarized in Tables 8.1 and 8.2.

Molecular profiling may eventually yield useful insights to establish the diagnosis with more certainty, as some molecular findings are distinctive for this neoplasm among the other cutaneous T-cell neoplasms. For example, approximately 75% of pcCD8-AECTC harbor either activating mutations of *JAK2* or inactivation of *SH2B3* (through rearrangements or deletions), both abnormalities contributing to the constitutive up-regulation of the JAK-STAT pathway signaling [5].

8.2.3 Differential Diagnosis

The differential diagnosis of $CD8^+$ neoplasms is based on clinical-pathological correlations and includes several other entities with very different clinical implications (Table 8.2): $CD8^+$ mycosis fungoides, Type D lymphomatoid papulosis, Generalized pagetoid reticulosis (Ketron-Goodman)

Distinguishing pcCD8-AECTCL from these conditions is critical, as they represent low-grade, indolent processes. In contrast to pcCD8-AECTCL, which necessitates aggressive management, these differential diagnoses can typically be managed conservatively.

Table 8.2 Differential diagnosis of pcCD8-AECTCL

	pcCD8-AECTCL	$CD8^+$ MF	Type D, LyP[a]	Pagetoid reticulosis Ketron Goodman
Lesions	Ulcerative and necrotic patches and plaques	Scaly patches and plaques	Papules, occasionally small plaques	Superficial scaly patches
Distribution	Widespread, often mucosa, palms, soles	Sun-protected areas of the lower trunk and upper legs	Widespread or agminated	Widespread
Course	Rapidly progressive	Chronic, slow progression	Waxing and waning	Chronic, slow progression
Pathology	Dense dermal and epidermal infiltrate, $CD3^+$ $CD8^+$ $CD7^+$, high proliferation rate CD30 negative	Superficial infiltrate with variable epidermotropism, $CD3^+$ $CD8^+$ $CD7^-$, low proliferation rate	$CD30^+$ lymphocytic infiltrate, often $CD8^+$	Epidermotropic infiltrate with pagetoid features, $CD3^+$ $CD8^+$ $CD7^-$

[a]Type E LyP also tends to be $CD8^+$, and shows CD30 expression with a dermal angiocentric pattern, but is not typically epidermotropic. DUSP22-mutated LyP, also positive for CD30, may be $CD8^+$ and shows both a dermal and an epidermotropic distribution with an increased proliferative rate. Finally, rare cases of primary cutaneous γδ T-cell lymphoma (pcGDTCL) may have an epidermotropic component, but their phenotypic profile is generally different from CD8-AECTCL

8.3 Primary Cutaneous γδ T-Cell Lymphoma (pcGDTCL)

8.3.1 Clinical Presentation

pcGDTCL demonstrates considerable variability in its clinical manifestations. Diagnosis hinges on the immunohistochemical detection of the δF1 (TCRδ-chain) chain on the lymphoma cells. The initial manifestation is often a swiftly enlarging skin tumor or a thick, ulcerated plaque. Within a brief period, patients develop additional tumors and plaques, most frequently occurring on the lower arms and legs—a presentation that notably deviates from MF [6]. Single lesions may present with extensive necrosis and ulceration, complicating differentiation from infectious cellulitis or pyoderma gangrenosum. Constitutional symptoms are also frequently observed, including hemophagocytic lymphohistiocytosis (HLH) in about 25% of cases.

The most commonly encountered immunophenotype is $CD3^{+}$, $CD2^{+}$, $CD4^{-}$, $CD5^{-}$, $CD56^{+/-}$, with cytotoxic markers expression (TIA-1, granzyme, and perforin) and a significant subset may express CD8 and CD30 and no evidence of EBV. Immunohistochemical testing for βF1 (negative) and δF1 (positive) is required to confirm the diagnosis. Rare cases may express both TCR βF1 and δF1, or none of these two markers [6]. At the molecular level, TCR rearrangements are usually seen for the TCRγ and/or the TCRδ gene, and the TCRβ gene is rearranged in selected cases [6]. Hence, the type of TCR gene that is rearranged is not useful for diagnosis.

On all biopsies of patients presenting with primary lymphoid skin tumors showing a loss of CD3 or double negativity for CD4 and CD8, additional IHC testing for γδ lymphoma is advisable to exclude pcGDTCL [7] (Fig. 8.2).

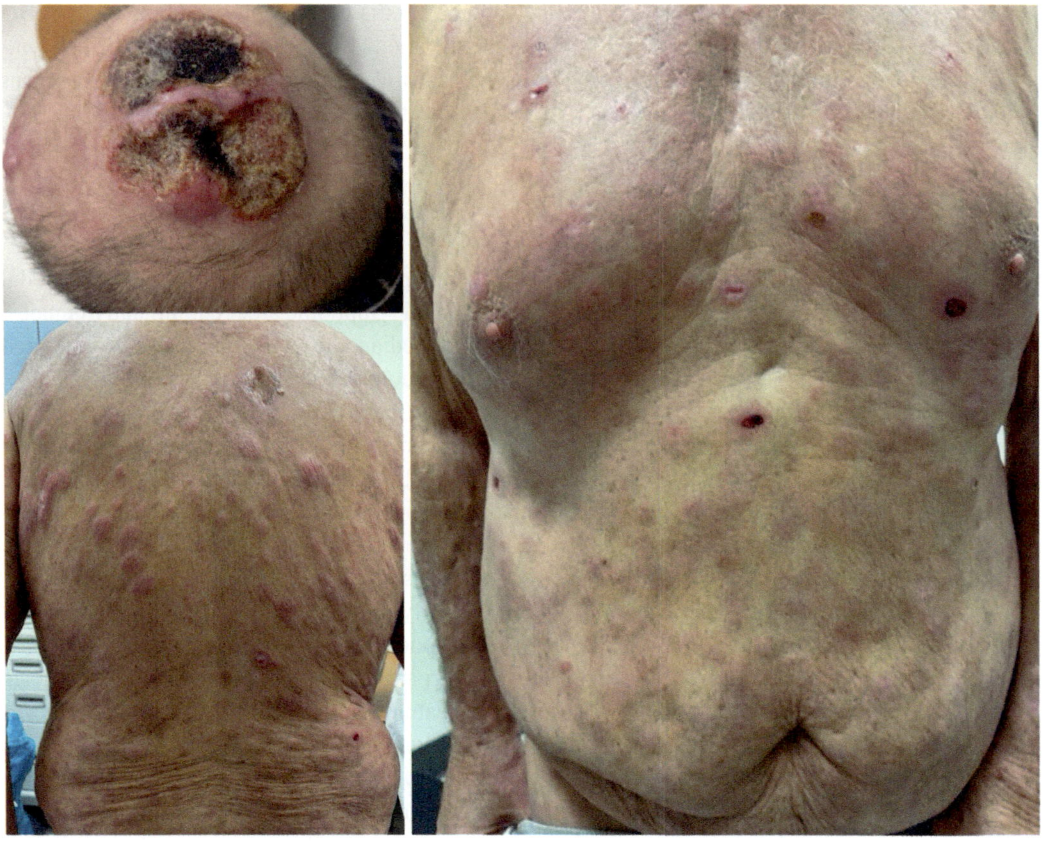

Fig. 8.2 Primary cutaneous γδ T-cell lymphoma (pcGDTCL) in a 72-year-old patient. The disease commenced with an ulcerated plaque on the scalp, swiftly progressing to involve the entire skin. Unfortunately, the patient succumbed to the lymphoma within 2 years from the initial presentation

8.3.2 Differential Diagnosis

While pcGDTCL is recognized in the WHO classification, well-characterized by immunohistochemical testing and depicted as a very rare aggressive lymphoma that should be segregated from the less aggressive subcutaneous panniculitis-like T-cell lymphoma (SPTCL) (with which it was originally lumped).

Clinicians often encounter difficulties in distinguishing the prototypical aggressive form from more indolent cutaneous lymphomas expressing γδTCR. Indeed, indolent forms of this lymphoma exist, as evidenced in recent studies [8–10]. These patients present with clinical features that mimic the aggressive variants but demonstrate less severe ulceration and respond favorably to treatments, achieving durable complete remission. Thus, the task of differentiating indolent from aggressive forms of pcGDTCL remains a significant challenge.

Discriminating between aggressive pcGDTCL and γδ mycosis fungoides (γδMF) is particularly challenging when patients present with skin lesions that resemble MF. Contrary to some literature that suggests comparable prognoses between γδMF and its classic TCR αβ form, our clinical experience points to a more unpredictable course for γδMF, with increased susceptibility to disease progression [11]. This complexity raises the possibility that γδMF, indolent pcGDTCL, and aggressive pcGDTCL could represent points along a clinical continuum, varying from low-grade, indolent diseases to high-grade, fatal lymphomas. Given this dynamic and uncertain landscape, we strongly advocate for regular clinical examinations for all patients with lymphomas featuring a γδTCR phenotype, as well as immediate evaluation of any new symptoms that may signify disease progression.

In a few rare instances, pcGDTCL must be differentiated from cutaneous metastases of γδ hepatosplenic lymphoma [12–14]. In such cases, identification of the primary tumor through comprehensive staging is typically straightforward, thereby aiding in the diagnostic process.

8.4 Cutaneous NK/T-Cell Lymphoma

NK/T-cell lymphoma typically presents as an Epstein-Barr virus (EBV)-related lymphoma predominantly affecting the nasal mucosa and is notably prevalent in Asian populations [15]. It characteristically manifests as nasal cavity infiltration and ulceration, leading to destructive tumoral infiltration into adjacent facial skin. However, variations of this lymphoma, referred to as "nasal-type" or "extranasal NK/T-cell lymphoma," have been described to manifest primarily in the skin, rather than the upper respiratory mucosal areas [16, 17]. Although this variant was previously recognized as a primary cutaneous entity, it has since been subsumed under "extranodal NK/T-cell lymphoma" in the upcoming 5th edition of the WHO classification [15] and "extranodal NK/T-cell lymphoma, nasal-type," in the International Consensus Classification (2022) [18] (Fig. 8.3).

8.4.1 Clinical Manifestations

Patients presenting with cutaneous extranodal NK/T-cell lymphoma are predominantly females, with a median age exceeding 50 years, although the lymphoma can manifest at any age [17, 19]. Clinical features include single or multiple tumors, indurated ulcers, erythematous nodules, and cellulitis-like or panniculitic lesions, almost always localized to the extremities or the head and neck region. The trunk is rarely affected in stage I disease.

This lymphoma variant is highly aggressive, with a poorer survival rate compared to its nasal counterpart [20, 21]. However, early diagnosis and treatment may offer a relatively better prognosis compared to other extranodal NK/T-cell lymphomas (median survival of 4 years vs. 3 months) [17].

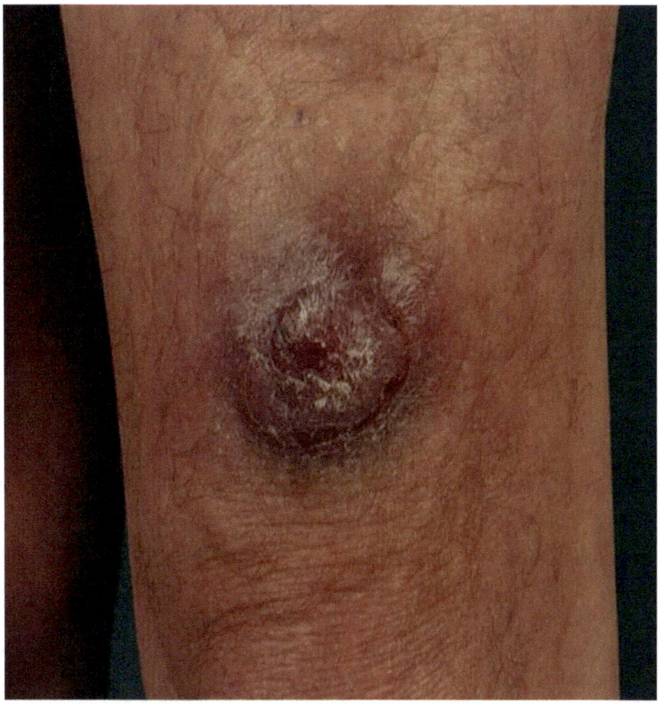

Fig. 8.3 Cutaneous NK/T-cell lymphoma, nasal type. The initial presentation featured a solitary, ulcerated tumor over the knee. Prompt administration of local radiotherapy and chemotherapy was initiated; however, despite these interventions, the disease disseminated to the lymph nodes, ultimately leading to the demise of the patient due to the lymphoma

8.4.2 Skin Biopsy

Histologically, the cutaneous presentation of extranodal NK/T-cell lymphoma is similar histologically to what is usually observed at other sites. There is tumor-associated vascular damage and destruction, angiocentricity, and often prominent necrosis. The tumor cells vary from small round cells to blastoid larger cells with prominent nucleoli, accompanied by apoptotic changes and mitoses in variable numbers, and commonly express CD56, cytotoxic markers (TIA-1, granzyme, and/or perforin) and EBV (EBER is virtually always positive), with variable expression of CD30 (30–40% of cases). Since a majority of cases are of NK histotype, the tumor cells lack surface CD3, although intracytoplasmic CD3 components (CD3ε and CD3ζ) are commonly detected by immunohistochemistry [22, 23]. In general, regardless of cell lineage (T or NK), the neoplastic cells are often positive for CD2, CD7, CD43, CD25 but negative for CD4, CD5, CD8, CD57, TCR βF1, and TCRγ. Of note, while most are in a germline configuration (indicating NK cells), a significant subset may exhibit rearranged TCRβ and/or γ locus (indicating a T-cell lineage). In this minority subset, surface T-cell marker expression is more variable, with occasional cases showing expression of CD4, CD8, CD5, commonly TCRδ^{+} (indicating a γδ phenotype), rarely βF1 and no expression of CD56. Proliferation is typically high (above 50%), irrespective of neoplastic cell size.

8.4.3 Differential Diagnoses

Extranasal cutaneous NK/T-cell lymphoma should be differentiated from secondary cutaneous involvement arising from systemic nodal or extranodal NK/T-cell lymphomas and from other cutaneous cytotoxic T-cell lymphoproliferative disorders (see Table 8.1). BPDCN may be considered, given it also expresses CD56. However, this aggressive skin neoplasm usually shows diffuse, medium-size blastoid cells devoid of an angiocentric tendency, which will often express TCL1, CD123, CD4, and BDCA2, with variable expression of TdT. They are negative for CD3 and negative for EBV. These features should enable clear distinction.

Notably, patients with a dominant extracutaneous tumor burden generally exhibit a worse prognosis than those with predominant skin involvement.

Distinction is also important from a subset of EBV-positive lymphoproliferative disorders presenting in the skin, such as hydroa vacciniforme lymphoproliferative disorder, the classic variant, which is a rare but indolent entity, usually limited to the skin, observed in children and young adults. Angioimmunoblastic T-cell lymphoma [24–26] or aggressive NK leukemia should also be considered in this group, but systemic features generally overshadow the cutaneous manifestations.

Of interest, cutaneous lesions from the very rare and likely related intravascular NK/T-cell lymphoma [27], which preferentially affects the skin and central nervous system, should also be included in the differential diagnosis (see Chap. 3). Lymphomatoid papulosis (LyP), type E (with its typical angiocentric growth pattern and necrotic skin lesions) is also in the differential, but LyP is negative for EBV and atypical cells are strongly, positive for CD30.

Finally, lower on the list, the possibility of a cutaneous peripheral T-cell lymphoma (PTCL, NOS) that is usually negative for EBV and rarely positive for CD56, is also to be considered. Non-neoplastic processes should always be kept in the differential, such as a fungal infection or a vasculitis.

8.5 Cutaneous Peripheral T-Cell Lymphoma, Not Otherwise Specified (cPTCL-NOS)

Cutaneous PTCL-NOS represents a heterogeneous group of cutaneous T-cell lymphomas that do not fit neatly into any specific diagnostic category, thus warranting a diagnosis of exclusion. The term "cutaneous PTCL-NOS" can be misleading as it implies a relationship with nodal PTCL-NOS, a disease that can be further subclassified based on its Th1-like and Th2-like phenotypes (Th2-like: GATA3$^+$ CCR4$^+$, and Th1-like CXCR3$^+$, TBX21$^+$) [28]. However, such detailed subclassification has not been performed for cutaneous PTCL-NOS, with the exception of one study suggesting that GATA3 positivity lacks prognostic significance [29]. A subset of primary cutaneous PTCL demonstrating a prominent T-follicular helper (T_{FH}) phenotype has been recently characterized, but it is too early to say if they will be considered a separate entity [1].

8.5.1 Clinical Presentation

Patients with cutaneous PTCL-NOS often present cutaneous manifestations as their sole initial clinical signs, and systemic involvement is considered secondary in approximately 50% of cases [30]. The remaining patients demonstrate simultaneous skin and systemic disease. Clinically, the presentation varies widely but is generally indistinguishable from other aggressive cutaneous lymphomas. About a third of the patients present with single lesions, such as tumors or ulcers, while the remainder display multiple lesions like nodules, plaques, ulcers, and purpuric lesions reminiscent of vasculitis [29].

The prognosis is generally poor; a study involving 29 patients classified as having cutaneous PTCL-NOS reported a 5-year survival rate of 61% and a median overall survival of 5.6 years [30]. Metastatic disease further escalated the mortality risk (Fig. 8.4).

8.5.2 Differential Diagnosis

This diagnosis is only made after the exclusion of numerous related and competing entities.

Patients with concurrent skin and systemic disease may more appropriately be diagnosed as having secondary cutaneous involvement, particularly as 15% of nodal PTCL-NOS patients are known to develop skin involvement [12]. Skin involvement is also noted in approximately 10% of T-PLL cases and may complicate differentiation from PTCL-NOS, especially in patients with leukemic blood involvement. Other T-cell LPD

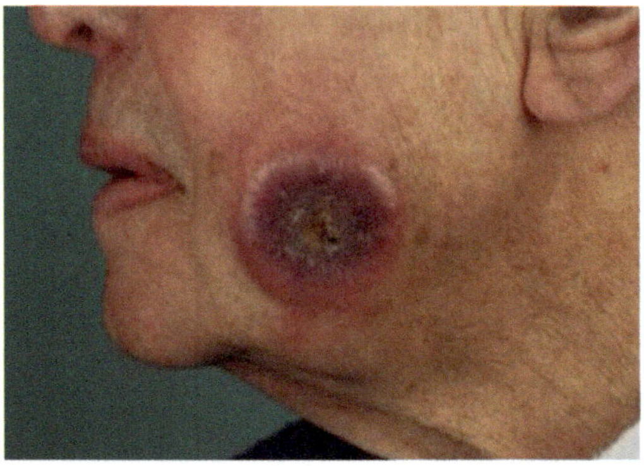

Fig. 8.4 Cutaneous peripheral T-cell lymphoma, not otherwise specified (cPTCL-NOS) in an 89-year-old male patient presenting with a solitary tumor on the face. Staging revealed involvement of the cervical and thoracic lymph nodes. Unfortunately, the patient passed away 8 months after the diagnosis, and the exact cause of death was not established

with skin involvement, such as NK/T-cell lymphoma, ATLL, and AITL should be ruled out.

Obviously, many cases previously categorized as "skin-only" PTCL-NOS might today be reclassified as specific types of primary cutaneous lymphomas or lymphoproliferations, such as pcGDTCL, and the rather less aggressive primary cutaneous anaplastic large cell lymphoma, or innocuous primary cutaneous $CD4^+$ small-medium lymphoproliferative disorder and T-cell-rich marginal zone lymphomas.

8.6 Imaging and Staging of Aggressive Cutaneous Lymphoma

Accurate staging is essential for patients suspected of having aggressive cutaneous lymphomas, irrespective of the size of the skin lesions. A multidisciplinary approach that incorporates imaging studies and possibly bone marrow biopsies is recommended to define the extent of the disease, unlike in other subtypes of cutaneous T-cell lymphomas.

Although bone marrow involvement has been reported [24] the routine use of bone marrow biopsy for staging purposes in this context has not been systematically studied. Thus, the decision to perform a bone marrow biopsy should be made on an individual basis, weighing the clinical implications and the patient's overall health status.

The intestine is a frequent extranodal site of involvement in both NK/T-cell lymphomas [31], and peripheral T-cell lymphoma, NOS [32]. Patients presenting with gastrointestinal symptoms may require additional diagnostic evaluations beyond routine PET/CT scans, which may not adequately visualize intestinal tumors due to physiological FDG uptake in the gut [33].

8.7 Therapy

Currently, there is no consensus on the optimal therapeutic strategy for aggressive cutaneous T-cell lymphomas. Treatment plans are often individualized, based on institutional protocols, extent of disease, and patient factors.

Radiotherapy directed at bulky tumors is frequently used, particularly for localized disease. Multiagent chemotherapy is commonly employed for systemic control, aligned with existing local guidelines. The choice of chemotherapeutic agents may vary, depending on the type of lymphoma and its associated features.

Allogeneic hematopoietic stem cell transplantation (alloHSCT) has been anecdotally reported to yield excellent outcomes in aggressive cutaneous T-cell lymphomas, although data are limited. The decision to proceed with HSCT should be based on a thorough evaluation of the risks and benefits, as well as the patient's overall condition and suitability for this intensive treatment modality.

References

1. Wang L, Rocas D, Dalle S, Sako N, Pelletier L, Martin N, et al. Primary cutaneous peripheral T-cell lymphomas with a T-follicular helper phenotype: an integrative clinical, pathological and molecular case series study. Br J Dermatol. 2022;187:970–80.
2. Nofal A, Abdel-Mawla MY, Assaf M, Salah E. Primary cutaneous aggressive epidermotropic CD8+ T-cell lymphoma: proposed diagnostic criteria

and therapeutic evaluation. J Am Acad Dermatol. 2012;67:748–59.
3. Guitart J, Martinez-Escala ME, Subtil A, Duvic M, Pulitzer MP, Olsen EA, et al. Primary cutaneous aggressive epidermotropic cytotoxic T-cell lymphomas: reappraisal of a provisional entity in the 2016 WHO classification of cutaneous lymphomas. Mod Pathol. 2017;30:761–72.
4. Goodlad JR, Cerroni L, Swerdlow SH. Recent advances in cutaneous lymphoma-implications for current and future classifications. Virchows Arch. 2023;482:281–98.
5. Bastidas Torres AN, Cats D, Out-Luiting JJ, Fanoni D, Mei H, Venegoni L, et al. Deregulation of JAK2 signaling underlies primary cutaneous CD8 aggressive epidermotropic cytotoxic T-cell lymphoma. Haematologica. 2022;107:702–14.
6. Guitart J, Weisenburger DD, Subtil A, Kim E, Wood G, Duvic M, et al. Cutaneous γδ T-cell lymphomas: a spectrum of presentations with overlap with other cytotoxic lymphomas. Am J Surg Pathol. 2012;36:1656–65.
7. Parekh V, Shim E-H, Knapp CF 3rd, Hughey L, Elmets CA, McKay K. Primary cutaneous T-cell lymphoma with coexpression of T-cell receptors αβ and γδ. Am J Dermatopathol. 2016;38:66–72.
8. Chen B-J, Wang RC, Jhuang J-Y, Chen S-W, Su Y-Z, Tseng C-E, et al. Primary cutaneous gamma/delta T-cell lymphoma in Taiwan: a series of six cases with frequent solitary presentation and relatively indolent behavior. J Cutan Pathol. 2022;49:350–7.
9. Galadari A, Ram-Wolff C, Al Hage J, Battistella M, Vignon-Pennamen MD, Rivet J, et al. Cutaneous gamma delta T-Cell lymphoma with indolent evolution: a series of five cases. J Eur Acad Dermatol Venereol. 2022;36:e715–7.
10. von Dücker L, Fleischer M, Stutz N, Thieme M, Witte M, Zillikens D, et al. Primary cutaneous gamma-delta T-cell lymphoma with long-term indolent clinical course initially mimicking lupus erythematosus profundus. Front Oncol. 2020;10:133.
11. Ferrier A, Soong L, Alabdulsalam A, Kunimoto B, Zhu X, Deschenes J, et al. Diagnosis of gamma/delta mycosis fungoides requires longitudinal clinical observation. J Am Acad Dermatol. 2021;85:1352–3.
12. Kawamoto K, Miyoshi H, Yanagida E, Yoshida N, Kiyasu J, Kozai Y, et al. Comparison of clinicopathological characteristics between T-cell prolymphocytic leukemia and peripheral T-cell lymphoma, not otherwise specified. Eur J Haematol. 2017;98:459–66.
13. Santonja C, Carrasco L, Pérez-Sáenz MLÁ, Rodríguez-Pinilla S-M. A skin plaque preceding systemic relapse of gamma-delta hepatosplenic T-cell lymphoma. Am J Dermatopathol. 2020;42:364–7.
14. Hocker TL, Wada DA, McPhail ED, Porrata LF, el-Azhary RA, Gibson LE. Relapsed hepatosplenic T-cell lymphoma heralded by a solitary skin nodule. J Cutan Pathol. 2011;38:899–904.
15. Alaggio R, Amador C, Anagnostopoulos I, Attygalle AD, Araujo IBO, Berti E, et al. The 5th edition of the World Health Organization Classification of haematolymphoid tumours: lymphoid neoplasms. Leukemia. 2022;36:1720–48.
16. Choi Y-L, Park J-H, Namkung J-H, Lee J-H, Yang J-M, Lee E-S, et al. Extranodal NK/T-cell lymphoma with cutaneous involvement: "nasal" vs. "nasal-type" subgroups—a retrospective study of 18 patients. Br J Dermatol. 2009;160:333–7.
17. Wu C-C, Takahashi E, Asano N, Miyata-Takata T, Takata K, Furukawa K, et al. Primary cutaneous NK/T--cell lymphoma of nasal type: an age-related lymphoproliferative disease? Hum Pathol. 2017;68:61–8.
18. Campo E, Jaffe ES, Cook JR, Quintanilla-Martinez L, Swerdlow SH, Anderson KC, et al. The International Consensus Classification of Mature Lymphoid Neoplasms: a report from the Clinical Advisory Committee. Blood. 2022;140:1229–53.
19. Gniadecki R, Rossen K, Ralfkier E, Thomsen K, Skovgaard GL, Jønsson V. CD56+ lymphoma with skin involvement: clinicopathologic features and classification. Arch Dermatol. 2004;140:427–36.
20. Au W-Y, Weisenburger DD, Intragumtornchai T, Nakamura S, Kim W-S, Sng I, et al. Clinical differences between nasal and extranasal natural killer/T--cell lymphoma: a study of 136 cases from the international peripheral T-cell lymphoma project. Blood. 2009;113:3931–7.
21. Vose J, Armitage J, Weisenburger D, International T-Cell Lymphoma Project. International peripheral T-cell and natural killer/T-cell lymphoma study: pathology findings and clinical outcomes. J Clin Oncol. 2008;26:4124–30.
22. Hong M, Lee T, Young Kang S, Kim S-J, Kim W, Ko Y-H. Nasal-type NK/T-cell lymphomas are more frequently T rather than NK lineage based on T-cell receptor gene, RNA, and protein studies: lineage does not predict clinical behavior. Mod Pathol. 2016;29:430–43.
23. Swerdlow SH. Cutaneous marginal zone lymphomas. Semin Diagn Pathol. 2017;34:76–84.
24. Chang SE, Lee SY, Choi JH, Sung KJ, Moon KC, Koh JK. Cutaneous dissemination of nasal NK/T-cell lymphoma with bone marrow, liver and lung involvement. Clin Exp Dermatol. 2002;27:120–2.
25. Sitthinamsuwan P, Pongpruttipan T, Bunyaratavej S, Karoopongse E, Kummalue T, Sukpanichnant S. Cutaneous involvement by colonic extranodal NK/T-cell lymphoma mimicking mycosis fungoides: a case report. J Cutan Pathol. 2011;38:1004–8.
26. Matsuura-Otsuki Y, Hanafusa T, Namiki T, Ueno M, Tokoro S, Igawa K, et al. Relapsed nasal extranodal NK/T-cell lymphoma with secondary cutaneous involvement presenting as a phlegmon-like lesion. Eur J Dermatol. 2016;26:630–1.
27. Quintanilla-Martinez L, Swerdlow SH, Tousseyn T, Barrionuevo C, Nakamura S, Jaffe ES. New concepts in EBV-associated B, T, and NK cell lymphoproliferative disorders. Virchows Arch. 2023;482:227–44.
28. Amador C, Greiner TC, Heavican TB, Smith LM, Galvis KT, Lone W, et al. Reproducing the molecular

subclassification of peripheral T-cell lymphoma-NOS by immunohistochemistry. Blood. 2019;134:2159–70.

29. Kempf W, Mitteldorf C, Battistella M, Willemze R, Cerroni L, Santucci M, et al. Primary cutaneous peripheral T-cell lymphoma, not otherwise specified: results of a multicentre European Organization for Research and Treatment of Cancer (EORTC) cutaneous lymphoma taskforce study on the clinicopathological and prognostic features. J Eur Acad Dermatol Venereol. 2021;35:658–68.
30. Tolkachjov SN, Weenig RH, Comfere NI. Cutaneous peripheral T-cell lymphoma, not otherwise specified: a single-center prognostic analysis. J Am Acad Dermatol. 2016;75:992–9.
31. van Vliet C, Spagnolo DV. T- and NK-cell lymphoproliferative disorders of the gastrointestinal tract: review and update. Pathology. 2020;52:128–41.
32. Zain JM, Hanona P. Aggressive T-cell lymphomas: 2021 Updates on diagnosis, risk stratification and management. Am J Hematol. 2021;96:1027–46.
33. Mao S, Diao C, Cao L. Primary small intestinal extranodal NK/T cell lymphoma, nasal type with kidney involvement: a rare case report and literature review. Diagn Pathol. 2022;17:75.

9 Primary Cutaneous T-Cell Lymphomas and Lymphoproliferative Diseases of Low Malignant Potential

Robert Gniadecki, Minakshi Taparia, Jean Deschenes, Jori Hardin, and Etienne Mahe

The category of primary cutaneous T-cell lymphomas and lymphoproliferative diseases with low malignant potential is defined more by prognostic considerations than by common clinical or histopathological features. This category encompasses a range of entities that are histopathologically diverse but share the commonality of generally favorable outcomes. Diseases from this category are "great mimickers" and may easily be misdiagnosed as aggressive malignancies, which can result in unnecessarily aggressive investigations and treatment, exposing the patient to undue toxicity and its associated morbidity.

The diseases included within this category are:

- Lymphomatoid papulosis (LyP)
- Primary cutaneous anaplastic large cell lymphoma (pcALCL)
- Primary cutaneous, subcutaneous panniculitis-like T-cell lymphoma (pcSPTCL)
- Primary cutaneous CD4$^+$ small-medium pleomorphic T-cell lymphoproliferative disease (pcCD4-LPD)
- Primary cutaneous acral CD8$^+$ T-cell lymphoproliferative disease (CD8-LPD)
- Hydroa vacciniforme lymphoproliferative disorder (HV-LPD)
- Benign CD30$^+$ intravascular lymphoproliferative disease (pcCD30-IVLPD)

There remains debate concerning the true nature of some of these entities. For instance, primary cutaneous CD4$^+$ small-medium pleomorphic lymphoproliferative disease may not represent a true malignancy but rather a clonal local expansion of T cells, with no metastatic potential. On the other hand, diseases such as pcALCL, pcSPTCL, or HV-LPD are unequivocally understood to have malignant potential, albeit with a generally indolent course.

R. Gniadecki (✉)
Division of Dermatology, University of Alberta, Edmonton, AB, Canada
e-mail: gniadeck@ualberta.ca

M. Taparia
Division of Hematology, University of Alberta Hospital, Edmonton, AB, Canada

J. Deschenes
Department of Pathology and Laboratory Medicine, Cross Cancer Institute, Edmonton, AB, Canada
e-mail: Jean.Deschenes@albertaprecisionlabs.ca

J. Hardin
Division of Dermatology, University of Calgary, Calgary, AB, Canada
e-mail: Jori.hardin@albertahealthservices.ca

E. Mahe
Department of Pathology & Laboratory Medicine, and Hematology & Hematological Malignancies, University of Calgary, Calgary, AB, Canada
e-mail: etienne.mahe@albertaprecisionlabs.ca

R. Gniadecki et al. (eds.), *Diseases of Blood and Skin*, https://doi.org/10.1007/978-3-031-65292-9_9

9.1 Lymphomatoid Papulosis (LyP)

9.1.1 Practice Essentials

- LyP is classified as a clinically benign variant of primary cutaneous CD30$^+$ lymphoproliferative disease.
- The hallmark is skin papules, which on biopsy show the presence of large, CD30$^+$ cells.
- The course is chronic, waxing and waning and recurrent.
- LyP may coexist with other malignant diseases, such as mycosis fungoides (MF) or nodal lymphomas.

9.1.2 Clinical Presentation

LyP is a clinically benign lymphoproliferative disorder characterized by the presence of CD30-positive T cells. It represents the benign end of a spectrum of CD30$^+$ lymphoproliferative disorders that show overlapping morphological, phenotypic, and molecular/genetic features, which also include primary cutaneous anaplastic large-cell lymphoma. CD30$^+$ cutaneous lymphoproliferative disorders account as a group for about 30% of all primary cutaneous lymphoproliferative disorders, after only MF and SS [1] and primary cutaneous CD4$^+$ small-medium pleomorphic T-cell lymphoproliferative disease (pcCD4-LPD).

This condition manifests as a chronic and recurrent skin disease. Typically, patients describe asynchronous episodes of erythematous papules primarily appearing on the trunk and extremities (Figs. 9.1 and 9.2). Over 3–4 weeks (usually) to 3–4 months (rarely), these papules ulcerate and eventually spontaneously resolve, leaving behind small varioliform scars. LyP affects both males and females across a wide age range, from as young as 4 to as old as 88 years [2]. In some instances, the clinical presentation of LyP may diverge from the typical papular morphology. It can manifest as small plaques, pustules, or even folliculocentric papules that resemble folliculitis [3]. In some patients with angiocentric lesions, atypical presentations may be observed, with larger ulcerated lesions and eschar-like scarring [4].

LyP may coexist with pcALCL in the same patient. In those cases, both lesions often share the same clone [5, 6]. Moreover, LyP is observed more frequently in patients with MF. Between 10% and 20% of patients with LyP develop MF, either synchronously or as a metachronous event (before or after LyP), and these lesions are also often clonally related [2]. It has been postulated that all three diseases—MF, LyP, and pcALCL—could arise from a common precursor T-cell clone that diverges into different pathways of differentiation [7–9].

Uncommonly, LyP may manifest in localized forms, presenting as agminated lesions, recurrent lesions confined to a single anatomical area, or solitary, recurring lesions [10]. Some evidence suggests that these uncommon forms may be associated with DUSP22-IRF4 rearrangement, a genetic alteration also found in a subset of nodal anaplastic large cell lymphomas [11, 12]. However, the prognostic implications of this rearrangement in LyP appear to be limited, as it does not seem to elevate the risk of progression to more aggressive forms of lymphoma.

Historical literature has reported a significantly elevated risk of secondary cancers, ranging from hematological malignancies to solid tumors, in patients with LyP [13, 14]. However, these studies did not adequately adjust for confounding factors such as age, smoking habits, and other comorbidities. More recent analyses indicate that the risk of secondary malignancy in LyP is relatively low, with the notable exception of cutaneous lymphomas like MF and ALCL. Additionally, the risk of Hodgkin disease appears to be elevated in LyP patients who also have coexisting MF [15].

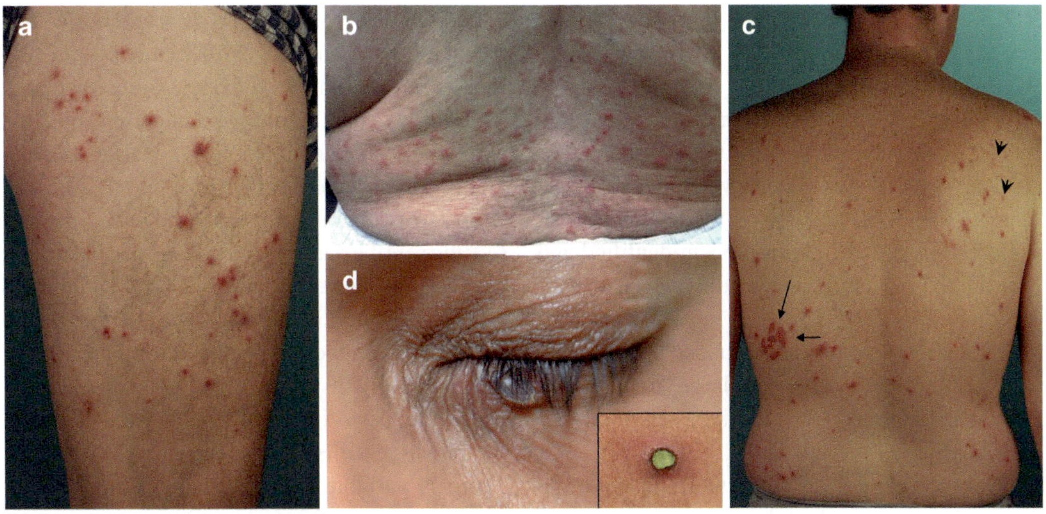

Fig. 9.1 Lymphomatoid papulosis (LyP). The classic presentation features widespread papules on the trunk and extremities (**a–c**). In some patients, the papules tend to ulcerate, as depicted in panel (**d**) with LyP involving the eyelids. Additionally, there is a heterogeneity of lesions, varying in size from relatively large, plaque-like elements (**c**, arrows) to very small, papular lesions (**c**, arrowheads)

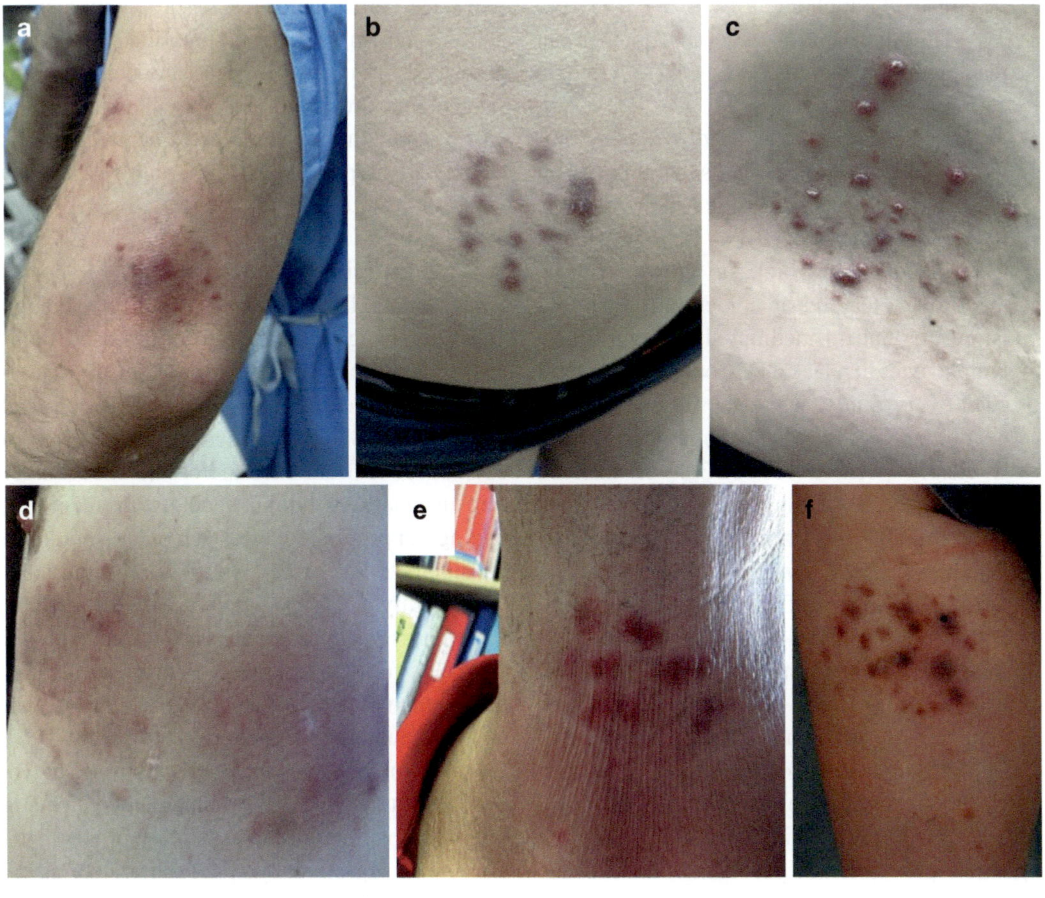

Fig. 9.2 Lymphomatoid papulosis (LyP) with agmination. Different clinical morphologies are shown in (**a-f**). Note the papules with a tendency to localize on a circumscribed, oval area of the skin. In some instances, the papules arise on areas of erythema, which, upon biopsy, may reveal epidermotropic atypical cells indistinguishable from mycosis fungoides (MF) (**a, d**)

9.1.3 Diagnostic Workup

9.1.3.1 Skin Biopsy

Histopathological examination of skin affected by LyP reveals an infiltrate in which most atypical large characteristic cells with Hodgkin-like features are CD30-positive. A few distinct histological subtypes of LyP have been identified and here are the most recognized subtypes [16–18]:

- Type A: Presents a wedge-shaped dermal infiltrate in which scattered large transformed lymphocytes are set in a mixed inflammatory background.
- Type B: Features an epidermotropic infiltrate that mimics the histological appearance of MF.
- Type C: Features a dermal infiltrate made of sheets of large, transformed lymphocytes, which closely resemble those seen in anaplastic large cell lymphoma.
- Type D: Represents an epidermotropic variant that predominantly displays $CD8^{+}$ cytotoxic cells.
- Type E: May be distinguished by its angioinvasive pattern, which explains that this variant often displays larger, necrotic lesions.
- LyP with DUSP22-IRF4 rearrangement: Characterized by a biphasic growth pattern, this subtype features an epidermotropic population of small to medium-sized cerebriform lymphocytes that lack CD30 or at most express CD30 very dimly, while the dermal component of larger atypical cells, often periadnexal is clearly positive for CD30. Of interest, DUSP22-IRF4 rearrangements are also seen in about 20% of primary cutaneous ALC, which may share some morphological features with this type of LyP.

Rare LyP will predominantly involve hair follicles, giving rise to the so-called folliculotropic or follicular variant, with its aforementioned typical clinical manifestation [19], and other rare cases show granulomatous histology. Other rare variants include the spindle cell LyP and the syringotropic variant LyP, which attacks the sweat ducts [18].

Among these subtypes, type A and C are most frequently encountered. While patients with type E tend to present with larger, more distinctly necrotic lesions, the overall clinical presentation and prognosis remain largely consistent across all histopathological subtypes.

In terms of immunophenotype and genotype, LyP mirrors the pattern seen in pcALCL. Typically, LyP cells are generally positive for CD4, though $CD8^{+}$ cells predominate in type D and E and occasionally in the DUSP22 variant. The atypical cells generally display cytotoxic markers (TIA-1, granzyme, perforin) and CD30. However, in type B, the large cells may be negative for CD30. There is variable loss of T-cell marker expression, including CD2, CD3, CD5, and most commonly CD7. A small subset of LyP is positive for CD56, estimated at 10% of cases and the large atypical cells may have some expression of CD15 in a subset of cases. Most cases are positive for T-cell receptor (TCR)-βF1, with a small subset showing TCRδ expression (especially described in type D). TCR monoclonal rearrangements are seen in a variable number of cases, depending on the type of sample and the density of atypical cells. Importantly, EBER is negative, as a rule.

9.1.3.2 Imaging and Staging

LyP is generally considered a clinically benign entity, thus negating the need for extensive diagnostic workup beyond dermatological assessment. Nonetheless, a comprehensive clinical examination should always be conducted to exclude concurrent MF and/or the exceedingly rare instances of lymph node involvement [2], and age-appropriate cancer screening should be considered to rule out any malignant comorbidity.

In cases where palpable lymphadenopathy is detected, further evaluation is warranted. This should include appropriate imaging studies, such as ultrasound or computed tomography (CT) scans, followed by a lymph node biopsy to ascertain the nature of the nodal enlargement. This is critical for ruling out the possibility of a concurrent, more aggressive lymphoproliferative disorder or for identifying the exceptional instances where LyP may have involved the lymph nodes [20–22].

9.1.4 Clinicopathological Correlations and Differential Diagnoses

The diagnosis of LyP is primarily established through a combination of histopathological examination of skin biopsies and the observation of characteristic clinical manifestations.

Given the morphological diversity of the histopathological subtypes of LyP and the general lack of specificity of CD30 expression (which is commonly expressed as an indicator of cell activation in reactive lymphoid populations), the differential diagnosis is accordingly broad. However, a few general statements can be made.

Type A LyP may be confused with Hodgkin lymphoma, but the expression of PAX5 (B-cell marker) is never seen in LyP.

Type B may be confused with mycosis fungoides, and clinical data confirming plaques and patches favor MF over LyP. When MF presents with papules instead of patches, they do not wax and wane as the typical LyP will do.

The differentiation of LyP type C and pcALCL should rely on clinical features. Unlike pcALCL, which often presents as a single, ulcerated tumor or plaque, LyP lesions are generally smaller (less than 1–2 cm), multiple, and undergo the characteristic cyclical evolution mentioned earlier. However, a minority of pcALCL may spontaneously regress. Also, multiple nodules rather than a single lesion are noted at presentation in about 20% of cases.

Type D LyP has already been alluded to in Chap. 8, and its $CD8^+$ epidermotropic infiltrate makes it a simulator of primary cutaneous aggressive epidermotropic $CD8^+$ T-cell lymphoma. The typical cyclical clinical presentation of LyP and its diffuse expression of CD30 are the two salient features enabling the paramount distinction to be made from aggressive lymphoma.

Type E LyP, with its angiocentricity, may simulate extranodal NK/T cell lymphoma, which is not uncommonly positive for CD30. The expression of EBER, almost universal in the latter and never seen in LyP, is a major distinguishing trait, along with the frequent expression of CD56 in NK/T cell lesions, rather unusual in LyP.

LyP with δF1 expression. Although rare cases of LyP may express the TCRδ (δF1), especially type D, and hence be mistaken for primary cutaneous γδ T-cell lymphoma, which is also negative for EBER, the latter lesion is only rarely positive for CD30 and commonly expresses CD56, in contradistinction to LyP. The clinical presentation, once again, will be a crucial clue to the right diagnosis. The reader is referred to Chap. 8 for more details.

LyP with DUSP22-IRF4 rearrangement is characterized by a biphasic growth pattern with an infiltrate of larger atypical often periadnexal strongly $CD30^+$ cells often contrasting with intraepidermal smaller cells, often dim or negative for CD30, hence raising the differential diagnosis of transformed mycosis fungoides. The clinical history pointing to preexisting MF-type patches and plaque is an important differential feature,

Folliculotropic LyP, with its clinical tendency to present with folliculitis or pustular lesions caused by the $CD30^+$ cells infiltrating around and within hair follicles, with secondary accumulation of mucin (mucinosis), intrafollicular neutrophils and/or eosinophils may easily be misdiagnosed clinically, and detection of the $CD30^+$ culprits is necessary to reach the right diagnosis. Granulomatous LyP, although rare, generates a differential diagnosis looking at inflammatory conditions, especially with cutaneous lupus erythematosus. More details are available below in this chapter.

It is important to remember that many neoplastic disorders, lymphoid and non-lymphoid, which commonly or only rarely involve the skin, may express CD30 in a subset of the neoplastic cell population. One can mention, in no specific order, pagetoid reticulosis, transformed MF, cutaneous aggressive T/NK-cell lymphomas, cutaneous follicle center lymphoma, systemic ALCL, classical Hodgkin lymphoma, adult T-cell leukemia/lymphoma, EBV-associated lymphoproliferation (B and T), follicular lymphoma and diffuse large B-cell lymphoma, mastocytosis, and related lesions, embryonal and nasopharyngeal carcinomas and angiosarcoma.

As mentioned before, a range of inflammatory or infectious conditions may also present with increased numbers of atypical CD30+ cells, further complicating the diagnostic landscape. In such scenarios, it is essential to note that inflammatory lymphocytes in benign conditions should exhibit a normal T-cell marker profile with no loss of T-cell antigen expression, no excess of CD56+ cells, scattered, non-clustered expression of CD30, no excess of cytotoxic marker expression within the larger CD30+ cells, and no molecular evidence of T-cell clonality, in general. Please see Table 9.1.

9.1.5 Therapy

The treatment approach for LyP is generally contingent upon the patient's symptoms and the extent of the disease manifestation. Given its benign course, some patients with a limited number of lesions may not require active intervention and can be followed through observation alone.

Topical corticosteroids, particularly those of medium to high potency, are often employed, especially when lesions exhibit pruritus. However, the therapeutic efficacy of corticosteroids varies among patients, and success in mitigating symptoms is not guaranteed.

Table 9.1 Inflammatory and infectious diseases which may mimic LyP [18, 23–26]

Infections
Nodular scabies
Molluscum contagiosum
Mycobacterial infections
Herpes simplex
Leishmaniasis
Syphilis
Inflammatory diseases
Pityriasis lichenoides and varioliformis acuta (PLEVA)
Atopic dermatitis
CD30+ intravascular lymphoproliferative disease (associated with skin trauma or inflammatory diseases)
Arthropod bite reaction
Pseudolymphomatous reaction to tattoo
Lymphoid cutaneous drug reactions (Chap. 11)

For patients presenting with more extensive disease, systemic therapy is typically considered. Low-dose methotrexate, administered at dosages of 15–25 mg weekly, is beneficial for a majority of these patients. In clinical experience, a partial response is seen in over 60% of individuals subjected to methotrexate therapy.

Phototherapy, involving narrow-band ultraviolet B (NB-UVB) or psoralen plus ultraviolet A (PUVA), has been explored as another treatment modality. However, available evidence suggests it is likely less effective than methotrexate for this condition. While phototherapy may reduce the number of active lesions, it does not appear effective in preventing disease relapses [27].

9.2 Primary Cutaneous CD30+ Anaplastic Large Cell Lymphoma (pcALCL)

9.2.1 Practice Essentials

- pcALCL is an indolent CD30+ lymphoma grouped with LyP in the family of primary cutaneous CD30+ lymphoproliferative diseases.
- The clinical picture is most commonly that of a solitary, rapidly growing ulcerated tumor.
- Dissemination to lymph nodes occurs in a small proportion of patients.
- Radiotherapy is the treatment of choice.

9.2.2 Clinical Presentation

The classic clinical manifestation of pcALCL often involves a swiftly enlarging, solitary, ulcerated tumor or a thick plaque (Fig. 9.3). This dominant lesion is frequently surrounded by smaller nodules or papular satellite formations.

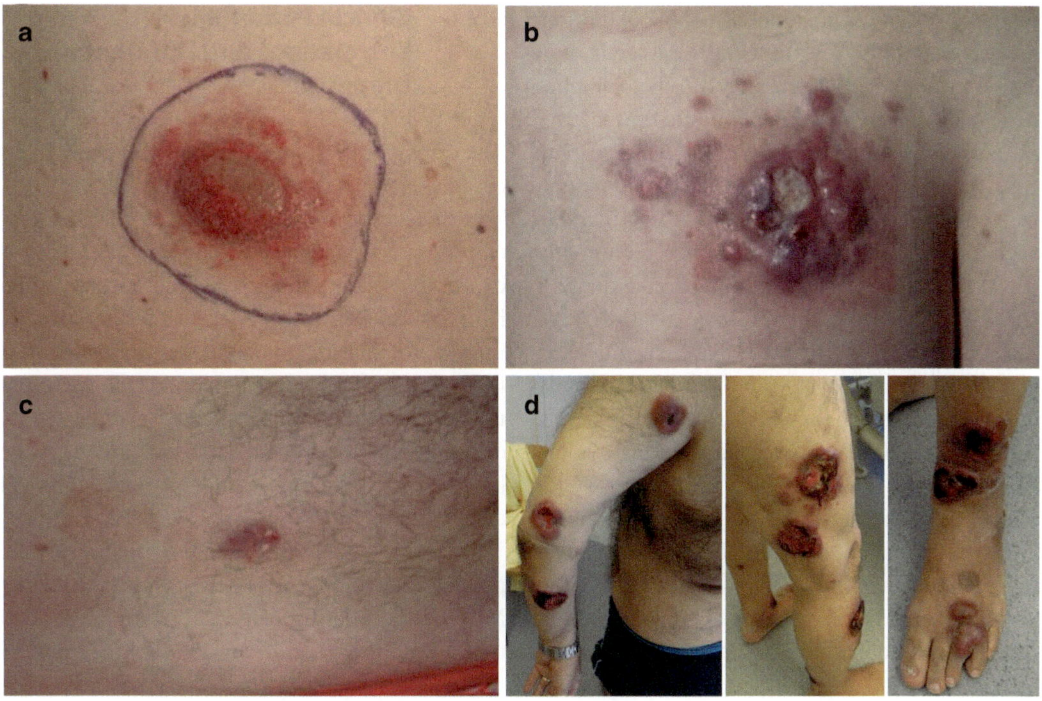

Fig. 9.3 Primary cutaneous CD30⁺ anaplastic large cell lymphoma (pcALCL). Solitary, rapidly growing, ulcerating tumors on the trunk (**a, b**). In some cases, the lesions are smaller and have a less aggressive appearance (**c**). Rarely, the patient may develop multiple, aggressive-looking tumors, which occasionally may metastasize to the lymph nodes, necessitating systemic chemotherapy (**d**, photos kindly provided by Dr. Tamra Osmanevic, Sweden)

Multifocal development of pcALCL is less common but can be particularly observed in patients who also have LyP. Overall, about 20% of patients with pALCL will demonstrate disease in two or more cutaneous sites.

Despite its alarming clinical appearance, pcALCL is generally an indolent malignancy, characterized by a tendency for spontaneous regression. In approximately one-third of cases, lesions have been observed to spontaneously disappear following traumatic events such as biopsy procedures. Remarkably, the 5-year survival rate for pcALCL surpasses 90% [27].

It is important to note that post-treatment relapses of the tumor may occur, either at the original site or at different cutaneous locations. However, these recurrent cutaneous manifestations do not seem to adversely affect the overall prognosis [2, 27].

A smaller subset of patients, constituting fewer than 5%, may experience lymph node involvement. When this occurs, the prognosis tends to be less favorable compared to cases restricted to cutaneous involvement alone [28]. Therefore, while pcALCL is generally characterized by a benign course, vigilance is required in managing and monitoring patients, particularly those showing signs of nodal involvement.

9.2.3 Diagnostic Workup and Staging

9.2.3.1 Skin Biopsy

The histopathological examination of skin biopsy samples from pcALCL lesions reveals a dense dermal infiltrate composed of pleomorphic, atypical large lymphoid cells. Pseudoepitheliomatous hyperplasia of the overlying epidermis has been typically observed in some cases. By definition, greater than 75% of these atypical cells will express CD30. The expression of other lymphocytic markers is more variable. While the majority of cases will be positive for $CD4^{+}/CD8^{-}$, some cases are $CD8^{+}/CD4^{-}$, $CD4^{+}/CD8^{+}$, or dual-negative cases ($CD4^{-}$ $CD8^{-}$). Pan-T-cell markers such as CD3, CD2, CD5, and most commonly CD7 may be lost. Anaplastic lymphoma kinase-1 (ALK-1) is absent in almost all cases. 40–50% of cases express CD15, CD25, cytotoxic markers, and CD45. EMA is typically negative, or only dimly focally positive, which is unlike systemic forms of ALCL. TCR rearrangement assays are abnormal in up to 90% of cases [29]. While TCRγ monoclonal rearrangement is commonly detected, TCRβ is frequently absent. This absence may reflect the lineage of ALCL, which is believed to originate from a more primitive lymphoid precursor compared to mature T-cell cutaneous lymphomas [9]. About 20% of pcALCL demonstrate rearrangement of the DUSP22-IRF4 gene at 6p25.3 [30], which may be associated with a specific epidermotropic histology, reminiscent of LyP cases that harbor the same underlying translocation. However, this marker is not associated with a significant clinical impact on outcome and hence is not useful in routine clinical practice.

9.2.3.2 Imaging and Staging

To exclude the possibility of cutaneous metastases from systemic ALCL and to identify uncommon cases of pcALCL with lymph node involvement, positron emission tomography-computed tomography (PET/CT) or comparable imaging modalities are recommended [27].

9.2.3.3 Additional Diagnostic Measures

While complete blood count and blood chemistry tests, including lactate dehydrogenase levels, are routinely conducted, their diagnostic utility in cases of skin-only disease is minimal. Bone marrow biopsies are generally not indicated unless there is clinical or imaging evidence suggesting systemic involvement. A lymph node biopsy is recommended in instances where abnormal lymph nodes are detected either clinically or through imaging.

9.2.4 Clinical Pathological Correlations and Differential Diagnoses

The primary differential diagnosis for pcALCL is cutaneous metastases from nodal ALCL.

Almost all cases of pcALCL are characteristically ALK-1 negative; hence, when it is expressed, an underlying systemic disease should be excluded. However, ALK-1 may be negative in systemic disease, and skin metastases from an underlying ALK–negative nodal ALCL are often indistinguishable from pcALCL, and therefore, differentiation between the two can only be made based on imaging studies and clinical correlation.

A further diagnostic challenge arises when pcALCL develops in patients with preexisting MF. Differentiating pcALCL from large cell transformation (LCT) of MF is of practical importance, as the former does not adversely impact the prognosis of MF, whereas the latter does [31, 32]. Both conditions may arise from the same cellular clone, rendering TCR rearrangement studies ineffective for differential diagnosis. Presently, there are no tests uniformly recognized as reliable that can be used to differentiate transformed MF from pcALCL. Therefore, the final diagnosis relies heavily on meticulous clinicopathological correlation [31, 32].

9.2.5 Therapy

pcALCL is sensitive to ionizing radiation and orthovolt or kilovolt radiotherapy produces complete remission in most cases. The doses of 30–40 Gy have been reported, but equally good results were obtained with lower doses of 16–20 Gy [27, 33]. Surgical excision of the tumor is a good option for unilesional disease. Patients with multiple cutaneous lesions or with pcALCL with LyP respond well to low-dose methotrexate (20–30 mg s.c. weekly).

For patients with extracutaneous disease, radiotherapy is suitable if just one regional lymph node is involved [28]. Anthracyclin-based chemotherapy (e.g., CHOP) and brentuximab vedotin also produced good outcomes for patients with lymph node involvement or extensive cutaneous disease [28, 34].

9.3 Primary Cutaneous Subcutaneous Panniculitis-Like T-Cell Lymphoma (pcSPTCL)

9.3.1 Practice Essentials

- pcSPTCL is an indolent lymphoma presenting as an infiltrate in the subcutaneous fat.
- There is an association with autoimmune diseases, especially lupus erythematosus.
- pcSPTCL may be difficult to distinguish from aggressive lymphomas presenting with panniculitic lesions, e.g., primary cutaneous γδT-cell lymphoma or cutaneous T-cell lymphoma, NOS.

9.3.2 Clinical Presentation

pcSPTCL is a mature, cytotoxic T-cell lymphoma developing in the subcutaneous fat [35]. Clinically, this lymphoma manifests as panniculitis, presenting as deep, palpable nodules, tumors, or areas of discoid induration. In the early phases of the disease, the overlying skin often appears erythematous and raised due to a concurrent inflammatory response. These lesions are frequently tender or painful upon palpation. However, as the disease progresses, the erythema tends to recede, and the skin surface may appear sunken or atrophic due to fat destruction from the neoplastic process.

Systemic symptoms such as low-grade fever, weight loss, or fatigue are commonly reported. It has been suggested that in certain cases, these systemic symptoms may be triggered by excessive production of interferon by the lymphoma cells [36]. The lesions can be multifocal and may appear in disparate regions of the body.

The incidence of pcSPTCL is twice as common in females as in males, and the median age of presentation is around 40 years. However, the age range is quite broad, extending from pediatric cases to the elderly population.

Generally, pcSPTCL follows an indolent course with an excellent prognosis. The reported 5-year survival rate exceeds 80%. Mortality is largely attributed to rare complications such as hemophagocytic lymphohistiocytosis (HLH) and is probably due to misdiagnoses of the aggressive cutaneous T-cell lymphomas as the clinically benign pcSPTCL.

Interestingly, approximately 25% of patients with pcSPTCL have a coexisting autoimmune disease, most frequently lupus erythematosus or inflammatory arthritis [37, 38]. This co-occurrence may explain some of the systemic symptoms as well as abnormal findings in blood tests, such as anemia, mild leukopenia, and elevated liver enzyme levels (Fig. 9.4).

9.3.3 Diagnostic Workup

9.3.3.1 Skin Biopsy

Standard punch biopsies often prove inadequate for diagnosing pcSPTCL, as they usually do not procure sufficient subcutaneous fat for accurate assessment. Therefore, deep incisional biopsies are the preferred method. An alternative approach is the "punch-in-punch" technique, wherein an initial biopsy is taken with a larger punch—typically 6 mm in diameter—followed by a deeper biopsy executed through the base of the first biopsy using a smaller, 4 mm punch to sample down to fat. In cases where patients present with multiple lesions, core needle biopsies can be employed.

Histological examination typically reveals an atypical lymphoid infiltrate predominantly affecting the subcutaneous fat, often in a pattern that mimics lobular panniculitis. This infiltrate may also extend into the deep dermis on occasion. A hallmark feature of pcSPTCL is the rimming of individual adipocytes by the neoplastic T cells.

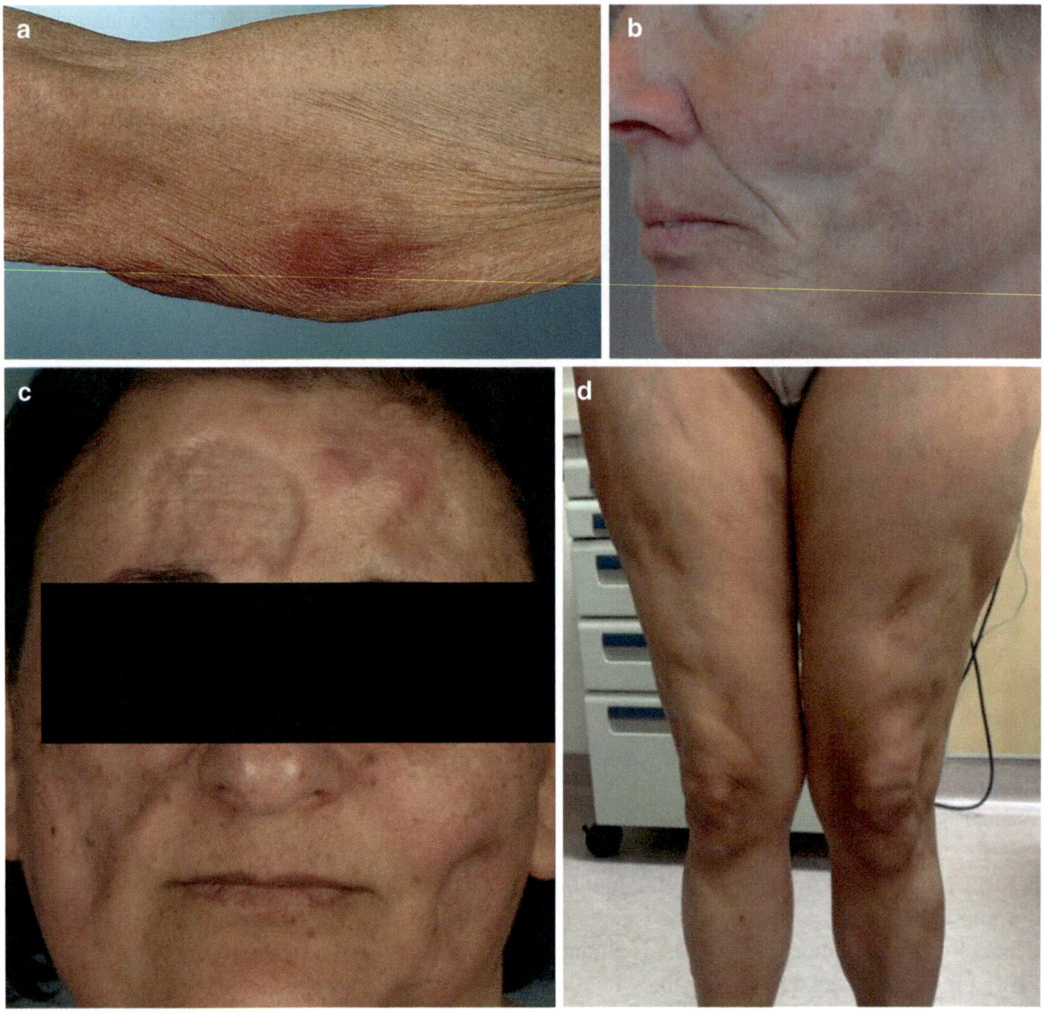

Fig. 9.4 Primary cutaneous subcutaneous panniculitis-like T-cell lymphoma (pcSPTCL). (**a**) Subcutaneous, painful nodule on the upper arm. Infiltration and destruction of the fat tissue often lead to areas of lipoatrophy, presenting as depressed areas of the skin, particularly in the face and the extremities (**b–d**)

The immunophenotypic profile generally aligns with that of a mature, cytotoxic T-cell, demonstrating positivity for CD3, CD8, and cytotoxic markers (TIA-1, granzyme, perforin), while typically being negative for CD4, CD30, CD56, and EBER. TCR (βF1) should be expressed, and its absence indicates an aggressive lymphoma. Loss of CD5 and/or CD7 is frequently observed, suggesting the abnormal nature of the infiltrating T cells.

The proliferation marker Ki-67 is focally positive, and its expression is particularly accentuated in the atypical cells rimming the adipocytes [39]. Plasmacytoid dendritic cells ($CD123^+$) and plasma cells are relatively scarce in the infiltrate, which is a differentiating feature from panniculitis of lupus erythematosus [40].

As expected for the mature T-cell neoplasm, TCRγ/TCRβ shows monoclonal rearrangement in most cases.

9.3.3.2 Autoimmune Markers

In spite of the well-documented coexistence of autoimmunity (lupus, rheumatoid arthritis) and pcSPTCL, data on serological markers in pcSPTCL patients are missing. In our experience, about 50% of patients will test positive for antinuclear antibodies, which usually comprise SSA/SSB antibodies. Specific lupus antibodies (anti-Smith, anti-dsDNA) are probably quite rare. All our lesional biopsies were negative in the direct immunofluorescence test.

9.3.4 Clinicopathological Correlations and Differential Diagnoses (Table 9.2)

9.3.4.1 Panniculitic Lupus Erythematosus Versus pcSPTCL

Differentiating between pcSPTCL and panniculitic lupus erythematosus is often challenging and may not always be straightforward. These two conditions could represent different stages of a continuum that initiates as immune-mediated panniculitis and culminates in neoplasm. In some cases, features of both conditions are evident in the same patient.

Testing for lupus antibodies is rarely useful in distinguishing between these two entities. This is because approximately half of patients with panniculitic lupus test negative for antinuclear antibodies (ANA) [41], and ANA positivity is common among healthy women. The presence of mucin, clusters of CD123$^+$ cells, abundant plasma cells, and granular components along with IgM deposits in blood vessels is more suggestive of lupus panniculitis [40, 42]. On the other hand, focally elevated levels of Ki-67 in atypical lymphocytes (often with "rimming" of the atypical adipocytes) lean toward a diagnosis of pcSPTCL [39]. In certain instances, the response to hydroxychloroquine can serve as a final diagnostic arbiter, as it is generally effective in treating lupus panniculitis but less so for pcSPTCL.

9.3.4.2 Panniculitic γδT-Cell Lymphoma Versus pcSPTCL

Panniculitic γδT-cell lymphoma (γδTCL) often manifests as panniculitis and was previously considered a subtype of pcSPTCL. However, it has been recognized that panniculitic γδTCL is markedly more aggressive and carries a much poorer prognosis compared to pcSPTCL. Therefore, accurate differentiation between these two conditions is paramount for appropriate prognostication and management. Panniculitis γδTCL often presents with ulcer-

Table 9.2 Histopathological differential diagnoses for pcSPTCL

	pcSPTCL	Primary cutaneous γδ T-cell lymphoma (panniculitic type pcGDTCL)	Panniculitis in lupus erythematosus	NK/T-cell lymphoma
Marked involvement of dermis	–	Variable	– (unless associated with lupus tumidus)	Variable
Clues	Adipocyte rimming	Adipocyte rimming	Clusters of dendritic cells, no adipocyte rimming, plasma cells may be abundant	Necrosis and angiocentric pattern, adipocyte rimming may be seen
Extracutaneous involvement	–	+	–	+
Ki67	Focal high	High (focal or diffuse)	Low to medium	High (>50%)
CD123	Few	Few	Clusters of CD123$^+$ cells	Few
TCRβ rearrangement	Usually present	May be present, generally negative	May be present, generally negative	Variable (commonly TCR germline)
βF1 IHC	+	Generally negative	+	Variable, majority negative
TCRδ IHC	–	+	+/– (minority of cells)	Variable, majority negative
CD56/EBER	–/EBER$^-$	Variable/EBER$^-$	Variable/EBER$^-$	Usually EBER$^+$

ated lesions, systemic symptoms, lymphadenopathy, anemia, and leukopenia. Additionally, HLH is more commonly associated with this type, occurring in up to 50% of cases [35].

Besides clinical features, immunohistochemical profiles overlap theand βF1 and δF1 staining is essential for accurate differential diagnosis (see Chap. 8).

9.3.4.3 Panniculitic NK/T-Cell Lymphoma

This lymphoma also presents with a clinical picture similar to that of panniculitic γδTCL. A critical distinguishing feature between these two aggressive, cytotoxic lymphomas is the positive staining for EBER, CD30, and CD56 in NK/T--cell lymphomas.

9.3.5 Imaging and Staging

Full staging (PET-CT or comparable imaging, bloodwork, lymph node biopsy from palpable lymph nodes) should be performed to rule out aggressive cytotoxic lymphoma masquerading as pcSPTCL. Moreover, panniculitic lesions avidly uptake [^{18}F]FDG, which helps to assess disease activity.

HLH should be ruled out in patients with systemic symptoms using an established diagnostic approach (cell blood count for cytopenias, liver panel, blood levels of ferritin, soluble IL-2 receptor, fibrinogen, and triglycerides, bone marrow biopsy) [43].

9.3.6 Therapy

Systemic corticosteroids are generally effective in treating pcSPTCL, as corroborated by several clinical studies [44]. While prospective studies are lacking, the common practice involves initiating treatment with medium doses, approximately 0.5 mg/kg of prednisone, until remission is achieved. The dose is then tapered to a maintenance dose ranging from 2.5 to 5 mg daily. The duration of treatment varies depending on the patient's response, typically 6 months to 2 years. In our experience, the addition of methotrexate 20–25 mg weekly s.c. helps to shorten the time to steroid discontinuation. However, methotrexate in monotherapy is rarely efficient.

For those patients whose clinical or histopathological findings overlap with lupus panniculitis, a trial of hydroxychloroquine, dosed at 200–400 mg daily, is often effective and exhibits minimal toxicity.

In instances of corticosteroid resistance, histone deacetylase (HDAC) inhibitors such as vorinostat and romidepsin have proven to be successful treatment alternatives [45, 46]. Cyclosporine has been used with success [47, 48]; however, we would advise caution given the often catastrophic effect of cyclosporine in other cutaneous lymphomas (Chap. 7).

9.4 Primary Cutaneous Small-Medium CD4$^+$ Lymphoproliferative Disease (pcCD4-LPD)

9.4.1 Practice Essentials

- pcCD4-LPD is a common, clinically benign, monoclonal lymphoproliferation of mature CD4$^+$ cells.
- The clinical manifestation is a solitary non-ulcerated nodule or plaque localized on the head, neck, upper trunk, and upper arms.
- The tumor may regress spontaneously after biopsy.
- Therapeutic options are watchful waiting, surgical excision, or radiotherapy.

pcCD4-LPD is characterized as a benign yet monoclonal proliferation of mature CD4$^+$ lymphocytes primarily localized to the dermis. Importantly, the term "lymphoproliferative disease" has supplanted the earlier nomenclature of "lymphoma" in the current WHO classification. This semantic shift reflects the evolving understanding of the disease's benign nature, specifically its absence of both local and systemic dissemination.

Despite the atypical appearance of the cells, the clinical course of pcCD4-LPD is more consistent with a benign tumor than with an aggressive lymphoma. Misdiagnosis can sometimes occur, leading to confusion with more aggressive forms of cutaneous lymphomas or even B-cell lymphomas. Such misinterpretations can subsequently result in overly aggressive therapeutic approaches, which are not only unnecessary but could also be potentially harmful.

9.4.2 Clinical Presentation

Small-medium pleomorphic lymphoproliferative disease, also known as pcCD4-LPD, typically manifests as a solitary, red or purple nodule or tumor. The peak incidence is observed in middle-aged adults, affecting both men and women. These lesions are characterized by a smooth, non-scaly surface and are generally devoid of any ulcerative tendencies. Most commonly, the nodules present as dome-shaped and symmetric, predominantly localized to the upper regions of the body, including the head, neck, torso, and upper arms [49, 50] (Fig. 9.5).

Interestingly, approximately one-third of pcCD4-LPD cases exhibit spontaneous regression, a phenomenon often observed following a diagnostic biopsy [51]. This self-limiting nature, combined with its relatively high incidence, arguably makes pcCD4-LPD one of the most common entities that has previously been classified under cutaneous T-cell "lymphomas," albeit it is now more accurately termed a lymphoproliferative disease.

9.4.3 Diagnostic Workup

The diagnosis of pcCD4-LPD is principally made through histopathological examination, as the clinical appearance of the lesions can be nondescript. A skin biopsy generally discloses a dermal infiltrate comprising small to medium-sized pleomorphic T cells, with fewer than 30% of large cells. While epidermotropism is generally absent, mild epidermotropism can occasionally occur and does not negate the diagnosis [52].

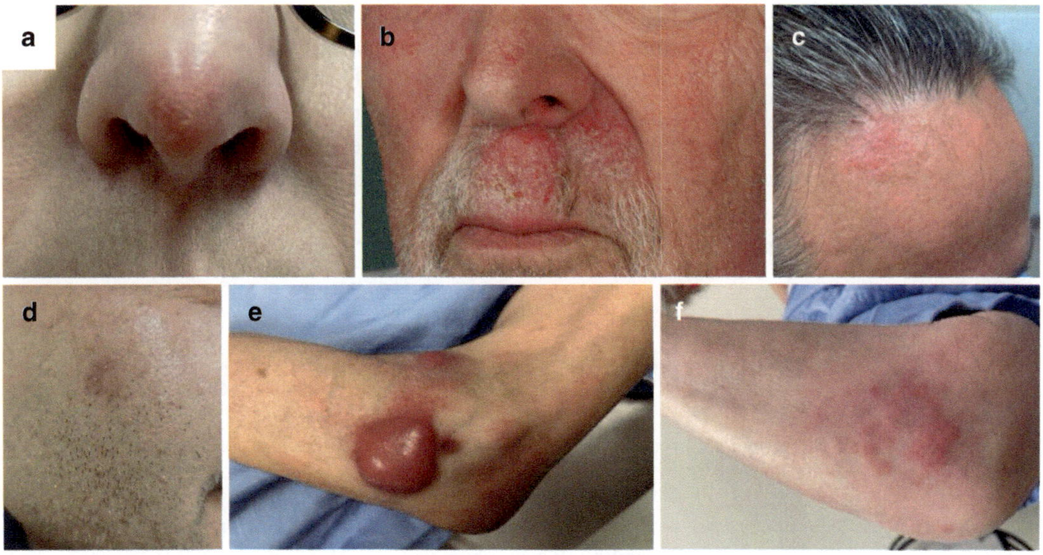

Fig. 9.5 Clinical spectrum of pcCD4-LPD. The lesions are most commonly located on the face (**a–d**) as nondescript papules (**a**), nodules (**b**), or plaques (**c, d**). The lesions are typically singular and do not exhibit a tendency to recur after removal. Additionally, we have encountered patients with larger, sometimes agminated lesions on the extremities that displayed histopathological features of pcCD4-LPD but recurred after surgical treatment, requiring radiotherapy for eradication (**e, f**). Whether these lesions can be classified as pcCD4-LPD or represent a separate clinical subtype remains to be determined

The immunophenotype typically reveals a mixture of predominant $CD4^+$ lymphocytes, with a minority reactive lymphoid population including $CD8^+$ T cells, histiocytes, plasma cells, and B cells. The $CD4^+$ cells have normal expression profiles of CD2, CD3, and CD5 with occasional loss of CD7. Follicular helper T-cell (T_{FH}) markers like programmed cell death protein 1 (CD279/PD-1), CD10, ICOS, BCL6, and CXCL13, are expressed, with the typical observation of clusters of lymphocytes, strongly positive for PD1. TCR gene rearrangements are usually monoclonal for both TCRβ and TCRγ. It is noteworthy that the neoplastic CD4 cells may functionally act like TFH cells, promoting B-cell proliferation and differentiation into plasma cells. Consequently, a subset of pcCD4-LPD cases may exhibit a prominent B-cell infiltrate, which can occasionally overshadow the neoplastic T cells, thereby mimicking primary cutaneous marginal zone B-cell lymphoma (pcMZL) [49, 52].

For patients presenting with a typical clinical picture and phenotype, which includes a solitary lesion localized in the upper regions of the body and a corroborative skin biopsy showing no loss of CD2, CD3, or CD5, and persistence of background reactive $CD8^+$ T cells, B cells, etc. Additional imaging and staging are generally not required, given the disease's benign clinical trajectory. However, a small percentage of patients may present with atypical clinical features, such as multiple lesions, localization below the waist, or on the distal extremities, or pathological features that overlap with pcMZL/LPD or even peripheral T-cell lymphoma with T_{FH} marker expression. In these instances, basic staging procedures could be considered to rule out underlying systemic leukemia or lymphoma. All patients should have a complete cutaneous and lymph node examination to ensure no other features of cutaneous lymphoma.

9.4.4 Clinicopathological Correlations and Differential Diagnoses

Primary cutaneous marginal zone lymphoma is the most common differential diagnosis, and clinical and pathological features may overlap largely in some patients. Table 9.3 summarizes the differentiating features between pcMZL and pcCD4-LPD. Although the presence of TCR or IgH monoclonality heavily suggests respectively pcCD4-LPD or pcMZL, there are cases of dual monoclonal TCR and IgG rearrangement [53].

Although T_{FH} phenotype is usual for pcCD4-LPD, patients who present with multifocal lesions composed of T cells with T_{FH} features may call for the differential diagnosis with systemic, nodal T-follicular helper cell lymphomas secondarily involving the skin. There are also descriptions of cases classified as "primary cutaneous peripheral T-cell lymphomas with a T-follicular helper phenotype" which present with multiple lesions and may have an aggressive course [54, 55]. Those patients should be staged and followed closely since a subset demonstrated

Table 9.3 Differential diagnosis of pcCD4-LPD

	pcCD4-LPD	pcMZL	Primary cutaneous peripheral T-cell lymphomas with a T-follicular helper phenotype
Lesions	Solitary, non-recurrent lesions	Solitary or multiple lesions, often recurrent course	Multiple lesions, often ulcerated
Localization	Upper body	Upper body	Multifocal, often lower extremities
Clinical course	Benign, lesions may regress spontaneously, no recurrence	Benign, chronic, recurrent	More aggressive, B-symptoms, systemic involvement
Reactive follicles in skin biopsy	−/+	+	−
PD-1	+ (rosettes of PD-1+ cells)	+	+
TCR monoclonality	+	−/+	+
IgH monoclonality	−/+	+	n/a

+ usually found, −/+ exceptional finding, n/a no information available a more aggressive course with systemic dissemination.

9.4.5 Therapy

Given the relatively nondescript presentation of pcCD4-LPD as a solitary pink nodule, most lesions are surgically excised in their entirety for diagnostic confirmation. Following excision, lesions do not generally recur, making additional therapy unnecessary, even if the excision is not complete.

In instances where the lesion does not regress post-biopsy, radiotherapy serves as a suitable alternative treatment option. Moreover, for smaller nodules and papules, topical or intralesional steroids have been observed to induce regression of the lesion, providing a less invasive treatment approach [49, 56].

9.5 Primary Cutaneous Acral CD8+ T-Cell Lymphoproliferative Disease (pcCD8-LPD)

9.5.1 Practice Essentials

- pcCD8-LPD is a clinically benign, monoclonal lymphoproliferation of mature CD8+ cells.
- The clinical manifestation is a solitary nodule or plaque, localized on the ears, nose, hands, or feet.
- Therapeutic options are surgical excision or radiotherapy.

9.5.2 Clinical Presentation

The initial description of this benign entity was a nodule on the ear, which histopathologically comprised a non-epidermotropic CD8+ lymphocytic infiltrate [57]. Subsequent reports described this entity as solitary pink papules or small nodules preferentially localized on the ears, the tip of the nose, or the acral skin of the hands and feet [58]. The patients are typically middle-aged males (>50 years of age). Lesions may be tender, growing slowly, and only rarely may achieve sizes exceeding 1 cm. Unlike the pcCD4-LPD, pcCD8-LPD may recur after treatment or reoccur in a different area of the skin [59] (Fig. 9.6).

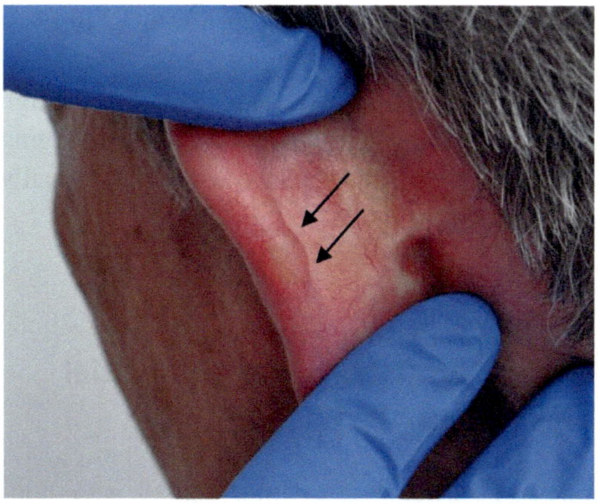

Fig. 9.6 A nondescript nodule on the ear representing primary cutaneous acral CD8+ T-cell lymphoproliferative disease (pcCD8-LPD)

9.5.3 Diagnostic Workup

Histopathological examination reveals a dense dermal infiltrate of intermediate-size slightly irregular lymphoid cells, often separated from the epidermis by a Grenz zone and sparing the dermal adnexa. They may occasionally extend into subcutaneous fat or show minor epidermotropism or Pautrier microabscess, and there is no necrosis [60]. They have an open chromatin with small nucleoli. Immunohistochemical staining typically demonstrates expression of CD3, CD8, TIA-1, and TCR-βF1, with a characteristic dot-like ("Golgi") expression pattern of CD68. Loss of CD2, CD5, and/or CD7 expression is commonly observed. Negative markers include CD56, CD30, and Epstein-Barr virus-encoded small RNA (EBER). The proliferation index in these lesions is generally low, but some cases with moderate proliferation have been reported. Rare cases express granzyme B. Clonal TCRγ and TCRβ rearrangements are detected in most cases [59].

Given the localized and clinically benign nature of pcCD8-LPD, no additional imaging studies or staging procedures are typically required.

9.5.4 Clinicopathological Correlations and Differential Diagnoses

The co-occurrence of a solitary, small, acral nodule and a dermal CD3+ CD8+ lymphocytic infiltrate is generally diagnostic for pcCD8-LPD. However, this rare and lesser-known condition is sometimes misdiagnosed as other types of CD8+ cutaneous lymphomas, necessitating a keen understanding of differential diagnoses (refer to Table 9.4 for summary).

Unilesional CD8+ MF may initially present in acral locations, resembling pcCD8-LPD that manifests as solitary plaques on the feet. Unlike CD4+ MF, this form may include some degree of epidermotropism. Pagetoid reticulosis typically localized to the feet, lacks the distinctive dermal infiltrate found in pcCD8-LPD. Meanwhile, CD8+ aggressive epidermotropic cutaneous T-cell lymphoma (pcCD8-AECTCL) characteristically presents with multiple lesions, more pronounced epidermotropism, and usually exhibits granzyme B expression with a higher proliferation rate. pcCD8-LPD can be further differentiated from CD8+ LyP by its lack of CD30 expression.

Patients with immunodeficiencies, both congenital and acquired, may develop cutaneous CD8 lymphoproliferations that present as multiple violaceous papules or nodules primarily localized to the extremities. These cases are Epstein-Barr virus (EBV)-negative, display a chronic and recurrent course, and may escalate into systemic lymphomas involving lymph nodes. In HIV-infected individuals, antiretroviral ther-

Table 9.4 Main differential diagnosis of CD8-LPD

	pcCD8-LPD	pcCD8-AECTCL	CD8+ MF	Immunosuppression-related CD8 lymphoproliferation	CD8+ PTL-NOS
Lesions	Pink papules, small nodules that do not ulcerate	Ulcerative and necrotic patches and plaques	Scaly patches and plaques	Multiple nodules and plaques	Large nodules, tumors, occasionally with ulceration. Solitary or multiple
Distribution	Ears, tip of the nose, hands, and feet	Widespread, often mucosa, palms, soles	Sun-protected areas of the lower trunk and upper legs, occasionally primary lesions on the feet	Mostly extremities, but can develop in any location	Any skin region, often the head and neck
Course	Slow growth, sometimes recurrent	Rapidly progressive	Chronic, slow progression	Chronic, progressive, resistant to therapy	Progressive, systemic involvement
Pathology	Dermal lymphocytic infiltrate with atypia and occasional blast-like cells, CD3+ CD8+ TIA-1+, CD68+, low or moderate proliferation rate. Occasional epidermotropism	Dense dermal and epidermal infiltrate, CD3+ CD8+ CD7+, cytotoxic markers, high proliferation rate	Superficial infiltrate with variable epidermotropism, CD3+ CD8+ CD7−, low proliferation rate	Granzyme B+ and TIA-1+, numerous histiocytes, otherwise like CD8-LPD	Granzyme B+ and TIA-1+, high proliferation rate, otherwise like CD8-LPD

apy often leads to the disappearance of such lesions [59].

Other differential diagnoses include skin-only peripheral T-cell lymphoma (PTL-NOS), which may manifest as a $CD8^+$ phenotype but with larger and more rapidly growing lesions. Furthermore, EBV-related lymphoproliferative disorders may present with a $CD8^+$ infiltrate, but these are usually seen in pediatric populations, feature a distinct clinical presentation, and are EBER positive, unlike pcCD8-LPD.

9.5.5 Therapy

Excision of the lesion is often curative; however, recurrences may occur in approximately 20% of patients. Radiotherapy has been used with success, but intralesional and topical corticosteroids seem to be less effective.

9.6 Hydroa Vacciniforme-Like Lymphoproliferative Disorder (HV-LPD)

9.6.1 Practice Essentials

- HV-LPD is an extremely rare form of EBV-related lymphoproliferative disease in children in Latin America and Asia.
- Clinical manifestations are distinctive: papules with vesicles on the face and sun-exposed areas that produce vacciniform (pox-like) scars.
- Histopathologically, it presents with T-cell-like phenotype or NK-like phenotype.
- HV-LPD may progress to systemic lymphoma.

9.6.2 Clinical Presentation

Hydroa vacciniforme-like lymphoproliferative disorder (HV-LPD) is an exceedingly rare cutaneous lymphoproliferative condition predominantly affecting children, with a median age of diagnosis at 8 years. Most prevalent in Latin America and Asia, this disorder is characterized by a chronic active EBV infection that primarily manifests on sun-exposed areas, such as the face.

Initially, patients develop necrotic, vesicular papules that resemble chickenpox lesions. These lesions often lead to ulcerations and produce pox-like scarring on the face [61, 62]. Over time, the condition may progress, presenting with facial edema and further ulcerations. Importantly, the disease has a protracted yet progressive course, eventually culminating in systemic lymphoma for 10 to 15 years. Accompanying symptoms may include systemic "B-symptoms" such as fever, night sweats, and weight loss, as well as lymphadenopathy, hepatosplenomegaly, and bone marrow infiltration.

HV-LPD is sometimes associated with mosquito bite allergies. When present, this association generally portends a more aggressive course and heightens the risk of developing hemophagocytic syndrome, a potentially life-threatening condition characterized by a hyperinflammatory response.

9.6.3 Diagnostic Workup

The definitive diagnosis of HV-LPD is primarily histopathological, often necessitating a skin biopsy. The biopsy specimen usually exhibits a lymphocytic infiltrate predominantly comprising $CD3^+$ $TIA1^+$ cells. These may express either a T-cell phenotype ($CD8^+$ $CD4^-$, or $CD4^+$ $CD8^-$) or NK/T-cell markers ($CD56^+$ $CD4^-$ $CD8^-$). While TCR rearrangement shows variable results, it is more frequently monoclonal in specimens demonstrating a T-cell histological type. The key diagnostic hallmark is the presence of EBER, which are identified via in situ hybridization.

Due to the progressive nature of HV-LPD and its potential to evolve into systemic lymphoma, comprehensive staging should be conducted. This typically involves imaging studies, including PET-CT scans, lymph node biopsies for those with palpable lymphadenopathy, and bone marrow examinations. Furthermore, a thorough hematologic workup, including a complete blood count and evaluation of lactate dehydrogenase levels, may be recommended. Moreover, patients should be monitored meticulously for potential disease progression and complications such as hemophagocytic syndrome.

9.6.4 Clinicopathological Correlations and Differential Diagnoses

The rarity of HV-LPD necessitates high clinical acumen for its diagnosis. Typical clinical presentations, such as pox-like facial scarring and facial edema, especially in children from Asian or Latin American backgrounds, often initiate the diagnostic process. A skin biopsy confirming an EBV-positive lymphoproliferative disorder is pivotal for diagnosis.

In the medical literature, it has been proposed that late-stage HV-LPD should be categorized as systemic EBV^{+} NK/T-cell lymphoma. This distinction underscores the importance of a comprehensive evaluation, as the disease may demonstrate different characteristics depending on its stage.

In terms of differential diagnosis, early-stage HV-LPD must be differentiated from other conditions with similar clinical manifestations. These include various photodermatoses such as polymorphic light eruption, actinic prurigo, and pellagra, as well as DNA repair deficiencies like xeroderma pigmentosum. Lupus erythematosus and porphyrias (erythropoietic protoporphyria) are additional conditions that may mimic the clinical features of HV-LPD.

The T-cell histological subtype of HV-LPD, in particular, presents its own set of diagnostic challenges. It needs to be carefully differentiated from other cutaneous lymphoproliferative diseases that can affect the face and result in skin scarring, such as LyP and folliculotropic MF.

9.6.5 Therapy

The therapeutic results are poor. Intensive sun protection may occasionally lead to the regression of skin lesions [62]. Allogeneic hematopoietic bone marrow transplant has produced satisfactory outcomes.

9.7 Benign CD30^{+} Intravascular Lymphoproliferative Disease (pcCD30-IVLPD)

9.7.1 Practice Essentials

- pcCD30-IVLPD is a clinically benign condition defined histopathologically as an accumulation of CD30^{+} lymphocytes inside cutaneous lymphatic vessels.
- pcCD30-IVLPD is a rare, accidental, histopathological finding in skin biopsies from inflammatory skin disease, sites of ulceration, or trauma.
- It mimics histopathologically intravascular lymphomas, from which it can be differentiated based on careful clinicopathological correlation.

The benign atypical intravascular CD30^{+} T-cell proliferation is not included in the current WHO classification (5th edition) of T-cell lymphomas [63]. Although for consistency with other clinically benign conditions we use the term "lymphoproliferative disease" it is not clear whether it is a true proliferation or an accumulation of reactive CD30^{+} cells accompanying different inflammatory skin diseases [22, 64]. pcCD30-IVLPD is probably not related to the family of CD30^{+} lymphoproliferative diseases (i.e., LyP and primary cutaneous anaplastic large cell lymphoma).

9.7.2 Clinical Presentation

pcCD30-IVLPD is fairly age-neutral and gender-neutral. It has been reported in both male and female patients, with ages ranging from 17 to 69 years. pcCD30-IVLPD is most often an incidental histopathological discovery rather than a clinically evident disorder. It has been identified in skin biopsies obtained for other reasons, such as in the context of inflammatory skin conditions like lichen sclerosus, or following trauma, as seen in cases involving pyogenic granulomas. The disease does not demonstrate a predilection for any specific anatomical region of the body.

9.7.3 Diagnosis and Clinicopathological Correlations

The biopsy specimen in cases of pcCD30-IVLPD reveals ectatic lymphatic vessels in the superficial dermis that are filled with medium- to large-sized lymphoid blasts. Notably, these vessels do not display signs of wall destruction. These blastic lymphocytes can also be observed in the adjacent tissue, where they coexist with various other cells such as histiocytes, plasma cells, and eosinophils. Immunohistochemical studies show that these large lymphocytes express not only CD30 but also common T-cell markers including CD2, CD3, CD4, and CD5. Occasionally, there may be a loss of CD7 expression. Anaplastic lymphoma kinase 1 (ALK-1), epithelial membrane antigen (EMA), CD56, CD20, CD79a, and EBER are negative. The TCR rearrangement pattern is characteristically polyclonal.

The main differential diagnoses for pcCD30-IVLPD are intravascular lymphomas and LyP type E [65]. Intravascular lymphomas are categorically different in that they are generally large B-cell or NK/T-cell lymphomas. Unlike pcCD30-IVLPD, they do not express the same array of T-cell or B-cell markers. Clinically, intravascular lymphomas present with more severe features, including painful panniculitic lesions, livedo racemosa, and skin necrosis with ulcerations.

LyP type E, on the other hand, exhibits atypical $CD30^{+}$ cells that are usually situated in the dermis but may occasionally invade the vessel wall, mimicking pcCD30-IVLPD. However, type E lesions are distinct from pcCD30-IVLPD in several key aspects. Specifically, they exhibit greater tissue necrosis, destruction of vessel walls, and microhemorrhages [22, 64].

9.7.4 Therapy

The lesions are usually biopsied or excised for diagnostic purposes, and no further therapy is necessary.

References

1. Willemze R, Cerroni L, Kempf W, et al. The 2018 update of the WHO-EORTC classification for primary cutaneous lymphomas. Blood. 2019;133(16):1703–14. Blood. 2019;134:1112.
2. Bekkenk MW, Geelen FA, van Voorst Vader PC, Heule F, Geerts ML, van Vloten WA, et al. Primary and secondary cutaneous CD30(+) lymphoproliferative disorders: a report from the Dutch Cutaneous Lymphoma Group on the long-term follow-up data of 219 patients and guidelines for diagnosis and treatment. Blood. 2000;95:3653–61.
3. Wagner G, Rose C, Klapper W, Sachse MM. Lymphomatoid papulosis. J Dtsch Dermatol Ges. 2020;18:199–205.
4. Kempf W, Kazakov DV, Schärer L, Rütten A, Mentzel T, Paredes BE, et al. Angioinvasive lymphomatoid papulosis: a new variant simulating aggressive lymphomas. Am J Surg Pathol. 2013;37:1–13.
5. de la Garza Bravo MM, Patel KP, Loghavi S, Curry JL, Torres Cabala CA, Cason RC, et al. Shared clonality in distinctive lesions of lymphomatoid papulosis and mycosis fungoides occurring in the same patients suggests a common origin. Hum Pathol. 2015;46:558–69.
6. Chott A, Vonderheid EC, Olbricht S, Miao NN, Balk SP, Kadin ME. The dominant T cell clone is present in multiple regressing skin lesions and associated T cell lymphomas of patients with lymphomatoid papulosis. J Invest Dermatol. 1996;106:696–700.
7. Gniadecki R, Lukowsky A, Rossen K, Madsen HO, Thomsen K, Wulf HC. Bone marrow precursor of extranodal T-cell lymphoma. Blood. 2003;102:3797–9.
8. Davis TH, Morton CC, Miller-Cassman R, Balk SP, Kadin ME. Hodgkin's disease, lymphomatoid papulosis, and cutaneous T-cell lymphoma derived from a common T-cell clone. N Engl J Med. 1992;326:1115–22.
9. Iyer A, Hennessey DC, Gniadecki R. Clonotype pattern in T-cell lymphomas map the cell of origin to immature lymphoid precursors. Blood Adv. 2022;6(7):2334–45.
10. Magro CM, Mo JH, Telang G. Localized lymphomatoid papulosis: unilesional lymphomatoid

papulosis, regional lymphomatoid papulosis, and persistent agmination of lymphomatoid papulosis. Clin Dermatol. 2022;40:622–38.
11. Karai LJ, Kadin ME, Hsi ED, Sluzevich JC, Ketterling RP, Knudson RA, et al. Chromosomal rearrangements of 6p25.3 define a new subtype of lymphomatoid papulosis. Am J Surg Pathol. 2013;37:1173–81.
12. Feldman AL, Oishi N, Ketterling RP, Ansell SM, Shi M, Dasari S. Immunohistochemical approach to genetic subtyping of anaplastic large cell lymphoma. Am J Surg Pathol. 2022;46:1490–9.
13. Cabanillas F, Armitage J, Pugh WC, Weisenburger D, Duvic M. Lymphomatoid papulosis: a T-cell dyscrasia with a propensity to transform into malignant lymphoma. Ann Intern Med. 1995;122:210–7.
14. Christensen HK, Thomsen K, Vejlsgaard GL. Lymphomatoid papulosis: a follow-up study of 41 patients. Semin Dermatol. 1994;13:197–201.
15. Kaul S, Belzberg M, Hughes J-DM, Mahadevan V, Khanna R, Bakhshi PR, et al. Comorbidities in mycosis fungoides and racial differences in co-existent lymphomatoid papulosis: a cross-sectional study of 580 patients in an Urban Tertiary Care Center. Medicines (Basel). 2019;7:1.
16. Quintanilla-Martinez L, Swerdlow SH, Tousseyn T, Barrionuevo C, Nakamura S, Jaffe ES. New concepts in EBV-associated B, T, and NK cell lymphoproliferative disorders. Virchows Arch. 2023;482:227–44.
17. Kempf W, Kerl K, Mitteldorf C. Cutaneous CD30-positive T-cell lymphoproliferative disorders-clinical and histopathologic features, differential diagnosis, and treatment. Semin Cutan Med Surg. 2018;37:24–9.
18. Kempf W. A new era for cutaneous CD30-positive T-cell lymphoproliferative disorders. Semin Diagn Pathol. 2017;34:22–35.
19. Kempf W, Kazakov DV, Baumgartner H-P, Kutzner H. Follicular lymphomatoid papulosis revisited: a study of 11 cases, with new histopathological findings. J Am Acad Dermatol. 2013;68:809–16.
20. Xerri L, Adélaïde J, Avenin M, Guille A, Taix S, Bonnet N, et al. Common origin of sequential cutaneous CD30+ lymphoproliferations with nodal involvement evidenced by genome-wide clonal evolution. Histopathology. 2019;74:654–62.
21. Ferrara G, Ena L, Cota C, Cerroni L. Intralymphatic spread is a common finding in cutaneous CD30+ lymphoproliferative disorders. Am J Surg Pathol. 2015;39:1511–7.
22. Samols MA, Su A, Ra S, Cappel MA, Louissant A Jr, Knudson RA, et al. Intralymphatic cutaneous anaplastic large cell lymphoma/lymphomatoid papulosis: expanding the spectrum of CD30-positive lymphoproliferative disorders. Am J Surg Pathol. 2014;38:1203–11.
23. Martinez-Escala ME, Sidiropoulos M, Deonizio J, Gerami P, Kadin ME, Guitart J. γδ T-cell-rich variants of pityriasis lichenoides and lymphomatoid papulosis: benign cutaneous disorders to be distinguished from aggressive cutaneous γδ T-cell lymphomas. Br J Dermatol. 2015;172:372–9.
24. Werner B, Massone C, Kerl H, Cerroni L. Large CD30-positive cells in benign, atypical lymphoid infiltrates of the skin. J Cutan Pathol. 2008;35:1100–7.
25. Kempf W. CD30+ lymphoproliferative disorders: histopathology, differential diagnosis, new variants, and simulators. J Cutan Pathol. 2006;33(Suppl 1):58–70.
26. Kempf W, Kazakov DV, Palmedo G, Fraitag S, Schaerer L, Kutzner H. Pityriasis lichenoides et varioliformis acuta with numerous CD30(+) cells: a variant mimicking lymphomatoid papulosis and other cutaneous lymphomas. A clinicopathologic, immunohistochemical, and molecular biological study of 13 cases. Am J Surg Pathol. 2012;36:1021–9.
27. Kempf W, Pfaltz K, Vermeer MH, Cozzio A, Ortiz-Romero PL, Bagot M, et al. EORTC, ISCL, and USCLC consensus recommendations for the treatment of primary cutaneous CD30-positive lymphoproliferative disorders: lymphomatoid papulosis and primary cutaneous anaplastic large-cell lymphoma. Blood. 2011;118:4024–35.
28. Melchers RC, Willemze R, Vermaat JSP, Jansen PM, Daniëls LA, Putter H, et al. Outcomes of rare patients with a primary cutaneous CD30+ lymphoproliferative disorder developing extracutaneous disease. Blood. 2020;135:769–73.
29. Ortiz-Hidalgo C, Pina-Oviedo S. Primary cutaneous anaplastic large cell lymphoma—a review of clinical, morphological, immunohistochemical, and molecular features. Cancers. 2023;15:4098.
30. Wada DA, Law ME, Hsi ED, Dicaudo DJ, Ma L, Lim MS, et al. Specificity of IRF4 translocations for primary cutaneous anaplastic large cell lymphoma: a multicenter study of 204 skin biopsies. Mod Pathol. 2011;24:596–605.
31. Fauconneau A, Pham-Ledard A, Cappellen D, Frison E, Prochazkova-Carlotti M, Parrens M, et al. Assessment of diagnostic criteria between primary cutaneous anaplastic large-cell lymphoma and CD30-rich transformed mycosis fungoides; a study of 66 cases. Br J Dermatol. 2015;172:1547–54.
32. Gao C, McCormack CJ, van der Weyden C, Twigger R, Buelens O, Lade S, et al. The importance of differentiating between mycosis fungoides with CD30-positive large cell transformation and mycosis fungoides with coexistent primary cutaneous anaplastic large cell lymphoma. J Am Acad Dermatol. 2021;84:185–7.
33. Jepsen ME, Gniadecki R. Treatment of primary cutaneous anaplastic large cell lymphoma with superficial x-rays. Dermatol Rep. 2015;7:5888.
34. Horwitz SM, Scarisbrick JJ, Dummer R, Whittaker S, Duvic M, Kim YH, et al. Randomized phase 3 ALCANZA study of brentuximab vedotin vs physician's choice in cutaneous T-cell lymphoma: final data. Blood Adv. 2021;5:5098–106.
35. Willemze R, Jansen PM, Cerroni L, Berti E, Santucci M, Assaf C, et al. Subcutaneous panniculitis-like T-cell lymphoma: definition, classification, and prognostic factors: an EORTC Cutaneous Lymphoma Group Study of 83 cases. Blood. 2008;111:838–45.

36. Burg G, Dummer R, Wilhelm M, Nestle F, Ott MM, Feller A, et al. A subcutaneous delta-positive T-cell lymphoma that produces interferon gamma. N Engl J Med. 1991;325:1078–81.
37. Magro CM, Kalomeris T, Dillard A. Autoimmune disease, including lupus panniculitis in association with panniculitic cell lymphomas. Clin Dermatol. 2023;41:680–91.
38. Pincus LB, LeBoit PE, McCalmont TH, Ricci R, Buzio C, Fox LP, et al. Subcutaneous panniculitis-like T-cell lymphoma with overlapping clinicopathologic features of lupus erythematosus: coexistence of 2 entities? Am J Dermatopathol. 2009;31:520–6.
39. Sitthinamsuwan P, Pattanaprichakul P, Treetipsatit J, Pongpruttipan T, Sukpanichnant S, Pincus LB, et al. Subcutaneous panniculitis-like T-cell lymphoma versus lupus erythematosus panniculitis: distinction by means of the periadipocytic cell proliferation index. Am J Dermatopathol. 2018;40:567–74.
40. Chen SJT, Tse JY, Harms PW, Hristov AC, Chan MP. Utility of CD123 immunohistochemistry in differentiating lupus erythematosus from cutaneous T cell lymphoma. Histopathology. 2019;74:908–16.
41. Ng PP-L, Tan SH, Tan T. Lupus erythematosus panniculitis: a clinicopathologic study. Int J Dermatol. 2002;41:488–90.
42. Arai S, Katsuoka K. Clinical entity of Lupus erythematosus panniculitis/lupus erythematosus profundus. Autoimmun Rev. 2009;8:449–52.
43. George MR. Hemophagocytic lymphohistiocytosis: review of etiologies and management. J Blood Med. 2014;5:69–86.
44. Guenova E, Schanz S, Hoetzenecker W, DeSimone JA, Mehra T, Voykov B, et al. Systemic corticosteroids for subcutaneous panniculitis-like T-cell lymphoma. Br J Dermatol. 2014;171:891–4.
45. Gleason L, Joffe D, Bhatti S, Cohen A, Banner L, Correia E, et al. Recalcitrant subcutaneous panniculitis-like T-cell lymphoma responsive to histone deacetylase inhibitor. Case Rep Oncol. 2022;15:1088–94.
46. Jothishankar B, Espinosa ML, Zain J, Parekh V, Di Raimondo C, Abdulla F. Complete response to romidepsin as monotherapy in treatment-resistant subcutaneous panniculitis-like T-cell lymphoma. JAAD Case Rep. 2020;6:1245–7.
47. Rojnuckarin P, Nakorn TN, Assanasen T, Wannakrairot P, Intragumtornchai T. Cyclosporin in subcutaneous panniculitis-like T-cell lymphoma. Leuk Lymphoma. 2007;48:560–3.
48. Chen R, Liu L, Liang YM. Treatment relapsed subcutaneous panniculitis-like T-cell lymphoma together HPS by Cyclosporin A. Hematol Rep. 2010;2:e9.
49. Surmanowicz P, Doherty S, Sivanand A, Parvinnejad N, Deschenes J, Schneider M, et al. The clinical spectrum of primary cutaneous CD4+ small/medium-sized pleomorphic T-cell lymphoproliferative disorder: an updated systematic literature review and case series. Dermatology. 2021;237:618–28.
50. Williams VL, Torres-Cabala CA, Duvic M. Primary cutaneous small- to medium-sized CD4+ pleomorphic T-cell lymphoma: a retrospective case series and review of the provisional cutaneous lymphoma category. Am J Clin Dermatol. 2011;12:389–401.
51. Beltzung F, Ortonne N, Pelletier L, Beylot-Barry M, Ingen-Housz-Oro S, Franck F, et al. Primary cutaneous CD4+ small/medium T-cell lymphoproliferative disorders: a clinical, pathologic, and molecular study of 60 cases presenting with a single lesion: a multicenter study of the French Cutaneous Lymphoma Study Group. Am J Surg Pathol. 2020;44:862–72.
52. Alberti-Violetti S, Torres-Cabala CA, Talpur R, Corti L, Fanoni D, Venegoni L, et al. Clinicopathological and molecular study of primary cutaneous CD4+ small/medium-sized pleomorphic T-cell lymphoma. J Cutan Pathol. 2016;43:1121–30.
53. Obiorah IE, Karrs J, Brown L, Wang H-W, Karai LJ, Pham TH-T, et al. Overlapping features of primary cutaneous marginal zone lymphoproliferative disorder and primary cutaneous CD4 + small/medium T-cell lymphoproliferative disorder: a diagnostic challenge examined by genomic analysis. Am J Surg Pathol. 2023;47:344–53.
54. Wang L, Rocas D, Dalle S, Sako N, Pelletier L, Martin N, et al. Primary cutaneous peripheral T-cell lymphomas with a T-follicular helper phenotype: an integrative clinical, pathological and molecular case series study. Br J Dermatol. 2022;187:970–80.
55. Battistella M, Beylot-Barry M, Bachelez H, Rivet J, Vergier B, Bagot M. Primary cutaneous follicular helper T-cell lymphoma: a new subtype of cutaneous T-cell lymphoma reported in a series of 5 cases. Arch Dermatol. 2012;148:832–9.
56. Virmani P, Jawed S, Myskowski PL, Horwitz S, Skripnik Lucas A, Moskowitz A, et al. Long-term follow-up and management of small and medium-sized CD4 T cell lymphoma and CD8 lymphoid proliferations of acral sites: a multicenter experience. Int J Dermatol. 2016;55:1248–54.
57. Petrella T, Maubec E, Cornillet-Lefebvre P, Willemze R, Pluot M, Durlach A, et al. Indolent CD8-positive lymphoid proliferation of the ear: a distinct primary cutaneous T-cell lymphoma? Am J Surg Pathol. 2007;31:1887–92.
58. Greenblatt D, Ally M, Child F, Scarisbrick J, Whittaker S, Morris S, et al. Indolent CD8(+) lymphoid proliferation of acral sites: a clinicopathologic study of six patients with some atypical features. J Cutan Pathol. 2013;40:248–58.
59. Kempf W, Petrella T, Willemze R, Jansen P, Berti E, Santucci M, et al. Clinical, histopathological and prognostic features of primary cutaneous acral CD8 T-cell lymphoma and other dermal CD8 cutaneous lymphoproliferations: results of an EORTC Cutaneous Lymphoma Group workshop. Br J Dermatol. 2022;186:887–97.
60. Hathuc VM, Hristov AC, Smith LB. Primary cutaneous acral CD8 T-cell lymphoma. Arch Pathol Lab Med. 2017;141:1469–75.

61. Quintanilla-Martinez L, Ridaura C, Nagl F, Sáez-de-Ocariz M, Durán-McKinster C, Ruiz-Maldonado R, et al. Hydroa vacciniforme-like lymphoma: a chronic EBV+ lymphoproliferative disorder with risk to develop a systemic lymphoma. Blood. 2013;122:3101–10.
62. Cho K-H, Lee S-H, Kim C-W, Jeon Y-K, Kwon I-H, Cho Y-J, et al. Epstein-Barr virus-associated lymphoproliferative lesions presenting as a hydroa vacciniforme-like eruption: an analysis of six cases. Br J Dermatol. 2004;151:372–80.
63. Alaggio R, Amador C, Anagnostopoulos I, Attygalle AD, Araujo IBO, Berti E, et al. The 5th edition of the World Health Organization classification of haematolymphoid tumours: lymphoid neoplasms. Leukemia. 2022;36:1720–48.
64. Kempf W, Keller K, John H, Dommann-Scherrer C. Benign atypical intravascular CD30+ T-cell proliferation: a recently described reactive lymphoproliferative process and simulator of intravascular lymphoma: report of a case associated with lichen sclerosus and review of the literature. Am J Clin Pathol. 2014;142:694–9.
65. Baum CL, Stone MS, Liu V. Atypical intravascular CD30+ T-cell proliferation following trauma in a healthy 17-year-old male: first reported case of a potential diagnostic pitfall and literature review. J Cutan Pathol. 2009;36:350–4.

Primary Cutaneous B-Cell Lymphomas and Lymphoproliferative Disorders

10

Robert Gniadecki, Minakshi Taparia, Jean Deschenes, Jori Hardin, and Etienne Mahe

Primary cutaneous B-cell lymphomas constitute a significant subset, approximately 25%, of all primary skin lymphomas. They comprise four major clinicopathological entities: primary cutaneous marginal zone lymphoma, primary cutaneous follicle center lymphoma, primary cutaneous diffuse large B-cell lymphoma, leg type, and B-cell lymphomas and lymphoid proliferations associated with immune deficiency and dysregulation (Table 10.1).

Clinically, patients present with cutaneous plaques, nodules, or tumors, which may occur as isolated or clustered lesions. Contrary to other dermatological conditions, these lesions usually lack epidermal change in the form of surface scaling, and necrotic ulcerations are notably infrequent or minimally prominent. The coloration spans a spectrum from pink to purple. The predilection for anatomical regions is apparent, with the upper torso, arms, and head being the most commonly afflicted sites.

Regarding the disease course, most primary cutaneous B-cell lymphomas are low-grade malignancies, thereby displaying a proclivity for

R. Gniadecki (✉)
Division of Dermatology, University of Alberta, Edmonton, AB, Canada
e-mail: r.gniadecki@ualberta.ca

M. Taparia
Division of Hematology, University of Alberta Hospital, Edmonton, AB, Canada
e-mail: mtaparia@ualberta.ca

J. Deschenes
Department of Pathology and Laboratory Medicine, Cross Cancer Institute, Edmonton, AB, Canada
e-mail: Jean.Deschenes@albertaprecisionlabs.ca

J. Hardin
Division of Dermatology, University of Calgary, Calgary, AB, Canada
e-mail: Jori.hardin@albertahealthservices.ca

E. Mahe
Department of Pathology & Laboratory Medicine, and Hematology & Hematological Malignancies, University of Calgary, Calgary, AB, Canada
e-mail: etienne.mahe@albertaprecisionlabs.ca

Table 10.1 Classification of primary cutaneous B-cell lymphoproliferative diseases

pcMZL/LPD (primary cutaneous marginal zone lymphoma/lymphoproliferative disorder)[a]
Class switched (IgG > IgA > IgE, including IgG4)—60–70% of cases
Non-class switched (IgM)—30–40% of cases
pcFCL (primary cutaneous follicle center lymphoma)
pcFCL, diffuse large cell type
pcDLBCL-LT (primary cutaneous diffuse large B-cell lymphoma, leg type)
B-cell LLP-IDD (lymphomas and lymphoid proliferations associated with immune deficiency and dysregulation), including EBV+ mucocutaneous ulcer

[a]In this book, we have adopted the term pcMZL/LPD, i.e., primary cutaneous marginal zone lymphoma/lymphoproliferative disorder, rather than the more widespread pcMZL (marginal zone lymphoma) to highlight the clinically benign nature of this disease and histopathological overlap with other benign lymphoproliferative diseases, such as primary cutaneous small-medium CD4 lymphoproliferative disease

R. Gniadecki et al. (eds.), *Diseases of Blood and Skin*, https://doi.org/10.1007/978-3-031-65292-9_10

localized cutaneous involvement without frequent dissemination to lymph nodes or extracutaneous tissues. This contrasts with nodal B-cell lymphomas, which often follow a more aggressive trajectory. Nonetheless, there are distinct exceptions to this general rule, such as primary cutaneous diffuse large B-cell lymphoma, leg type (pcDLBCL-LT), which tends to exhibit a more aggressive course and could manifest with disseminated lesions. Similarly, expansive lesion distribution has been documented in cases of immunodeficiency-associated B-cell lymphomas and lymphoproliferative diseases (B-cell LLP-IDD) [1].

10.1 Primary Cutaneous Marginal Zone B-Cell Lymphoma/Lymphoproliferative Disease (pcMZL/LPD)[1]

10.1.1 Practice Essentials

- Non-ulcerating smooth, dome-shaped plaques and nodules with a predilection to the upper torso and upper arms, less commonly in the head and neck area.
- The prognosis is excellent, but pcMZL/LPD may have a chronic, recurrent course.
- Therapy: observation, radiotherapy, intralesional rituximab, surgical excision.

10.1.2 Clinical Manifestations and Disease Course

Primary cutaneous marginal zone lymphoma/lymphoproliferative disorder (pcMZL/LPD) predominantly affects young to middle-aged adults and exhibits a subtle male predominance. pcMZL/LPD was reported to have slightly lower incidence than the primary cutaneous follicular lymphoma (pcFCL) [2], however, in our center pcMZL/LPD is the most common primary cutaneous B-cell lymphoma, with a 2-fold higher incidence than pcFCL. Clinically, patients typically present with cutaneous manifestations characterized by pink, violaceous, or reddish-brown nodules and plaques (Fig. 10.1). These lesions are primarily localized to the head and neck region, upper torso, and arms. It's noteworthy that the lesions lack both ulceration and surface scaling. Lesions may regress spontaneously after the biopsy and a subset of patients with pcMZL/LPD may experience a gradual resolution of untreated lesions over years.

From a prognostic standpoint, pcMZL/LPD is associated with an excellent outcome, with a 5-year overall survival rate exceeding 95%. Nonetheless, a small subset of patients, accounting for less than 4% of all cases, may experience a more aggressive course of the disease, manifesting as lymph node involvement [3]. Given the generally favorable prognosis, clinicians must distinguish pcMZL/LPD from other forms of cutaneous lymphoma and nodal marginal zone lymphoma to avoid unnecessary aggressive treatments and to provide accurate prognostication.

10.1.3 Diagnosis and Staging

10.1.3.1 Skin Biopsy

There is a dense, bottom-heavy, nodular, or diffuse lymphocytic infiltrate in the dermis with a Grenz zone. The nodular structures may contain reactive germinal centers. The appearance of neoplastic B-cells varies from monocytoid and centrocyte to small cells resembling small-cell lymphoma. Plasma cells may be arranged in prominent clusters at the periphery of the main lesion (especially in class-switched patients).

The non-class switched pcMZL/LPD (IgM^+) shows more similarity to systemic extracutaneous marginal zone lymphoma and arises in the background of chronic inflammation of Th1 type. The malignant cells are more prominent, producing dense sheets or nodules in the dermis and often involve the subcutis. The plasma cells are arranged more diffusely in the neoplastic infil-

[1] In this book we have adopted the term pcMZL/LPD, i.e., primary cutaneous marginal zone lymphoma/lymphoproliferative disorder rather than the more widespread pcMZL (marginal zone lymphoma) to highlight the clinically benign nature of this disease and histopathological overlap with other benign lymphoproliferative diseases, such as promary cutaneous small-medium CD4 lymphoproliferative disease (pcCD4-LPD).

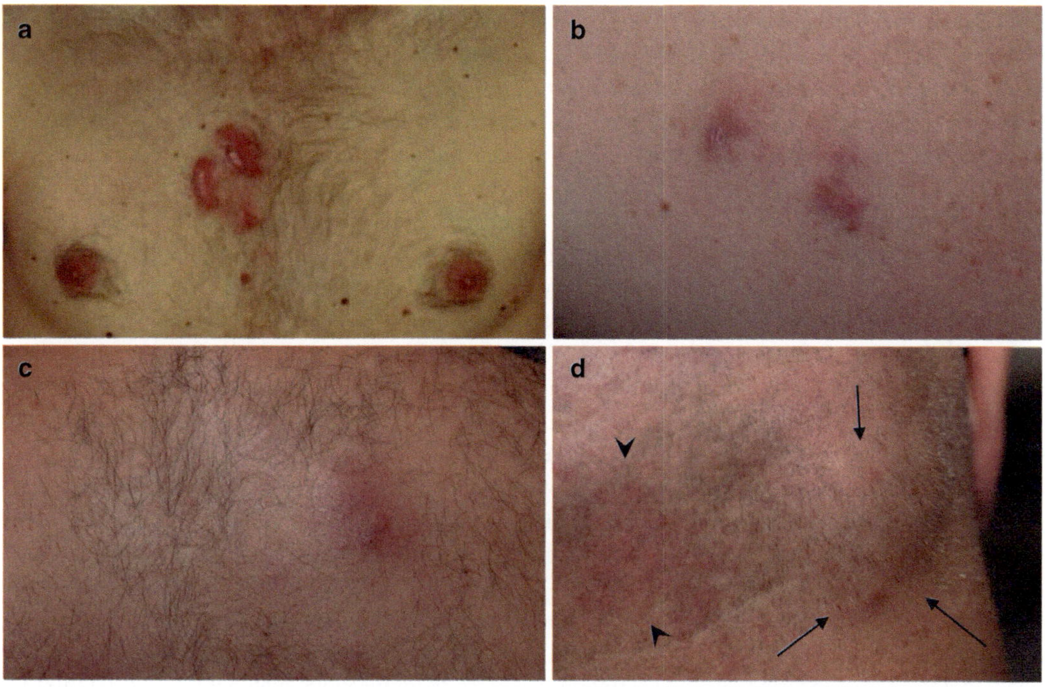

Fig. 10.1 Primary cutaneous marginal zone lymphoma. (**a**) Nodular, agminate lesions on the chest, (**b, c**) papules and patches on the upper trunk, (**d**) superficial lesions manifested as red patches (arrowheads) and deeper nodular lesions in the subcutis (arrows) on the scalp and neck

trate. The T-cells, which are less abundant in this subtype, are a more even mixture of CD4$^+$ and CD8$^+$ T-cells.

In the class-switched type, representing the majority of the cases, the disease arises in the setting of chronic Th2-type inflammation, and the malignant cells comprise only a subset of the infiltrate; they show variable distribution patterns, ranging from dense nodules to sparse perivascular infiltrate. The biopsy tends to be dominated by reactive T-cells (often T_{FH} phenotype, often mostly CD4$^+$, with fewer CD8$^+$ T-cells), reactive B-cells (occasionally forming germinal centers), and eosinophils. When determined by IHC, the heavy chains are of IgG or, less commonly, of IgA and rarely IgE subtypes.

Immunohistochemistry shows that the neoplastic cells express common B-cell markers (CD20, CD79a, PAX5) and Bcl-2 but not Bcl-6 or CD10 (except in reactive germinal centers). This profile differentiates pcMZL/LPD from follicular lymphoma (pcFCL). There is often κ or λ restriction in plasma cells. CD5 and cyclin D1 are negative. Ki67 stains proliferating cells at the periphery of the germinal centers. The isotype of class-switched pcMZL/LPD is often IgG4 (representing about 35% of all pcMZL/LPD cases). Immunoglobulin heavy chain rearrangement is monoclonal.

10.1.3.2 Other Investigations

Serology for *Borrelia burgdorferi* should be considered in areas where *Borrelia* is found. There is a link between *B. burgdorferi* infection and marginal zone lymphoma and appropriate antibiotic treatment may lead to the resolution of the disease [4–6].

Complete blood cell count with differential and a comprehensive blood chemistry measurement are recommended, although they rarely contribute to important findings. In selected patients (e.g., plasma cell-rich infiltrates), serum electrophoresis can be considered to exclude a monoclonal gammopathy.

10.1.3.3 Bone Marrow Biopsy

In one study [7, 8] 2/82 patients with pcMZL/LPD showed bone marrow involvement. However, those results were not confirmed, and bone marrow biopsy was not indicated [7, 9].

10.1.3.4 Imaging

Per consensus recommendations, adequate imaging is required to confirm the disease is primarily a skin-based neoplasm. It should include a contrast-enhanced computed tomography (CT) scan, with or without positron emission tomography (PET), or a whole-body integrated PET/CT. At a minimum, imaging should focus on the chest, abdomen, and pelvis. Additionally, for cases involving skin lesions in the head and neck area, imaging of the neck should also be performed [7].

Despite these recommendations, it is important to note that most pcMZL/LPD cases are confined to the skin, rendering extensive imaging often superfluous in the absence of other alarming signs. Such imaging is generally negative and does not influence therapeutic decisions [10].

10.1.4 Differential Diagnosis

As seen in Table 10.2, primary cutaneous marginal zone lymphoma/lymphoproliferative disorder (pcMZL/LPD) may overlap in clinical and histopathological features with other B-cell lymphomas, notably primary cutaneous follicle center lymphoma (pcFCL). Because of its polymorphous features and its diverse cell types, pcMZL/LPD should be distinguished from small medium pleomorphic $CD4^+$ lymphoproliferative disease. (see Table 10.3).

Indeed, class-switched pcMZL/LPD may display a histopathological presentation rich in T follicular helper (T_{FH}) cells, making it hardly distinguishable from CD4-LPD. While the presence of monoclonal T-cell receptor (TCR) in the absence of B-cell monoclonality is very helpful for differentiation, it should be noted that up to 35% of marginal zone lymphomas, both nodal and extranodal, may also exhibit monoclonal TCR [11–13] while a subset of pc$CD4^+$ LPD may lack TCR gene rearrangement [14, 15]. Finding a B-cell monoclonal population (either detected by IgH rearrangement or demonstrated by monotypic plasma cells), with no accompanying evidence of a clonal T-cell population (TCR rearrangements absent) will favor pcMZL/LPD over pcCD4-LPD, in the right pathological and clinical context, and the reverse is also true. One should nevertheless consider that B-cell clonal populations, especially monotypic plasma cells, may also occur in pcCD4-LPD, and they will generate conflicting interpretations if there is concurrent T-cell clonality by TCR rearrangement studies. In fact, overlap cases are increasingly detected and reported, highlighting the common immune dysregulation and exaggerated immune stimulation shared by these two apparently related but distinct lesions [14].

Primary cutaneous MZL/LPD is generally more polymorphous than pcFCL, with a mixture of B-cells, T-cells, and germinal centers, with scattered or clustered plasma cells. Bcl-6 and CD10 are usually negative in these LPDs (except in reactive germinal centers), further helping in the distinction with follicular lymphoma (pcFCL). There is often κ or λ restriction in plasma cells, which is rarely observed in pcFCL. Bcl2 is uniformly positive in pcMZL/LPD but often negative in pcFCL. Clinical features may also contribute to the differential diagnosis.

Another differential diagnosis to consider is cutaneous infiltration by chronic lymphocytic leukemia/small lymphocytic lymphoma (CLL/SLL). This can resemble pcMZL/LPD, particularly when the lymphoma presents with a predominance of small B-cells and lacks plasma cells. The typical phenotype of CLL/SLL ($CD5^+$, $CD23^+$, $CD20^{dim}$, $LEF1^+$) should make this distinction relatively easy in combination with appropriate clinical data.

pcMZL/LPD may mimic benign conditions such as benign B-cell predominant or mixed B/T-cell cutaneous lymphoid hyperplasia, pseudolymphomatous folliculitis, and tumid lupus erythematosus/Jessner lymphocytic infiltrate (Chap. 11).

Table 10.2 Comparison of key features of cutaneous B-cell lymphomas

Disease	Characteristic clinical features	Key IHC profile	Differential diagnosis
pcMZL/LPD	Young adults. Papules and plaques on the upper torso, arms, and head	CD20⁺ CD79a⁺, Bcl-2⁺, Bcl-6⁻, CD10⁻, fragmented CD21⁺ follicular dendritic cell networks, the majority (up to 75%) show an isotype switched phenotype (IgG, commonly IgG4, less commonly IgA, IgE), remaining non-switched isotype (IgM⁺)	IgG4-related disease Pseudolymphoma Metastatic MZL Plasma cell neoplasm or other low-grade B cell lymphoma (e.g., SLL/ CLL), pcFCL, pcCD4-LPD, the cutaneous spread of angioimmunoblastic T-cell lymphoma
pcFCL	Plaques or tumors on the head and neck, less commonly upper torso	CD20⁺, CD79a⁺, Bcl-6⁺, Bcl-2$^{-/\text{dim a}}$, CD10$^{-/+}$, MUM-1⁻, cIgM⁻, FOXP1⁻ Remnants of CD21+ FDC networks	Metastatic nodal FCL, pcDLBCL-LT, reactive follicular hyperplasia, pcMZL/LPD
pcDLBCL-LT	Plaques and tumors on lower legs in elderly women	CD20⁺, CD79a⁺, Bcl-2⁺⁺⁺, Bcl-6$^{+/-}$, CD10⁻, MUM-1⁺, c-Myc⁺, EBV⁻, cIgM⁺	Secondary skin involvement by nodal FCL, blastoid mantle cell lymphoma
		No remnants of CD21⁺ follicular dendritic cell networks	pcFCL with diffuse large cell features, any cutaneous LPD with aggressive features, EBV$^{+/-}$ (DLBCL, plasmablastic lymphoma, B-cell lymphoblastic lymphoma)
EBV⁺ mucocutaneous ulcer	Immunosuppressed or elderly patients. Sharply demarcated ulcer	EBV⁺ in large B cells, (CD20$^{+/-}$, PAX5 $^{+/\text{dim}}$, MUM1⁺, OCT2+, BOB1⁺, CD45$^{+/-}$, CD30⁺, CD15$^{+/-}$)	Herpes simplex ulcers. Classic Hodgkin lymphoma, EBV⁺ diffuse large B cell lymphoma, pcALCL, lymphomatoid granulomatosis, IDD-associated EBV⁺ B-cell LPD
IDD-associated B-cell lymphomas and lymphoid proliferations (varying from polymorphous LPD to EBV$^{+/-}$DLBCL)	Papules, nodules or ulcerated plaques in immunosuppressed patients	Generally EBV⁺, variable IHC depending on polymorphous or monomorphic character and cell make-up	Immunodeficiency associated CD8⁺ T-cell lymphoproliferative disease, histiocytoses. EBV⁺ mucocutaneous ulcer, pcDLBCL-LT
B-cell pseudolymphoma	Pink nodules or plaques, often in the face or upper trunk	CD20⁺ CD79a⁺, admixed T-cells, intact CD21⁺ follicular dendritic cell networks and germinal centers, polytypic plasma cells	pcMZL/LPD, pcFCL, follicular hyperplasia

[a]Most cases are negative for t(14;18), CD10 expression and Bcl-2, but a minority are positive (see Table 10.6)

Table 10.3 Key points in differential diagnosis

	Clinical features	Phenotypic profile and key histopathological features
pcMZL/LPD	One or several papules, nodules or plaques: upper torso, less commonly head and neck. Recurrent	Bcl-2$^+$, Bcl-6$^-$, CD10$^-$ commonly isotype switched phenotype (IgG, often IgG4), remaining IgM$^+$, commonly monoclonal plasma cells, polyclonal TCR rearrangement, monoclonal IgH rearrangement
pcFCL	Nodules or plaques: head and neck, upper torso	Bcl-2$^{-/+}$/Bcl-6$^+$ CD10$^{-/+}$ MUM1/c-Myc-
pcDLBCL-LT	Tumors, legs, progressive	High mitotic and proliferative activity, Bcl-2+ Bcl-6$^{+/-}$ MUM-1/c-Myc$^+$
CD4-LPD (B-cell rich)	Single nodule or papule: head and neck, upper torso	No κ/λ restriction, polyclonal IgH rearrangement, monoclonal TCR, rarely monoclonal plasma cells

In benign pseudolymphomas, one generally encounters well-formed, reactive germinal centers, a well-demarcated network of CD21$^+$ follicular dendritic cells, and proliferating cells confined to these germinal centers. In contrast, pcMZL/LPD, besides often showing monotypic plasma cells or having molecularly confirmed monoclonal B-cell population, typically shows disrupted and disorganized networks of follicular dendritic cells.

10.1.4.1 pcMZL/LPD, Plasma-Cell Rich

A subset of pcMZL/LPD may have numerous admixed or even a dominant component of plasma cells (plasmacytic or lymphoplasmacytic subtypes). Those plasma cells may express IgG4, which may raise the possibility of IgG4-related skin disease [16]. Although immunophenotyping will often confirm monotypic plasma cells or monoclonal B-cells in pcMZL/LPD and so rule out a polyclonal process such as IgG4-RD, the diagnosis can be further ascertained (in cases with equivocal features) by considering the specific histopathological features of IgG4-RD and measuring the plasma levels of IgG4 (see Chap. 15). In Castleman's disease (see Chap. 15) the dermal infiltrate may contain sheets of proliferating mature plasma cells, but the infiltrate is usually polytypic and often aggregates in the secondary lymphoid structures [17]. However, rare cases, especially HHV8$^+$, may have monotypic features (see Table 10.4).

Cutaneous plasmacytosis mainly affects Asian males and presents as widespread pigmented plaques on the trunk and head [18].

Table 10.4 Diseases in the skin with prominent plasma cell infiltration which may mimic pcMZL/LPD

Malignant
Myeloma (cutaneous plasmacytoma) (Chap. 4)
Erdheim-Chester disease (Chap. 12)
Cutaneous lymphoplasmacytic lymphoma (Waldenström)
Inflammatory
IgG4-related disease (Chap. 15)
Castleman's disease (Chap. 15)
Cutaneous plasmacytosis (Chap. 4)
Angioplasmacellular pseudolymphoma
Pretibial lymphoplasmacytic plaque
Pseudolymphomatous angiokeratoma of children
Zoon balanitis
Syphilis
Lyme disease (*Borrelia* sp.)

Angioplasmacellular pseudolymphomas, mainly seen in children, can present as pretibial lymphoplasmacytic plaques or acral pseudolymphomatous angiokeratoma (APACHE) [19]. These usually manifest as benign-looking grouped papules or plaques on distal extremities. Similar lesions, papular or polypoid have been described in adults [20, 21]. The term "primary cutaneous angioplasmacellular pseudolymphoma" is used to underscore the plasma cell-rich infiltrate and the presence of high endothelial venules (HEV)-like vessels [19, 21]. Lymphoplasmacytic lymphoma (Waldenstrom macroglobulinemia) may secondarily involve the skin and be difficult to distinguish from non-class switched marginal zone lymphoma (IgM$^+$). Clinical correlation and testing for the MYD88 L265P molecular abnormality will resolve the issue in dubious cases (see Table 10.5).

Table 10.5 Differential diagnosis of pcMZL/LPD with abundant plasma cells

	pcMZL/LPD	Lymphoplasmacytic lymphoma	Castleman's disease	IgG4-related disease
Serum hypergammaglobulinemia	Usually absent	Present (IgM M-protein)	Present (polyclonal)	Present (elevated IgG4 levels)
Infiltrate	Dermal infiltrate around vessels and adnexa, plasma cells at the periphery	Monotonous lymphocytes, lymphoplasmacytoid cells and plasma cells	Secondary lymphoid structures, lymphocytes, sheets of proliferating mature plasma cells, eosinophils. Hyalinized sclerotic collagen. No atypia	Secondary lymphoid structures, dense lymphoplasmacytic infiltration with IgG4-positive plasma cells
Clonal B-cell population detected by IgH rearrangement studies	Present	Present	Absent	Absent
Immunophenotyic profile	See Tables 10.2 and 10.3	$CD20^+$, $BCL2^+$ variable CD138 and $MUM1^+$ $BCL6/CD10^-$ IgM^+, κ or λ	Plasma cells usually polytypic, but subset (esp. $HHV8^+$) may show monotypic atypical $HHV8^+$ cells	Normal phenotype of plasma cells. $IgG4^+$ plasma cell counts are elevated

10.1.5 Treatment

For the management of primary cutaneous marginal zone lymphoma/lymphoproliferative disorder (pcMZL/LPD), several first-line therapeutic options are recommended, including radiotherapy, surgical excision, and intralesional rituximab [7, 22]. The likelihood of relapse tends to be higher in patients presenting with multifocal skin involvement, with the rate exceeding 50%, according to some studies [3].

Radiotherapy remains an effective option, achieving a complete response in up to 99% of cases [23]. The typical dosage is between 20 and 30 Gy, although lower doses of 12–16 Gy can also be considered when prioritizing cosmetic outcomes [24]. While local recurrences are not uncommon, they are rarely observed within the radiation field based on our clinical experience. When such recurrences occur, they tend to be at the periphery of the radiation area, suggesting the possibility of insufficient treatment margins. Margins ranging from 0.5 to 5 cm have thus been recommended based on lesion size and demarcation [23].

Intralesional rituximab has well-established efficacy and is generally administered in weekly cycles consisting of three 10 mg injections, a regimen that may be repeated monthly [25]. Approximately two-thirds of patients achieve a complete response after 2–3 cycles. However, it's worth noting that tumor cells may downregulate surface CD20 expression, thereby rendering them less sensitive to this treatment modality [26]. In most patients, intralesional rituximab will exert systemic effects with pronounced B-cell lymphopenia.

10.2 Primary Cutaneous Follicle Center Lymphoma (pcFCL)

10.2.1 Practice Essentials

- Solitary or clustered tumors, nodules, or plaques, in a similar distribution as pcMZL/LPD (head and neck, upper trunk).
- Very good prognosis (>95% 5-year survival).
- Full staging is required because approximately 10% of patients have bone marrow involvement.
- Therapy: radiotherapy, intralesional rituximab, surgical excision.

10.2.2 Clinical Manifestations and Disease Course

The clinical manifestations of pcFCL resemble those of pcMZL/LPD. Clinically, patients usually present with isolated or grouped papules, nodules, or plaques predominantly located on the head, neck, and upper torso (Fig. 10.2). A unique characteristic of pcFCL is the tendency for the skin infiltrates to cluster in a more circumscribed, agminated pattern. For instance, agminated, papular pcFCL appearing on the face may simulate rosacea. In some cases, a central tumor may be encircled by smaller nodules or papules, a pattern somewhat akin to primary cutaneous anaplastic large cell lymphoma. In rare instances, the lesions may become more widespread, covering large skin surfaces such as the back. Historically, this manifestation has been termed "reticulohistiocytoma of the dorsum" or "Crosti lymphoma" [27].

Spontaneous regression of pcFCL is an uncommon event. Generally, the disease carries an excellent prognosis, with a 5-year overall disease-specific survival rate exceeding 95%. However, a minority of patients—fewer than 10%—may experience a more aggressive course with the potential for spread to lymph nodes and bone marrow [8, 28]. Notably, pcFCL cases on the distal extremities, particularly those on the lower leg, may have a worse prognosis with an elevated risk for systemic dissemination.

10.2.3 Diagnostic Workup and Staging

10.2.3.1 Skin Biopsy

The histopathology of primary cutaneous follicle center lymphoma (pcFCL) typically shows a dermal, bottom-heavy lymphocytic infiltrate composed largely of centrocytes, which are often large and

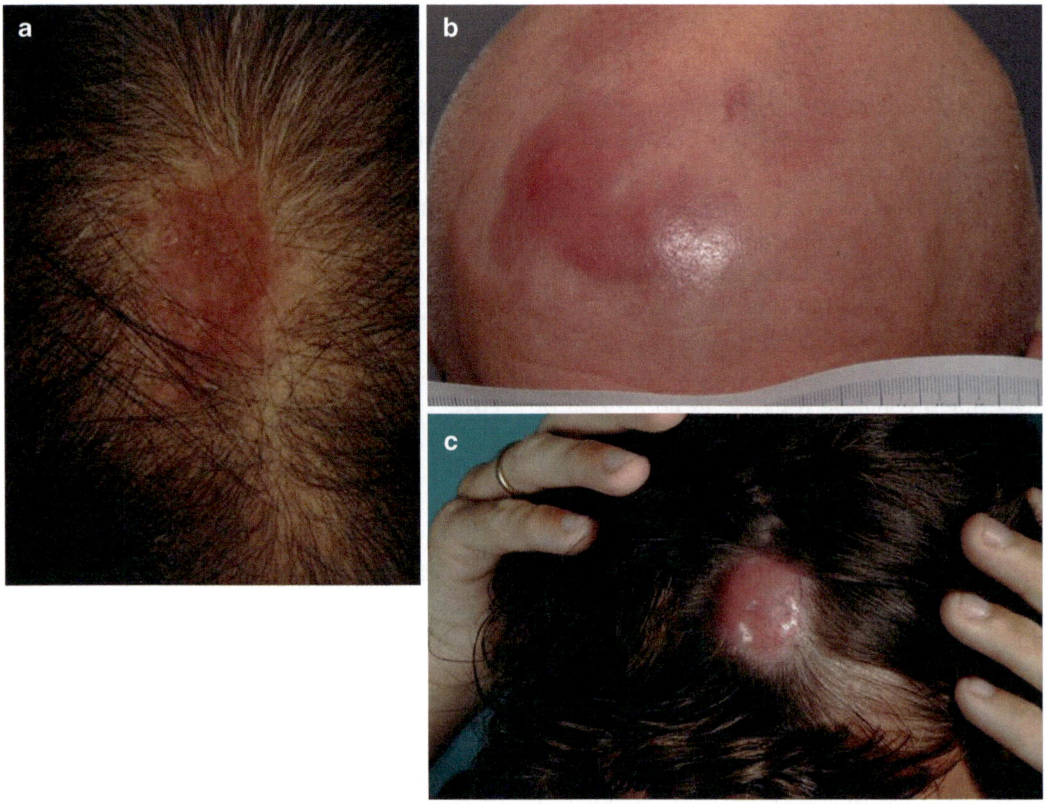

Fig. 10.2 Primary cutaneous follicular lymphoma. (**a**) An infiltrated plaque on the scalp, (**b**) regional involvement of the scalp, (**c**) a nodule on the scalp

only rare bona fide centroblasts. The atypical cells are arranged in an ill-defined nodular (follicular), diffuse, or mixed pattern. Rare variants with spindle cell features are described. Immunophenotypically, these cells express pan-B-cell markers (CD20, CD79a, CD19, and PAX5), along with germinal center cell markers (Bcl-6, LMO2, HGAL, and MEF2B). Of interest, these neoplasms often contain abundant background T cells.

A key distinguishing feature of pcFCL from its nodal counterpart, follicular center lymphoma (FCL), is the lack of Bcl-2 expression in most cases of pcFCL. A small subset has however been reported to be positive for Bcl-2 (very often dimly, but convincingly in approximately 10–25% of cases [15, 29]. The t(14;18) cytogenetic abnormality has been identified in 10–40% of pcFCL [29]. Also, in comparison with the nodal counterpart, CD10 expression is observed much less commonly, as it is reported in less than 25% of cases, mostly those with a follicular growth pattern. MUM1, CD5, CD23, and Cyclin D1 are typically negative, further helping to differentiate this cutaneous variant from other lymphomas. In doubtful cases, monoclonal B-cell populations may be demonstrated by IgH gene rearrangement studies in most, but not all, cases.

10.2.3.2 Imaging

Imaging studies (contrast-enhanced CT scans with or without whole-body positron emission tomography) should be performed to rule out systemic involvement [7].

10.2.3.3 Bone Marrow Biopsy

Bone marrow biopsy should be considered on a case-by-case basis. Bone marrow involvement is present in 5–10% of patients and is a negative prognostic factor. Bone marrow biopsy should be contemplated in patients with atypical clinical presentation (e.g., localization on the leg), large skin tumor burden, or immunosuppressed individuals who have a worse prognosis and higher risk of extracutaneous spread [7]. In our center we order PET/CT scans for patients diagnosed with pcFCL, and our results concur with the results of others that the risk of extracutaneous involvement is low (<5%) [10]. We consider bone marrow biopsies only for patients with abnormal imaging indicating extracutaneous involvement.

10.2.3.4 Other Investigations

Complete blood cell count with differential and comprehensive blood chemistry (including lactate dehydrogenase levels).

10.2.4 Differential Diagnosis

The differentiation of primary cutaneous follicle center lymphoma (pcFCL) from other cutaneous B-cell lymphomas and pseudolymphomas should rely on a combination of clinical, imaging and pathological features and is important for appropriate clinical management (Table 10.3).

Reactive follicular hyperplasia is to be distinguished from pcFCL by a combination of morphological and immunophenotypic features (well-circumscribed polymorphous follicles with dense, orderly, $CD21^+$ dendritic cell nodules, abundant tingle-body macrophages, high Ki67) and demonstration of a polyclonal B cell population by molecular or flow cytometric methods if required (see Chap. 11).

The distinction between pcFCL and secondary skin involvement from systemic nodal follicular lymphoma (FCL) is crucial. Given that the clinical presentations of primary cutaneous and nodal FCL can be quite similar, imaging studies become vital, along with a distinct set of expressed markers for differential diagnosis (key features are summarized in Table 10.6). However, it should be noted that the lines between pcFCL and nodal FCL can blur in some instances. For example, CD10 may be negative in up to 40% of nodal FCL cases and could be positive in approximately 25% of pcFCL cases [30, 31]. Moreover, clear Bcl-2 positivity and *BCL-2* t (14,18) translocations have been found in 10–25% and 10–40% of pcFCL cases [15, 31, 32]. Conversely, nodal FCLs with high proliferative activity may sometimes lose Bcl-2 expressions and simulate pcFCL [33]. On the other hand, a combination of strong Bcl-2 and CD10 expression should seriously raise the possibility of secondary involvement by a systemic follicular lymphoma, since

Table 10.6 Key features differentiating primary cutaneous and metastatic follicular lymphomas

	pcFCL	Secondary cutaneous involvement from nodal FCL
Imaging	No systemic involvement	Nodal and/or bone marrow involvement
Bcl-2	Negative, but weak positive, patchy seen in a significant variable number of cases; 10–25% may show stronger staining (>50% of cells)	Positive in most cases
CD10	Rarely positive in follicular pattern, negative in diffuse pattern (overall <25% of cases are positive)	Positive in most cases
Bcl-6	Positive	Positive
Ki67	Often above 30%	Often below 30%
BCL2 rearrangement/t(14;18)	Occasionally positive (10–40%)	Usually positive (approx. 85%)
BCL6 rearrangements	Generally negative	May be positive

this remains very rare in cases of pcFCL [33]. Given these complexities, imaging studies are strongly recommended for all cases of cutaneous FCL, especially if the IHC profile deviates from the standard expected pattern.

The differential diagnosis with pcDLBCL-LT is discussed below. The distinction from pcMZL/LPD was previously mentioned; also see Tables 10.2 and 10.3.

10.2.5 Treatment

First-line therapies are radiotherapy, surgical excision, or intralesional rituximab for small lesions in sensitive areas [7, 22]. Patients with generalized cutaneous lesions have been treated with systemic rituximab or rituximab-CHOP combination chemotherapy [34]. Approximately 30% of patients relapse after treatment, but the presence of a cutaneous relapse does not affect prognosis.

10.3 Primary Cutaneous Diffuse Large B-Cell Lymphoma (Leg Type), pcDLBCL-LT

10.3.1 Practice Essentials

- The most aggressive type of primary cutaneous B-cell lymphoma, extracutaneous dissemination in 50% of patients
- Elderly (commonly female) or immunosuppressed patients
- Tumors and ulcerations of the lower leg
- 5-year survival rate of 55%
- Treatment with radiotherapy and systemic chemotherapy

10.3.2 Clinical Manifestations and Disease Course

PcDLBCL-LT tends to localize to lower extremities as a single tumorous lesion or as multiple, even bilateral nodules, plaques, and tumors. Despite the name, pcDLBCL can be found in other body areas than the legs, although this is rather uncommon (<15% of all cases). The course is progressive and half of the patients develop extracutaneous disease, most commonly in inguinal lymph nodes [29, 35]. pcDLBCL-LT has a peak incidence in elderly individuals, particularly females (seventh decade of life or older), and can rarely develop in a setting of immunosuppression, e.g., in patients treated with anti-tumor necrosis factor-α agents [36] (Fig. 10.3).

10.3.3 Diagnostic Workup and Staging

10.3.3.1 Skin Biopsy

Biopsy reveals a monotonous proliferation of centroblast-like or immunoblast-like cells filling the dermis and extending to the subcutis. Malignant cells strongly express CD20, CD79a, and Bcl-2 and commonly express Bcl-6 (about

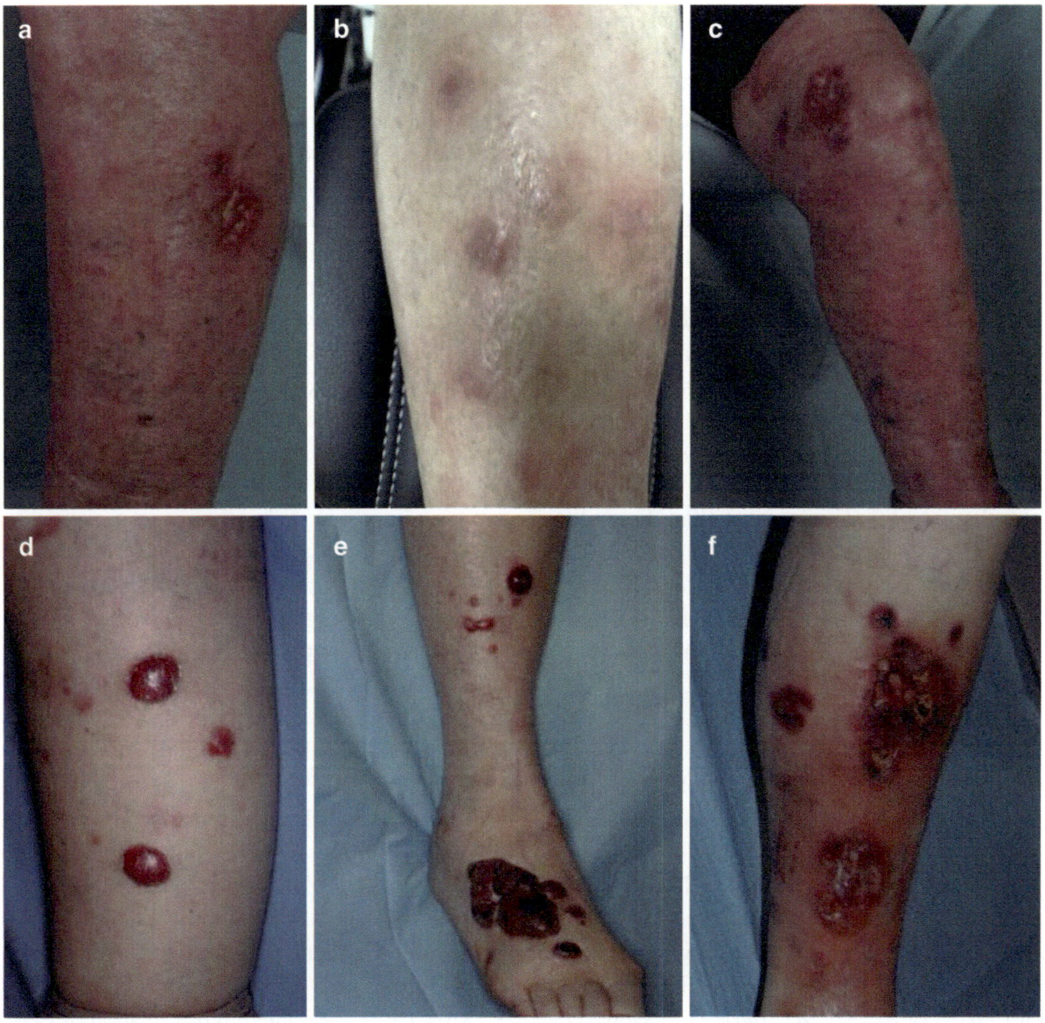

Fig. 10.3 Primary cutaneous large B-cell lymphoma, leg type. (**a**) A single ulcerated plaque on the lower leg, (**b–d**) multiple plaques and nodules. The lesions vary from a single nodule, (**e, f**) large tumors with or without ulceration

60% of cases), but CD10, TdT, EBER-ISH, CD5, and CD30 are generally negative. MUM-1 and FOXP1 are typically positive.

A subset of cases, however, deviate from this typical profile and show expression of CD10 or absent, dim, or minimal expression of MUM1 and/or Bcl-2, emphasizing the need for a careful correlation of all parameters, including clinical presentation to obtain the best diagnostic assessment [37]. Additionally, c-Myc is expressed in >60% of patients [38] and cytoplasmic IgM is positive and may be accompanied by IgD in up to half the cases [29]. A clonal B cell population may be demonstrated by molecular IgH rearrangement testing in most, if not all, cases.

10.3.3.2 Staging

Patients should be staged according to current guidelines for nodal diffuse large B-cell lymphoma with comprehensive blood work (including lactate dehydrogenase) and imaging.

10.3.3.3 Prognostic Factors

In primary cutaneous diffuse large B-cell lymphoma (pcDLBCL-LT), several negative prognostic factors have been identified, including advanced age, immunosuppression, elevated levels of lactate dehydrogenase (LDH), and the presence of extracutaneous disease.

Approximately 50% of pcDLBCL cases display a double expressor status (concurrent IHC expression of c-Myc and Bcl-2), but its impact on survival remains unclear [38, 39].

The same applies to the impact of double hit/triple hit (DH/TH) status (at the cytogenetic level, regarding *MYC*, *BCL2*, and *BCL6* rearrangements) on the prognosis of pcDLBCL-LT. Although *MYC* translocations are common in pcDLBCL-LT, DH/TH status is seen in only a minority of patients, ranging from 2% to 15% [38–40]. Many consider that cases with double-hit status are best classified as high-grade B-cell lymphomas [37]. This suggests that the molecular and prognostic landscape of pcDLBCL-LT differs from that of its nodal counterpart and that research is still ongoing to delineate its diagnostic outlines against other aggressive B-cell lymphomas.

10.3.4 Differential Diagnosis

Differentiating primary cutaneous diffuse large B-cell lymphoma (pcDLBCL-LT) from other cutaneous B-cell lymphomas, especially pcFCL with similar large-cell morphology, is critical for appropriate clinical management. The expression of c-Myc, Bcl-2, MUM1, intracytoplasmic IgM, and Bcl-6 can serve as valuable diagnostic clues. For instance, primary cutaneous follicle center lymphoma (pcFCL) is typically negative for Bcl-2, CD10, and c-Myc, and Bcl-6-positive, with no expression of MUM1 (see Tables 10.2 and 10.3).

Furthermore, pcDLBCL-LT must be distinguished from systemic B-cell lymphomas with secondary skin involvement. Intravascular diffuse large B-cell lymphoma, including its skin-only variant, can be differentiated by its characteristic intravascular neoplastic cells rather than a diffuse infiltration pattern seen in pcDLBCL. Additionally, Epstein-Barr Virus (EBV) positivity can help in differentiating pcDLBCL-LT from conditions like lymphomatoid granulomatosis and immunodeficiency-associated B-cell lymphoproliferative diseases.

10.3.5 Treatment

The pcDLBCL-LT should be treated with systemic chemotherapy such as R-CHOP followed by local RT 36–40 Gy [23]. However, many patients are elderly and fragile, and good disease control can be obtained with rituximab monotherapy, surgery, and/or radiotherapy [41, 42].

The efficacy of radiotherapy seems to be lower than other primary cutaneous B-cell lymphomas (complete response ≅ 80%, relapse rate >50%). Extracutaneous progression will eventually take place in 30% of responders [7]. Rituximab monotherapy leads to complete responses in less than 50% of patients.

10.4 Lymphomas and Lymphoid Proliferations Associated with Immune Deficiency and Dysregulation (LLP-IDD)

10.4.1 Practice Essentials

- B-cell LLP-IDD develops in a setting of immunosuppressive or immunomodulatory treatments, in patients with inborn errors of immunity or acquired immunodeficiency, or in elderly patients in whom the immune system is impaired due to immunosenescence.
- Most cases are related to reactivation of EBV.
- Clinical manifestations are heterogeneous, ranging from papules, plaques, and skin nodules to large ulcers (EVB$^+$ mucocutaneous ulcer). Lymph nodes and parenchymatous organs may be involved.
- Prognosis ranges from excellent to aggressive disease.

The emergence of cutaneous B-cell lymphoproliferative diseases in the milieu of compromised immune states underscores the profound influence of immune homeostasis on lymphoid cell behavior. As described in the current 5th edition of the World Health Organization Classification of Haematolymphoid Tumours (WHO-HAEM 5), the assessment and classification of LLP-IDD necessitate a comprehensive approach, harmonizing histological diagnosis, viral pathogenesis, and the clinical backdrop of immunodeficiency [43].

A critical component in the diagnostic algorithm is the histological examination, ensuring that the tissue's morphology adheres to established criteria. Beyond morphological assessment, discerning the role of oncogenic viruses is pivotal. Notably, while EBV is frequently implicated in these lymphoproliferative disorders in the setting of immune compromise, a proportion of patients do not demonstrate evidence of oncogenic viral involvement.

The third and equally significant determinant is the clinical milieu of immunodeficiency or immune dysfunction. This can be as diverse as the iatrogenic immunosuppression seen the post-transplant setting or with cytotoxic therapies, inherent immune defects as seen in inborn errors of immunity, immunodeficiencies related to HIV, immune dysfunction associated with systemic malignancies, polychemotherapy, the effect of CAR-T cell therapy and/or the use of immune checkpoint inhibitors, and finally, immunosenescence, which represents the natural waning of immune robustness with age.

Navigating this triad of considerations, histological characteristics, viral association, and the nature of immunodeficiency, aids in precisely categorizing lymphoid proliferation and facilitates tailored clinical management.

10.4.2 Clinical Manifestations

The clinical presentation of cutaneous LLP-IDD can be remarkably heterogeneous, reflecting the underlying complexity of immune dysregulation and viral involvement. Unlike other more uniform skin lymphomas, skin manifestations in this setting may show a spectrum of abnormalities. Patients may present with various forms of lymphoid infiltrations, such as papules, plaques, nodules, or tumors. These lesions are often multiple and can be distributed regionally or spread across different areas of the skin. One particular subtype that stands out among LLP-IDD is the Epstein-Barr Virus positive (EBV^+) mucocutaneous ulcer. This is recognized as a recurring pattern within the spectrum of EBV-associated lymphoproliferative diseases (Fig. 10.4).

10.4.3 Skin Biopsy

The histopathological evaluation of biopsies in LLP-IDD is complex due to the highly variable pattern/mixture of cell populations, the presence of prominent reactive T-cell populations, and the presence of immunoblastic and/or Hodgkin-like cells, which raise the possibility of diffuse large B-cell lymphoma (DLBCL) or classical Hodgkin lymphoma [44]. Expression of CD15 and CD30 are not rare. Aberrant or lost/decreased expression of plasma cell markers and/or B-cell markers are common, further increasing diagnostic confusion. Many cases of "primary Hodgkin lymphoma of the skin" in fact represent IDD-associated lymphoid proliferations (e.g., EBV^+ mucocutaneous ulcer). IgH and TCR rearrangement patterns can also be variable, sometimes showing dual monoclonal rearrangements, and must be considered cautiously within the broader histopathological context [29]. In patients with immunosuppression and/or immune dysfunction, clinicians should be aware of the possibility of a potentially easily reversible LLP-IDD even in cases where the skin lesions appear malignant. EBV testing through EBER in situ hybridization is the gold standard for the detection of EBV in cases that contain the virus, although some cases may be EBV-negative.

A comprehensive clinical history remains essential for accurate diagnosis and management [29].

10.4.4 Other Investigations, Staging, and Imaging

The diagnostic and classification difficulties in patients with LLP-IDD call for extensive testing, which should be tailored to the individual patient. When the cause of immunodeficiency is unclear, testing for humoral and cellular immunodeficiencies may be needed (see Chap. 16). LLP-IDD

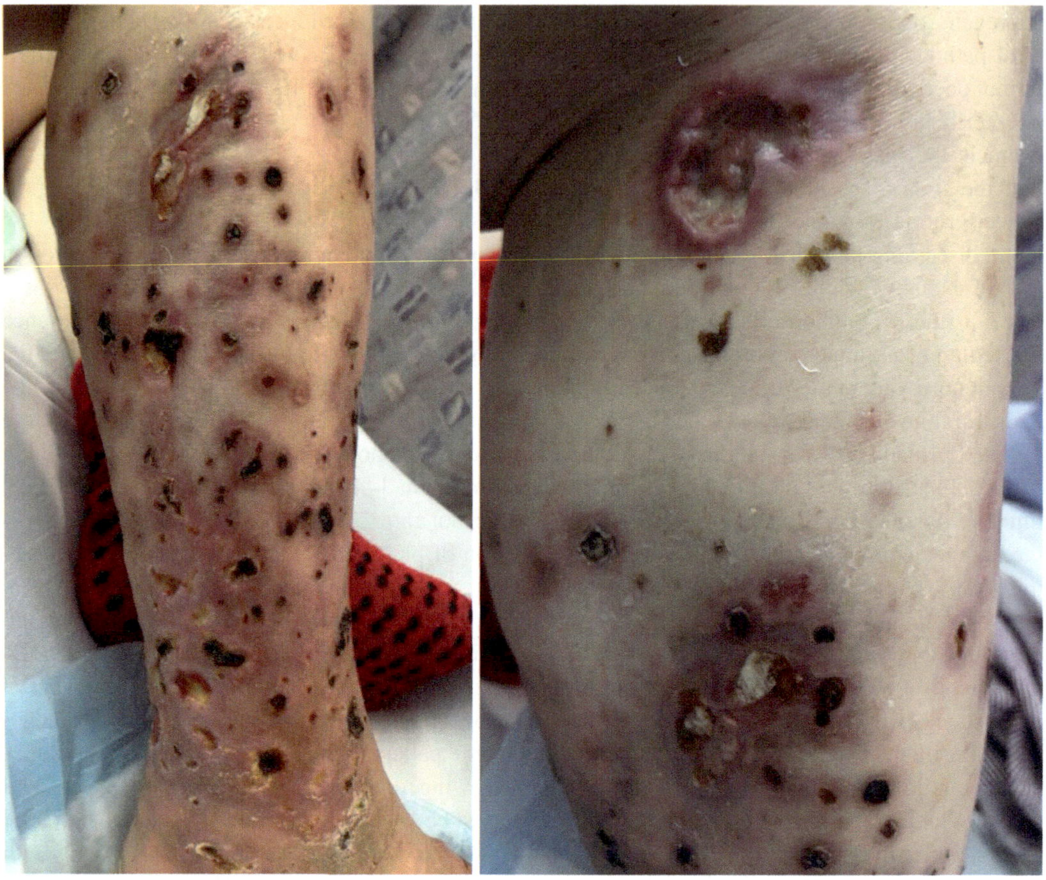

Fig. 10.4 Immune deficiency/dysfunction-associated lymphoid proliferation in a patient with Hodgkin lymphoma. The manifestations are heterogenous comprising superficial and deep skin ulcers and infiltrated plaques on the lower legs

may involve lymph nodes, bone marrow, and internal organs (especially the gut), which will be detected using appropriate imaging techniques.

10.4.5 Common Patterns of LLP-IDD in the Skin

10.4.5.1 EBV$^+$ Mucocutaneous Ulcer [45]

EBV$^+$ mucocutaneous ulcer is a solitary and sharply demarcated ulcer that may develop on the oro-pharyngeal mucosa, the skin, and the gastro-intestinal tract (especially colon and rectum), usually in a setting of immunosenescence or iatrogenic immunosuppression (e.g., methotrexate, azathioprine, cyclosporin), including bone marrow or solid organ transplantation [46]. The course is variable, from self-limited, waxing and waning to chronic and progressive, causing considerable distress and suffering. However, most have a benign course and may disappear after discontinuation or disappearance of the underlying causal factor responsible for the immune deficiency. Spontaneous regression happens in about 25% of cases. Surgical excision, intralesional rituximab, or radiation may be effective [47]. The histopathology resembles classical Hodgkin lymphoma but the differential diagnosis of EBV$^+$ mucocutaneous ulcer includes EBV$^+$ DLBCL, pcALCL, and lymphomatoid granulomatosis [45].

10.4.5.2 Methotrexate-Induced ID-LPD

Methotrexate (sometimes in combination with anti-TNF-α agents) is the most common cause of LLP-IDD [44, 48]. EBV-associated cutaneous DLBCL has a high rate of spontaneous regression after discontinuation of methotrexate, but nodal and bone marrow involvement is not infrequent [48, 49].

10.4.5.3 Age-Related EBV-Associated B-Cell Lymphoproliferative Disorders [50]

Although the peak incidence is at the age of 90, it is now acknowledged that so-called "age-related" EBV^+ B-cell LPD may develop in much younger individuals (>50 years) and is part of the LLP-IDD spectrum. Although some cases are mostly skin-based, lymphadenopathy is common (≅50% of patients), sometimes involving the lungs, tonsils, and stomach. Histopathology varies along a spectrum, ranging from EBV-positive DLBCL. Survival is poor in patients with extracutaneous involvement.

10.4.5.4 Post-Transplant Lymphoproliferative Disorder

Post-transplant lymphoproliferative disorder (PTLD) is a significant concern after solid organ transplantation and, less commonly, hematopoietic stem cell transplantation, comprising 21% of all cancers that occur post-transplantation [51] and occurring in 1–16% of solid organ transplant recipients. The risk of developing PTLD correlates with the level and duration of the immunosuppression required (itself modulated depending on the type of transplant) and also with the EBV serological status of the patient (EBV-naïve patients who acquire the virus at transplantation (primary infection) are at highest risk for developing PTLD). However, cutaneous involvement is relatively uncommon, varying from about 5% to 20% of all PTLD cases [1, 52, 53], with about 0.7 cutaneous PTLD/1000 solid organ transplants per year [54]. The skin manifestations can vary widely, ranging from nodules and tumors to ulcers and agminated papules [52, 55].

Histopathologically, PTLD presents with a broad spectrum of features. It may appear as plasmacytic or follicular hyperplasia, polymorphic lymphoproliferative disease, or even manifest as a bona fide histologically recognized lymphoma subtype, such as Hodgkin lymphoma or diffuse large B-cell lymphoma (DLBCL) [56, 57]. Many cases are associated with EBV infection, and extranodal sites are frequently affected. Isolated skin involvement is a rare occurrence.

Management of PTLD often involves reducing the level of immunosuppression. This approach can result in cure rates ranging from 25% to 50% [58].

References

1. Tran H, Nourse J, Hall S, Green M, Griffiths L, Gandhi MK. Immunodeficiency-associated lymphomas. Blood Rev. 2008;22:261–81.
2. Suárez AL, Pulitzer M, Horwitz S, Moskowitz A, Querfeld C, Myskowski PL. Primary cutaneous B-cell lymphomas: part I. Clinical features, diagnosis, and classification. J Am Acad Dermatol. 2013;69:329.e1–13; quiz 341–2.
3. Servitje O, Muniesa C, Benavente Y, Monsálvez V, Garcia-Muret MP, Gallardo F, et al. Primary cutaneous marginal zone B-cell lymphoma: response to treatment and disease-free survival in a series of 137 patients. J Am Acad Dermatol. 2013;69:357–65.
4. Travaglino A, Varricchio S, Pace M, Russo D, Picardi M, Baldo A, et al. Borrelia burgdorferi in primary cutaneous lymphomas: a systematic review and meta-analysis. J Dtsch Dermatol Ges. 2020;18:1379–84.
5. Qin Y, Wang Y. Penicillin in Borrelia burgdorferi-negative primary cutaneous marginal zone lymphoma: a case series and literature review. Acta Derm Venereol. 2022;102:adv00668.
6. Ferreri AJM, Govi S, Ponzoni M. Marginal zone lymphomas and infectious agents. Semin Cancer Biol. 2013;23:431–40.
7. Senff NJ, Noordijk EM, Kim YH, Bagot M, Berti E, Cerroni L, et al. European Organization for Research and Treatment of Cancer and International Society for Cutaneous Lymphoma consensus recommendations for the management of cutaneous B-cell lymphomas. Blood. 2008;112:1600–9.
8. Senff NJ, Kluin-Nelemans HC, Willemze R. Results of bone marrow examination in 275 patients with histological features that suggest an indolent type of cutaneous B-cell lymphoma. Br J Haematol. 2008;142:52–6.
9. Quereux G, Frot AS, Brocard A, Leux C, Renaut J-J, Dreno B. Routine bone marrow biopsy in the initial evaluation of primary cutaneous B-cell lymphoma does not appear justified. Eur J Dermatol. 2009;19:216–20.

10. Kheterpal MK, Dai J, Geller S, Pulitzer M, Ni A, Myskowski PL, et al. Role of imaging in low-grade cutaneous B-cell lymphoma presenting in the skin. J Am Acad Dermatol. 2019;81:970–6.
11. Edinger JT, Kant JA, Swerdlow SH. Cutaneous marginal zone lymphomas have distinctive features and include 2 subsets. Am J Surg Pathol. 2010;34:1830–41.
12. Evans PAS, Pott C, Groenen PJTA, Salles G, Davi F, Berger F, et al. Significantly improved PCR-based clonality testing in B-cell malignancies by use of multiple immunoglobulin gene targets. Report of the BIOMED-2 concerted action BHM4-CT98-3936. Leukemia. 2007;21:207–14.
13. Obiorah IE, Aguilera NS, Gru A, Courville EL. Isolated light chain-restricted germinal centers are common in follicular hyperplasia by ultrasensitive in situ hybridization. Am J Surg Pathol. 2023;47:694–700.
14. Obiorah IE, Karrs J, Brown L, Wang H-W, Karai LJ, Pham TH-T, et al. Overlapping features of primary cutaneous marginal zone lymphoproliferative disorder and primary cutaneous CD4 + small/medium T-cell lymphoproliferative disorder: a diagnostic challenge examined by genomic analysis. Am J Surg Pathol. 2023;47:344–53.
15. Beltzung F, Ortonne N, Pelletier L, Beylot-Barry M, Ingen-Housz-Oro S, Franck F, et al. Primary cutaneous CD4+ small/medium T-cell lymphoproliferative disorders: a clinical, pathologic, and molecular study of 60 cases presenting with a single lesion: a multicenter study of the French Cutaneous Lymphoma Study Group. Am J Surg Pathol. 2020;44:862–72.
16. Brenner I, Roth S, Puppe B, Wobser M, Rosenwald A, Geissinger E. Primary cutaneous marginal zone lymphomas with plasmacytic differentiation show frequent IgG4 expression. Mod Pathol. 2013;26:1568–76.
17. Zapata-Salazar NA, Gómez-Flores M, Ocampo-Candiani J, Chavez-Alvarez S. Cutaneous manifestations of Castleman disease: histopathological characteristics and review of literature. Am J Dermatopathol. 2021;43:926–31.
18. Gutierrez RA, Jacobson R, Dawson A, Haemel A, North J. Cutaneous and systemic plasmacytosis with concurrent lymphoid hyperplasia. J Cutan Pathol. 2023;50:379–82.
19. Fernandez-Flores A, Suarez Peñaranda JM, De Toro G, Alvarez Cuesta CC, Fernández-Figueras MT, Kempf W, et al. Expression of peripheral node addressins by plasmacytic plaque of children, APACHE, TRAPP, and primary cutaneous angioplasmacellular hyperplasia. Appl Immunohistochem Mol Morphol. 2018;26:411–9.
20. Okada M, Funayama M, Tanita M, Kudoh K, Aiba S, Tagami H. Acral angiokeratoma-like pseudolymphoma: one adolescent and two adults. J Am Acad Dermatol. 2001;45:S209–11.
21. Mitteldorf C, Palmedo G, Kutzner H, Kauer F, Prestin M, Schuster C, et al. Diagnostic approach in lymphoplasmacytic plaque. J Eur Acad Dermatol Venereol. 2015;29:2206–15.
22. Menzer C, Rendon A, Hassel JC. Treatment of indolent cutaneous B-cell lymphoma with intralesional or intravenous rituximab. Cancers. 2022;14:4787.
23. Specht L, Dabaja B, Illidge T, Wilson LD, Hoppe RT, International Lymphoma Radiation Oncology Group. Modern radiation therapy for primary cutaneous lymphomas: field and dose guidelines from the International Lymphoma Radiation Oncology Group. Int J Radiat Oncol Biol Phys. 2015;92:32–9.
24. Neelis KJ, Schimmel EC, Vermeer MH, Senff NJ, Willemze R, Noordijk EM. Low-dose palliative radiotherapy for cutaneous B- and T-cell lymphomas. Int J Radiat Oncol Biol Phys. 2009;74:154–8.
25. Peñate Y, Hernández-Machín B, Pérez-Méndez LI, Santiago F, Rosales B, Servitje O, et al. Intralesional rituximab in the treatment of indolent primary cutaneous B-cell lymphomas: an epidemiological observational multicentre study. The Spanish Working Group on Cutaneous Lymphoma. Br J Dermatol. 2012;167:174–9.
26. Lozzi GP, Coletti G, Peris K. Persistent CD20-negative primary cutaneous marginal zone lymphoma/lymphoproliferative disorder after treatment with intralesional rituximab therapy. J Am Acad Dermatol. 2008;59:S110–2.
27. Berti E, Alessi E, Caputo R, Gianotti R, Delia D, Vezzoni P. Reticulohistiocytoma of the dorsum. J Am Acad Dermatol. 1988;19:259–72.
28. Senff NJ, Hoefnagel JJ, Jansen PM, Vermeer MH, van Baarlen J, Blokx WA, et al. Reclassification of 300 primary cutaneous B-cell lymphomas according to the new WHO-EORTC classification for cutaneous lymphomas: comparison with previous classifications and identification of prognostic markers. J Clin Oncol. 2007;25:1581–7.
29. Swerdlow SH, Quintanilla-Martinez L, Willemze R, Kinney MC. Cutaneous B-cell lymphoproliferative disorders: report of the 2011 Society for Hematopathology/European Association for Haematopathology workshop. Am J Clin Pathol. 2013;139:515–35.
30. Servitje O, Climent F, Colomo L, Ruiz N, García-Herrera A, Gallardo F, et al. Primary cutaneous vs secondary cutaneous follicular lymphomas: a comparative study focused on BCL2, CD10, and t(14;18) expression. J Cutan Pathol. 2019;46:182–9.
31. Zhou XA, Yang J, Ringbloom KG, Martinez-Escala ME, Stevenson KE, Wenzel AT, et al. Genomic landscape of cutaneous follicular lymphomas reveals 2 subgroups with clinically predictive molecular features. Blood Adv. 2021;5:649–61.
32. Szablewski V, Ingen-Housz-Oro S, Baia M, Delfau-Larue M-H, Copie-Bergman C, Ortonne N. Primary cutaneous follicle center lymphomas expressing BCL2 protein frequently harbor BCL2 gene break and may present 1p36 deletion: a study of 20 cases. Am J Surg Pathol. 2016;40:127–36.

33. Masir N, Campbell LJ, Goff LK, Jones M, Marafioti T, Cordell J, et al. BCL2 protein expression in follicular lymphomas with t(14;18) chromosomal translocations. Br J Haematol. 2009;144:716–25.
34. Wang S, Perlmutter JW, Johnston J, Nugent Z, Wiseman M. Rituximab treatment of primary cutaneous follicle center lymphoma: a retrospective review. J Cutan Med Surg. 2022;26:604–12.
35. Willemze R, Cerroni L, Kempf W, Berti E, Facchetti F, Swerdlow SH, et al. The 2018 update of the WHO-EORTC classification for primary cutaneous lymphomas. Blood. 2019;133:1703–14.
36. Fujimi A, Nagamachi Y, Yamauchi N. Primary cutaneous diffuse large B-cell lymphoma, leg type, in a patient with rheumatoid arthritis undergoing etanercept therapy. Mod Rheumatol Case Rep. 2021;5:195–9.
37. Schrader AMR, de Groen RAL, Willemze R, Jansen PM, Quint KD, van Wezel T, et al. Cell-of-origin classification using the Hans and Lymph2Cx algorithms in primary cutaneous large B-cell lymphomas. Virchows Arch. 2022;480:667–75.
38. Menguy S, Frison E, Prochazkova-Carlotti M, Dalle S, Dereure O, Boulinguez S, et al. Double-hit or dual expression of MYC and BCL2 in primary cutaneous large B-cell lymphomas. Mod Pathol. 2018;31:1332–42.
39. Schrader AMR, Jansen PM, Vermeer MH, Kleiverda JK, Vermaat JSP, Willemze R. High incidence and clinical significance of MYC rearrangements in primary cutaneous diffuse large B-cell lymphoma. Leg Type Am J Surg Pathol. 2018;42:1488–94.
40. Lucioni M, Pescia C, Bonometti A, Fraticelli S, Moltrasio C, Ramponi A, et al. Double expressor and double/triple hit status among primary cutaneous diffuse large B-cell lymphoma: a comparison between leg type and not otherwise specified subtypes. Hum Pathol. 2021;111:1–9.
41. Heinzerling LM, Urbanek M, Funk JO, Peker S, Bleck O, Neuber K, et al. Reduction of tumor burden and stabilization of disease by systemic therapy with anti-CD20 antibody (rituximab) in patients with primary cutaneous B-cell lymphoma. Cancer. 2000;89:1835–44.
42. Zehnder M, Amarov B, Abrunhosa-Branquinho AN, Maiwald-Urosevic M, Mühleisen B, Saulite I, et al. Radiotherapy as a treatment option for local disease control in primary cutaneous diffuse large B-cell lymphoma, leg type. Dermatology. 2022;238:967–76.
43. Alaggio R, Amador C, Anagnostopoulos I, Attygalle AD, Araujo IBO, Berti E, et al. The 5th edition of the World Health Organization classification of haematolymphoid tumours: lymphoid neoplasms. Leukemia. 2022;36:1720–48.
44. Momose S, Tamaru J-I. Iatrogenic immunodeficiency-associated lymphoproliferative disorders of B-cell type that develop in patients receiving immunosuppressive drugs other than in the post-transplant setting. J Clin Exp Hematop. 2019;59:48–55.
45. Gru AA, Jaffe ES. Cutaneous EBV-related lymphoproliferative disorders. Semin Diagn Pathol. 2017;34:60–75.
46. Roberts TK, Chen X, Liao JJ. Diagnostic and therapeutic challenges of EBV-positive mucocutaneous ulcer: a case report and systematic review of the literature. Exp Hematol Oncol. 2015;5:13.
47. Ikeda T, Gion Y, Yoshino T, Sato Y. A review of EBV-positive mucocutaneous ulcers focusing on clinical and pathological aspects. J Clin Exp Hematop. 2019;59:64–71.
48. Hoshida Y, Xu J-X, Fujita S, Nakamichi I, Ikeda J-I, Tomita Y, et al. Lymphoproliferative disorders in rheumatoid arthritis: clinicopathological analysis of 76 cases in relation to methotrexate medication. J Rheumatol. 2007;34:322–31.
49. Koens L, Senff NJ, Vermeer MH, Willemze R, Jansen PM. Methotrexate-associated B-cell lymphoproliferative disorders presenting in the skin: a clinicopathologic and immunophenotypical study of 10 cases. Am J Surg Pathol. 2014;38:999–1006.
50. Shimoyama Y, Asano N, Kojima M, Morishima S, Yamamoto K, Oyama T, et al. Age-related EBV-associated B-cell lymphoproliferative disorders: diagnostic approach to a newly recognized clinicopathological entity. Pathol Int. 2009;59:835–43.
51. Teras LR, DeSantis CE, Cerhan JR, Morton LM, Jemal A, Flowers CR. 2016 US lymphoid malignancy statistics by World Health Organization subtypes. CA Cancer J Clin. 2016;66:443–59.
52. Salama S, Todd S, Cina DP, Margetts P. Cutaneous presentation of post-renal transplant lymphoproliferative disorder: a series of four cases. J Cutan Pathol. 2010;37:641–53.
53. Seçkin D. Cutaneous lymphoproliferative disorders in organ transplant recipients: update 2014. G Ital Dermatol Venereol. 2014;149:401–8.
54. Seçkin D, Barete S, Euvrard S, Francès C, Kanitakis J, Geusau A, et al. Primary cutaneous posttransplant lymphoproliferative disorders in solid organ transplant recipients: a multicenter European case series. Am J Transplant. 2013;13:2146–53.
55. Ferreira MCC, Arai Seque C, Enokihara MMSES, Batista MD, Tomimori J, Porro AM. Post-transplant lymphoproliferative disorder with cutaneous involvement: a series of four cases. Clin Transplant. 2021;35:e14162.
56. Dierickx D, Habermann TM. Post-transplantation lymphoproliferative disorders in adults. N Engl J Med. 2018;378:549–62.
57. Dharnidharka VR, Green M, Webber SA, Trappe RU. Post-transplant lymphoproliferative disorders. Springer Nature; 2021.
58. Benkerrou M, Durandy A, Fischer A. Therapy for transplant-related lymphoproliferative diseases. Hematol Oncol Clin North Am. 1993;7:467–75.

11 Cutaneous Lymphoid Hyperplasias Mimicking Malignancies in the Skin

Robert Gniadecki, Minakshi Taparia, Jean Deschenes, Jori Hardin, and Etienne Mahe

11.1 Practice Essentials

- Cutaneous lymphoid hyperplasia (CLH) is a benign, reactive proliferation of B or T cells resulting in lesions clinically and histopathologically mimicking cutaneous lymphomas.
- Clinically, the lesions are nodules or plaques, clinically indistinguishable from cutaneous B-cell lymphomas, mycosis fungoides (MF), and other malignancies.
- Common triggers of CLH are skin infections, drugs, contact allergens and irritants.

R. Gniadecki (✉)
Division of Dermatology, University of Alberta, Edmonton, AB, Canada
e-mail: gniadeck@ualberta.ca

M. Taparia
Division of Hematology, University of Alberta Hospital, Edmonton, AB, Canada

J. Deschenes
Department of Pathology and Laboratory Medicine, Cross Cancer Institute, Edmonton, AB, Canada
e-mail: Jean.Deschenes@albertaprecisionlabs.ca

J. Hardin
Division of Dermatology, University of Calgary, Calgary, AB, Canada
e-mail: Jori.hardin@albertahealthservices.ca

E. Mahe
Department of Pathology & Laboratory Medicine, and Hematology & Hematological Malignancies, University of Calgary, Calgary, AB, Canada
e-mail: etienne.mahe@albertaprecisionlabs.ca

Cutaneous lymphoid hyperplasia (CLH) is a benign dermal condition characterized by the reactive proliferation of lymphocytes, resulting in the formation of lymphoid follicles within the skin. Also referred to as pseudolymphoma due to its histological resemblance to malignant lymphomas, CLH nonetheless maintains a benign course. Accurate diagnosis can be challenging owing to its variable clinical manifestations, which can mimic a range of other dermatological disorders.

The clinical features of CLH can be remarkably heterogeneous, making it a condition that is often subject to diagnostic dilemmas. Patients may present with cutaneous lesions ranging from erythematous macules and papules to larger plaques and nodules. These lesions can be singular or multiple and can be located on various anatomical regions including, but not limited to, the face, trunk, and extremities. While the lesions are usually asymptomatic, some patients may report pruritus or mild discomfort.

CLH often appears as a skin response triggered by various factors such as drugs, infections, toxic substances, systemic conditions like connective tissue diseases, persistent antigen exposure, and co-occurring malignant conditions, including skin tumors and T-cell lymphomas.

Given its varying presentations, the differential diagnosis for CLH is extensive and includes conditions such as cutaneous lymphoma, drug

R. Gniadecki et al. (eds.), *Diseases of Blood and Skin*, https://doi.org/10.1007/978-3-031-65292-9_11

reactions, lupus erythematosus (especially tumid lupus), Jessner's lymphocytic infiltrate, reticular erythematous mucinosis, and other benign reactive processes. A comprehensive clinical history, along with histopathological examination, is pivotal in differentiating CLH from another morphological look-alike. Immunohistochemical staining is often employed to characterize the lymphocytic infiltrate, helping to confirm a diagnosis of CLH.

CLH may be categorized based on the predominant cell type present in the lymphoid infiltrate:

- **B-cell CLH**: Characterized by a predominance of B lymphocytes in the dermal infiltrate. It may present as localized or disseminated skin lesions. This is the most common type of CLH.
- **T-cell CLH**: The infiltrate is predominantly composed of T lymphocytes. Similar to B-cell CLH, the presentation can range from localized to more disseminated forms.
- **Combined CLH**: The lesions in combined CLH contain balanced amounts of both T and B lymphocytes in the infiltrate, thereby complicating the diagnosis further by introducing elements of both B-cell and T-cell CLH.

Mitteldorf and Kempf proposed another diagnostically functional classification based on cell types, morphology, etiology as well as main diagnostic pattern, which we reproduce below [1]:

1. Nodular pseudolymphomas
   - Nodular B-cell pseudolymphoma
   - *Borrelia*-associated nodular B-cell pseudolymphoma
   - Nodular T-cell and mixed pseudolymphoma
   - Nodular $CD30^+$ pseudolymphoma
2. Pseudo-T-cell lymphomas (simulating mycosis fungoides or other CTCLs)
   - Lymphomatoid contact dermatitis
   - Lymphomatoid drug reaction
   - Actinic reticuloid
   - $CD8^+$ T-cell pseudolymphoma in immunodeficiency
   - Infections as simulators of T-cell lymphomas
     - *Borrelia*-associated T-cell pseudolymphoma
     - Leishmaniasis-associated T-cell pseudolymphoma
     - Herpes virus-associated T-cell pseudolymphoma
     - Syphilis-associated pseudolymphoma
     - Other infections as simulators of CTCL
   - Inflammatory dermatosis as simulators of CTCL
3. Other pseudolymphomas
   - T-cell rich angiomatoid pseudolymphoma
     - Acral pseudolymphomatous angiokeratoma (APA)
     - T-cell-rich angiomatoid polypoid pseudolymphoma (TRAPP)
     - Primary cutneous angioplasmocellular hyperplasia
     - Lymphoplasmacytoid plaque (LPP)
   - Cutaneous plasmocytosis
   - Benign atypical intravascular ($CD30^+$) lymphoproliferation

11.2 Clinical Features (Fig. 11.1)

11.2.1 B-cell CLH

Usually manifests mostly as solitary, rarely multiple erythematous to violaceous papules, plaques, or nodules. Lesions are usually deeper and do not extend to the epidermis and therefore scaling of the skin is not seen. They frequently involve the upper torso, head, and neck, mimicking the distribution of primary cutaneous marginal zone lymphoma or $CD4^+$ lymphoproliferative disease (pcCD4-LPD) [2].

Known triggers of B-cell CLH are listed in Table 11.1. A special case of B-cell CLH is lymphocytoma cutis associated with *Borrelia* infection. It is relatively frequent, occurring in around 1% of *Borrelia* infections in Europe [3]. Clinical presentation typically involves a purplish plaque or nodule located on anatomical regions such as the earlobes, nipples, areolas, or scrotum. Regional lymph node enlargement is also frequently observed.

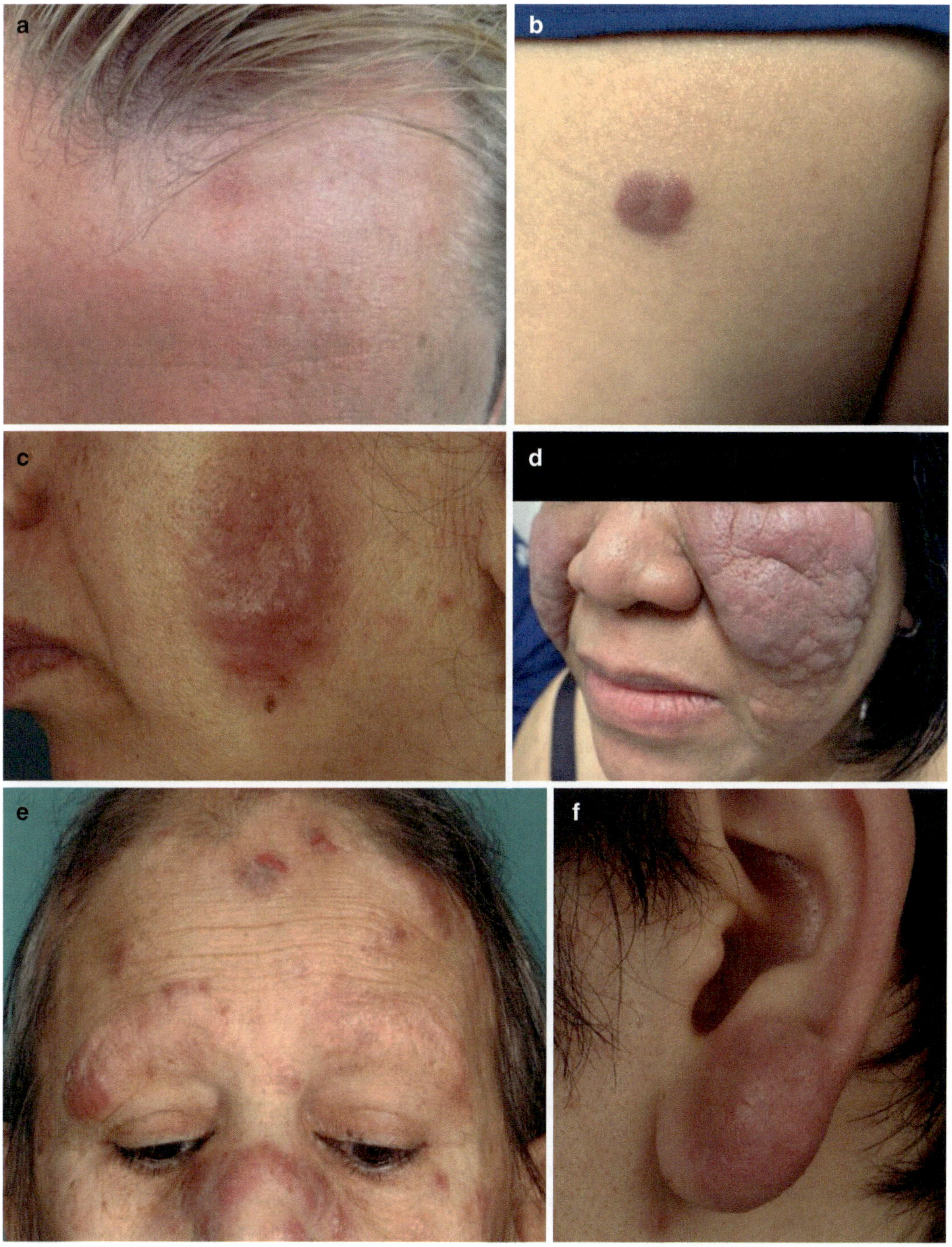

Fig. 11.1 Clinical spectrum of cutaneous lymphoid hyperplasias. The lesions exhibit a range from flat plaques (**a**), papules, and nodules (**b, c**) to florid tumorous lesions (**d, e**). While the face appears to be the most common location, lymphoid hyperplasias may occur in any region of the skin. (**f**) *Borrelia burgdorferi* should be considered as a potential cause of earlobe lymphocytoma

Table 11.1 Common triggers of CLH (From [1, 2])

	Comment
Infections	Mostly B-cell
Borrelia	
Syphilis	
Bacterial folliculitis	
Molluscum contagiosum	
Herpes simplex	
Infestations	T cell (often $CD30^{+}$)
Scabies	
Insect bites	
Medications, e.g.:	Both B cell and T cell
Phenytoin	Antidepressants (fluoxetine) associated with B cell CLH and may progress to clonal disease indistinguishable from pcMZL/LPD
Carbamazepine	
Valproate	
Angiotensin-converting enzyme (ACE) inhibitors	
Contact allergens (mostly metals: nickel, gold)	Majority T cell (lymphomatoid contact dermatitis)
Medicinal leech (*Hirudo medicinalis*)	B cell
Tatoos	Majority T cell
Comorbid to other diseases	B-cell CLH, probably driven by hyperactive or neoplastic T_{FH} cells
Lupus erythematosus	
Angioimmunoblastic T-cell lymphoma	

Clonality, defined by IgH gene rearrangement studies, is observed in 20–30% of analyzed cases and some of those lesions may further evolve into an indolent B-cell lymphoma or lymphoproliferation (e.g., pc MZLPD), underscoring the relationship between those conditions [4].

11.2.2 T-Cell and Combined CLH

T-cell and combined CLH types are less prevalent and present similarly to their B-cell counterpart, but may additionally feature erythroderma and generalized lymphadenopathy. The lymphocytic infiltrate may involve the epidermis; therefore, the lesions may look more superficial and scaly than in B-cell CLH. Combined B- and T-cell CLH cases are relatively rare, and their clinical presentation is largely indistinguishable from other types of CLH.

11.3 Diagnostic Workup

11.3.1 Skin Biopsy

The cornerstone for diagnosing CLH resides in the histopathological examination of a skin biopsy. The histological spectrum of CLH may differ depending on its subtype—B cell, T cell, or combined—but certain universal features are routinely observed.

The most salient histological feature of B-cell CLH is a dense dermal infiltrate of lymphocytes, which may extend into the subcutaneous adipose tissue. The infiltrate is top-heavy, generally consists of both small and large lymphocytes, and contains well-circumscribed, polarized, reactive germinal centers, hallmark features of a benign lymphoproliferative process. These centers are delineated by a mixture of large, activated lymphocytes known as centroblasts and of smaller "cleaved" lymphocytes (centrocytes), associated with tingle body macrophages [2]. In B-cell CLH the epidermis is usually not involved. Besides lymphocytes, the infiltrate may also contain other inflammatory cells like plasma cells, histiocytes, and eosinophils. The relative abundance and spatial arrangement of these cells may provide valuable insights into the etiological underpinnings of the CLH, such as whether it is drug-induced (abundant eosinophils) or related to an infection.

In B-cell CLH, there is a preponderance of B cells that are CD20-positive, while T-cell CLH predominantly features CD3-positive T cells. Germinal centers are positive for Bcl-6 and CD10 and negative for Bcl-2 and have a high proliferative rate (Ki67) and there are tight nodular arrays of dendritic cells, positive for CD21 and CD23. κ and λ staining shows polytypic plasma cells. $CD123^+$ plasmacytoid dendritic cells are typically found in small clusters around the germinal centers [1].

Although the major histopathological features of CLH are localized to the dermis, some cases may also exhibit concurrent epidermal alterations, especially the T-cell CLH. These could range from acanthosis and spongiosis to interface dermatitis. T-cell processes show expression of T-cell markers CD2, CD3, CD5, and CD7, although loss of CD7 is common in reactive T-cell populations. CD4 and CD8 show a mixture of both $CD4^+$ and $CD8^+$ cells.

Combined B- and T-cell CLH will display a heterogeneous population of both B and T cells.

11.3.1.1 Molecular Studies

Importantly, in general, the presence of polyclonal immunoglobulin gene rearrangement studies in B-cell CLH and polyclonal T-cell receptor gene rearrangement studies in T-cell CLH serve as molecular markers to help distinguish these benign conditions from their malignant equivalents. One should remember that these molecular studies are adjunct studies, with imperfect sensitivity and specificity, that can only be used in correlation with morphological, clinical, and phenotypic data.

In cases of B-cell CLH, molecular analyses target the gene rearrangements of the immunoglobulin heavy (IgH) and light chains (κ and λ). The observation of a polyclonal pattern in these gene rearrangements clearly favors a non-neoplastic B cell. By opposition, B-cell neoplasm will usually be accompanied by specific IgH chain gene rearrangements, indicating monoclonality.

T-cell CLH warrants a similar molecular approach, specifically targeting the clonal and specific rearrangements in the T-cell receptor (TCR) genes. The TCR comprises α, β, γ, and δ loci, but the current PCR-based methods used for TCR gene rearrangement analysis will specifically assess the β and γ loci. A polyclonal pattern of TCR gene rearrangement (or weak positivity of TCRβ with polyclonal TCRγ) will support the non-neoplastic diagnosis of T-cell CLH.

As mentioned above, in some cases, hyperplastic infiltrates will show a monoclonal pattern. Those patients have a higher rate of lymphoma progression [5].

11.3.2 Clinicopathological Correlations and Differential Diagnoses

There are multiple differential diagnoses for CLH (Table 11.2) [1].

Table 11.2 Diseases that mimic CLH [1, 5]

B-cell CLH	Zoon balanitis
	Actinic prurigo
	Primary cutaneous Marginal zone B-cell lymphoma (Chap. 10)
	Primary cutaneous Follicle center B-cell lymphoma (Chap. 10)
	Rosai-Dorfman disease (Chap. 13)
	Castleman's disease (Chap. 15)
	IgG4-related disease (Chap. 15)
	Kimura disease (Chap. 15)
	B-cell lymphoproliferative diseases associated with immunodeficiency (Chap. 10)
T-cell CLH	$CD4^+$ small/medium-sized T-cell lymphoproliferative disorder (pcCD4-LPD) (Chap. 9)
	Actinic reticuloid
	Mycosis fungoides (MF) (Chap. 7)
	Primary cutaneous marginal zone B-cell lymphoma (pcMZL/LPD), T-cell rich variant (Chap. 10)
	Lymphomatoid papulosis (Chap. 9)
	$CD8^+$ pseudolymphoma in immunodeficiency (Chap. 9)
	Subcutaneous panniculitis-like T-cell lymphoma (Chap. 9)
	Hypereosinophilic syndrome (Chap. 13)
	Cutaneous leishmaniasis
	Secondary syphilis
	Pigmented purpuric dermatosis

11.3.2.1 B-cell CLH vs Primary Cutaneous Marginal Zone Lymphoma/ Lymphoproliferative Disorder (pcMZL/LPD)

Primary cutaneous pcMZL/LPD often presents as red-to-bluish nodules or papules, primarily on the upper torso and arms, which are indistinguishable from B-cell CLH based solely on clinical appearance. Histopathologically, pcMZL/LPD features monotypic plasma cells in a significant number of cases (32). Neoplastic cells are positive for B-cell markers, accompanied by often abundant T cells, but they generally have a normal phenotypic profile A light chain restriction is evident in approximately 85% of pcMZL/LPD cases and clonal B cells detected with IgH rearrangement assays are observed in 60–70% of cases.

11.3.2.2 B-cell CLH vs pcFCL

Primary cutaneous follicle center lymphoma (pcFCL) presents as nodular lesions in the same distribution as pcMZL/LPD and B-cell CLH. Whereas B-CLH usually exhibits highly proliferative, well-defined follicles (with Ki67 close to 100%) showing a polymorphous germinal center population with tingle-body macrophages and intact mantle zones, only about 20% of pcFCL cases exhibit tingible-body macrophages. Additionally, the follicular dendritic cell networks in pcFCL are usually irregular and fragmented. The proliferative activity in the neoplastic follicles is moderately elevated (usually between 30% and 70%) and not as tightly restricted to germinal centers as in B-cell CLH and Bcl-6 expression is seen both within and outside the atypical follicles, with variable expression of CD10 (often negative) and Bcl-2 (dim and variable). Finally, clonal B-cell populations are more frequently detected in pcFCL, either by flow cytometry or by molecular pathology.

11.3.2.3 T-Cell CLH vs Mycosis Fungoides (MF) and pcCD4-LPD

T-cell CLH can clinically and histopathologically simulate MF and is sometimes referred to as pseudo-MF. The most common causes of pseudo-MF are lymphomatoid contact dermatitis, lymphomatoid drug reaction, and a photosensitive disease, actinic reticuloid. Sometimes, skin infections (*Borrelia*, *Leishmania*, *Herpes simplex*, *Herpes zoster*, pox viruses, fungal infections) induce T-cell CLH with a pattern of pseudo-MF. Partial loss of CD7 expression can take place in pseudo-MF, and should not be taken as evidence of a neoplastic lymphoid population [5].

Lymphomatoid contact dermatitis, lymphomatoid drug reaction, and actinic reticuloid are often $CD8^+$ and histologically show more spongiosis or eosinophilic infiltration as compared with MF. The lymphocytes show exocytosis into the epidermis and Pautrier-type microabscess formation is not observed, or is minimal, and cytological atypia and hyperchromasia are features that are more commonly observed in MF.

$CD4^+$ LPD may be very similar to pcMZL/LPD and CLH, but the T-cell population in this T-cell LPD will be predominantly made up of $CD4^+$ cells, with typical phenotypic features, including expression of PD1 and CD30 (see Chap. 10). Most cases of pcCD4-LPD will show a monoclonal pattern T-cell rearrangement by molecular TCR studies. In doubt, monoclonal results favor pcCD4-LPD.

11.3.2.4 Infectious Disorders of the Skin

The amastigote-negative, lymphocytic-rich variant of cutaneous leishmaniasis can mimic lymphoproliferative disorders like lymphoma. Typically, leishmaniasis displays a granulomatous inflammation interspersed with plasma cells and lymphocytes, which can be mistaken for granulomatous MF [1, 6].

Similarly, varicella zoster virus (VZV) and herpes simplex virus (HSV) infections can also mimic MF. These conditions may present with lymphocyte-rich infiltrates but lack typical herpes virus-induced epithelial changes and have been termed “herpes incognito” [7].

11.3.3 Therapy

As CLH is a benign reactive process, the primary therapeutic objective is to alleviate symptoms and prevent potential complications.

Identification and elimination of the trigger will help to prevent recurrences. In asymptomatic patients or cases where the clinical and histopathological features of CLH are indolent, a conservative approach of observation and regular follow-up may be sufficient. This strategy involves monitoring patients for any changes in the size, appearance, or symptoms of the skin lesions, as well as conducting periodic re-evaluations to exclude the possibility of an underlying malignant process. Especially, the patients who have shown T-cell or B-cell monoclonality in the biopsy should be monitored because it is believed that they may progress and develop a cutaneous lymphoma [5].

Topical or intralesional corticosteroids can be effective in reducing pruritus, erythema, and induration. In some cases, topical calcineurin inhibitors (e.g., tacrolimus, pimecrolimus) may be employed as an alternative or adjuvant to corticosteroids, particularly in patients with contraindications or side effects to corticosteroid therapy. For localized, persistent, or cosmetically unacceptable CLH lesions, surgical excision may be considered.

Radiotherapy can be employed as an adjuvant or alternative to surgery in cases where complete excision is not feasible or in patients with contraindications to surgery.

In patients with disseminated lesions, systemic therapy with hydroxychloroquine, methotrexate, or azathioprine has been utilized.

References

1. Mitteldorf C, Kempf W. Cutaneous pseudolymphoma—a review on the spectrum and a proposal for a new classification. J Cutan Pathol. 2020;47:76–97.
2. Khalil S, Donthi D, Gru AA. Cutaneous reactive B-cell lymphoid proliferations. J Cutan Pathol. 2022;49:898–916.
3. Berglund J, Eitrem R, Ornstein K, Lindberg A, Ringér A, Elmrud H, et al. An epidemiologic study of lyme disease in southern Sweden. N Engl J Med. 1995;333:1319–27.
4. Schöllkopf C, Melbye M, Munksgaard L, Smedby KE, Rostgaard K, Glimelius B, et al. Borrelia infection and risk of non-Hodgkin lymphoma. Blood. 2008;111:5524–9.
5. Sarantopoulos GP, Palla B, Said J, Kinney MC, Swerdlow SM, Willemze R, et al. Mimics of cutaneous lymphoma: report of the 2011 Society for Hematopathology/European Association for Haematopathology Workshop. Am J Clin Pathol. 2013;139:536–51.
6. Tomasini C, Moneghini L, Barbui AM. Chronic amastigote-negative cutaneous leishmaniasis: a clinical, histopathologic and molecular study of 27 cases with emphasis on atypical and pseudolymphomatous presentations. J Cutan Pathol. 2017;44:530–7.
7. Böer A, Herder N, Blödorn-Schlicht N, Falk T. Herpes incognito most commonly is herpes zoster and its histopathologic pattern is distinctive! Am J Dermatopathol. 2006;28:181–6.

12 Histiocytoses

Robert Gniadecki, Minakshi Taparia, Jean Deschenes, Jori Hardin, and Etienne Mahe

The histiocytoses are hyperproliferations of dendritic cells or macrophages. Histiocytoses are currently classified into five groups (L, C, H, M, R groups) reflecting histopathological features and the cell of origin. Table 12.1 provides a simplified overview of histiocytoses, including those disease entities that are most commonly associated with skin manifestations [1].

R. Gniadecki (✉)
Division of Dermatology, University of Alberta, Edmonton, AB, Canada
e-mail: gniadeck@ualberta.ca

M. Taparia
Division of Hematology, University of Alberta Hospital, Edmonton, AB, Canada

J. Deschenes
Department of Pathology and Laboratory Medicine, Cross Cancer Institute, Edmonton, AB, Canada
e-mail: Jean.Deschenes@albertaprecisionlabs.ca

J. Hardin
Division of Dermatology, University of Calgary, Calgary, AB, Canada
e-mail: Jori.hardin@albertahealthservices.ca

E. Mahe
Department of Pathology & Laboratory Medicine, and Hematology & Hematological Malignancies, University of Calgary, Calgary, AB, Canada
e-mail: etienne.mahe@albertaprecisionlabs.ca

12.1 Langerhans Cell Histiocytosis

12.1.1 Practice Essentials

- LCH is a clonal proliferation of Langerhans cells in various organs with frequent involvement of the skin.
- Isolated skin involvement is seen in 10% of adult patients.
- The most common cutaneous manifestations are eroded papules or plaques on the face or in intertriginous areas, but skin signs are pleiotropic and not specific.
- LCH may be associated with secondary hematological and solid cancers.

Langerhans cell histiocytosis (LCH) is a rare disorder characterized by the clonal proliferation of Langerhans cells in various tissues and organs, including the skin. LCH is included among the "L-group" of the revised classification of histiocytic disorders and is grouped along with Erdheim-Chester disease (ECD) [1].

LCH is further subclassified based on the organ involvement and association with other malignancies:

- Single system LCH: In this type of LCH, the disease is limited to a single organ or system, such as the skin, bone, or lungs. Isolated skin involvement with LCH in adults is uncommon

R. Gniadecki et al. (eds.), *Diseases of Blood and Skin*, https://doi.org/10.1007/978-3-031-65292-9_12

Table 12.1 Classification of histiocytoses associated with skin manifestations

Group	Disease		Main skin manifestations
L group (Langerhans cell and indeterminate histiocytoses)	Langerhans cell	LCH with isolated skin involvement	Ulcerated papules and plaques
		Multisystem LCH with organ involvement	
		LCH associated with myeloproliferative disorder	
	Erdheim-Chester disease	Erdheim-Chester disease (ECD)	Palpebral xanthoma-like lesions, often symmetric
	Mixed LCH/ECD	Mimics LCH, ECD or both	Features of both LCH (about 60% of patients) and ECD (about 35% of patients)
		ECD rarely follows LCH, but either precedes or happens concurrently	
	Indeterminate cell histiocytosis	Most commonly isolated cutaneous disease in healthy adults	Pleomorphic
		But rare pediatric cases and rare cases with bone or eye involvement	Pink-red papules or nodules Unifocal, or disseminated without Accompanying pain, pruritus or mucosal finding
C-group (cutaneous and mucocutaneous)	Xanthogranulomas primarily localized in the skin	Adult xanthogranuloma (AXG)	Solitary yellowish nodule or plaque
		Generalized eruptive histiocytosis (GEH)	Numerous flesh-color or red macules
		Progressive nodular histiocytosis (PNH)	Numerous superficial lesions similar to GEH and deep, fibrotic lesions
	Cutaneous histiocytoses with significant systemic involvement	XD (Xanthoma disseminatum)	Disseminated brown papules and nodules on the flexor surfaces and around the eyes
		Necrobiotic xanthogranuloma (NXG)	Indurated xanthomatous plaques with ulceration and telangiectasias
	Multicentric reticulohistiocytosis (MRC)		"Coral beads" red, papular lesions on the dorsal hands and face
R-group	Cutaneous Rosai-Dorfman disease (RDD)[a]		Painless nodules and papules on the torso, head, and neck
	Systemic Rosai-Dorfman disease	Nodal classical RDD with skin involvement	
		Extranodal RDD	
		Neoplasia-associated RDD	
		Immune disease-associated RDD	

(continued)

Table 12.1 (continued)

Group	Disease		Main skin manifestations
H-group (hemophagocytic syndrome)	Primary HLH (Hemophagocytic lymphohistiocytosis)	HLH due to monogenic mutations	Nonspecific rash, exanthem, panniculitis
	Secondary HLH	HLH induced by infection	
		Malignancy-associated HLH	
		HLH associated with autoimmune diseases	
M-group (malignant histiocytoses, MH)	Primary cutaneous malignant histiocytosis		Tumors
	Primary MH	Primary MH of the bone, lymph node, digestive system, CNS, or other	
	Secondary MH	MH due to leukemia, lymphoma, or other hematological malignancy	

[a]Cutaneous RDD is sometimes included in the C-group

(5–10% of all LCH cases) and tends to occur more commonly as part of multisystem disease (20–50%).

- Multisystem LCH that affects two or more organs or systems in the body. The most common organs involved in multisystem LCH are the bones, skin, and lymph nodes, but it can also affect the liver, spleen, lungs, and other organs.
- LCH associated with myeloproliferative disorder/myelodysplastic syndrome.

Twenty percent (20%) of patients with ECD also have LCH lesions, both diseases have clonal mutations involving the mitogen-activated protein kinase (MAPK) pathway in more than 80% of cases, and they both share similar clinical manifestations, such as diabetes insipidus or neurodegenerative diseases. It will then come as no surprise that LCH can coexist with ECD. Such cases are classified as mixed histiocytoses (i.e., characterized by the presence of both Langerhans and non-Langerhans cells) [1].

12.1.2 Clinical Manifestations

12.1.2.1 Skin Manifestations

The disease most frequently manifests during early childhood, although it is worth noting that new cases can emerge in adults, constituting up to 10% of total occurrences. The cutaneous symptoms are quite variable. Among the most prevalent are erythematous papules, which may sometimes be accompanied by vesicles that can evolve into a central crust or erosion. These skin lesions are commonly found on the scalp, face, trunk, and extremities and can either be solitary or multiple. Areas prone to friction or rubbing, such as the groin, inner thighs, and genital region, are often characteristic locations for these lesions (Fig. 12.1).

In more severe instances, these skin lesions may progress to ulceration and secondary infection. Moreover, in extreme cases, the lesions can coalesce to form large, scaly, or eroded plaques. While it is exceedingly rare, mucosal involvement has been documented [2]. Nails may occasionally be involved, showing pustular lesions, longitudinal grooving and splitting of the nail, hyperkeratosis, onycholysis, or paronychia [3].

12.1.2.2 Other Manifestations

The distribution and severity of skin lesions in LCH can vary widely depending on the individual and the subtype of the disease. Some common systemic manifestations of LCH include:

- Bone involvement: bone pain, swelling, and fractures.
- Pulmonary involvement: cough, shortness of breath, and chest pain. Pulmonary involve-

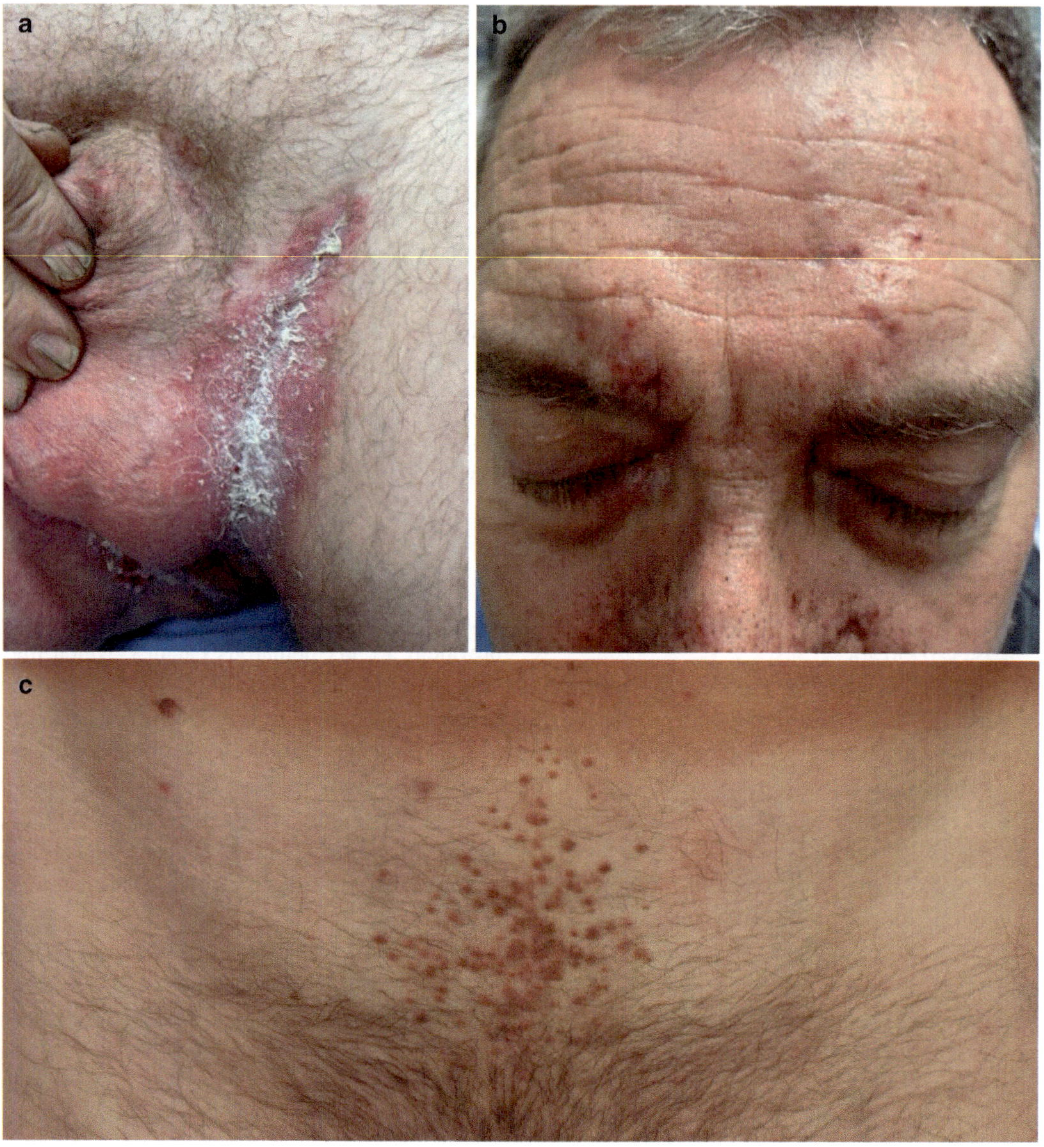

Fig. 12.1 Langerhans cell histiocytosis of the skin. (**a**) Infiltrated plaque in the perianal area. Note nail dystrophy, which may accompany cutaneous LCH. (**b**) Erosive papules on the face. (**c**) Confluent, scaly papules in the genital area

ment can result in lung nodules, cysts, and fibrosis, with lung function impairment.

- Liver and spleen: hepatomegaly and/or splenomegaly, cysts, fibrosis.
- Lymph nodes: enlargement of lymph nodes, particularly in the neck and groin areas.
- Central nervous system: headaches, seizures, neurologic deficits, and behavioral changes.
- Endocrine manifestations: pituitary (diabetes insipidus), thyroid gland, and adrenal glands.
- Concomitant cancer: Numerous studies consistently demonstrated a higher prevalence of additional cancers in LCH, such as myeloid and myeloproliferative neoplasms, lymphomas and solid organ malignancies, particularly lung and thyroid cancer [2].

12.1.3 Histopathology and Molecular Features

In the biopsy specimen, the presence of neoplastic Langerhans cells is identified by their unique "coffee-bean" or "folded-paper" morphology, attributed to intracytoplasmic Birbeck granules. Alongside these Langerhans cells, other immune cells, like T cells and eosinophils, are often part of the infiltrate.

Immunohistochemical staining confirms the positivity of the atypical cells for CD1a, S-100, CD207 (langerin, associated with Birbeck granules), Cyclin D1 and CD68, but negative for CD163 and OCT-2 in the vast majority of cases [4].

Genetic investigations have revealed that up to 80% of Langerhans cell histiocytosis cases show mutually exclusive, clonal somatic mutations that result in constitutive activation of the MAPK pathway, specifically the RAS-RAF-MEK-ERK cascade. The most commonly identified mutation involves *BRAF* V600E, noted overall in 55–60% of cases, and especially common in patients with cutaneous involvement (estimated at 75% of cases). In cases negative for *BRAF* mutations, other mutations, most commonly *MAP2K1* [1], but also *ARAF*, *NRAS*, and *KRAS*, as well as alternative *BRAF* mutations have also been noted in these neoplasms [4]. Next-generation sequencing (NGS) may be considered to ascertain the mutational status of the MAPK pathway for a given lesion and confirm the potential efficacy of BRAF or MEK inhibitors. One should remember that these somatic abnormalities are also identified in ECD, Rosai-Dorfman(-Destombes) disease, juvenile xanthogranuloma, as well as other histiocytic and non-histiocytic neoplasms.

Histopathological features of LCH may display similarities with other histiocytic disorders such as ECD, Rosai-Dorfman disease (RDD), or juvenile xanthogranuloma (Table 12.2). These similarities may manifest in the same biopsy or appear in biopsies obtained from different anatomical locations [2]. Given that mutations in the MAPK pathway are observed across these disorders, some researchers propose that these diseases could be different manifestations originating from a common precursor cell undergoing various differentiation processes.

Table 12.2 Immunohistochemical differentiation between LCH, ECD, and RDD

Marker	LCH	ECD	RDD[a]
CD68	+[b]	+	+
CD163	(−)[c]	+	+[d]
CD1a	+	(−)	(−)
CD207 (Langerin)	+	(−)	(−)
Factor XIIIa	(−)	+	−/+[e]
S100	+	−/+[f]	+
Cyclin D1	+	+/−	+
OCT2	(−)[c]	(−)	+

[a]CD68 has a dot-like discrete staining pattern in LCH
[b]May be focally positive for CD30 and have abundant IgG4+ plasma cells
[c]A small (less than 10%) subset of LCH may be positive for CD163 and OCT2
[d]About 10% of RDD are negative for CD163
[e]S-100 is positive in about 20–30% of ECD disease
[f]About 30% of RDD diseases are positive for Factor XIII a

12.1.4 Workup

For patients who initially present with skin lesions histopathologically diagnosed as LCH, the initial workup includes *BRAF* mutation status (ideally, MAPK pathway analysis by NGS should be considered for *BRAF* wild-type cases) and whole body PET/CT scan to rule out systemic involvement (Table 12.3).

Other investigations depend on the individual symptoms and signs. MRI can be considered to rule out CNS and pituitary lesions. Bone marrow biopsy is usually performed in patients with cytopenias. Endoscopy to rule out gastrointestinal involvement in patients with evidence of malabsorption.

12.1.5 Differential Diagnosis

The differential diagnosis of cutaneous LCH includes several other conditions that can present with similar skin lesions. Besides the possibility of other histiocytic lesions that may involve the

Table 12.3 Suggested initial workup in patients with LCH

Blood work	
	Complete blood count with differential count
	Metabolic panel including electrolytes
	Liver and kidney function test
	C-reactive protein
	Hormonal assessment: TSH, free T4, morning serum cortisol
	Serum osmolarity
	Lipid profile
Urine	
	Urinalysis
	Morning urine osmolarity
Genetic	
	BRAF-V600 genotype in lesional tissue
	Consider next-generation sequencing for BRAF negative cases
Imaging	
	PET/CT imaging

skin, some of the common differential diagnoses include:

- Inflammatory dermatoses: Skin lesions in LCH can resemble those seen in other inflammatory dermatoses, such as psoriasis, eczema, and lichen planus. Facial LCH can resemble actinic keratoses or rosacea.
- Skin infections: intertrigo, tinea, candidiasis.
- Skin malignancies, e.g., extramammary Paget disease, actinic keratoses, squamous cell carcinoma.

12.1.6 Treatment

The management of cutaneous LCH is tailored to the specific circumstances of the patient, considering factors like the severity and extent of the disease as well as any systemic manifestations. While some isolated cases of cutaneous LCH may resolve on their own without medical intervention, more aggressive or symptomatic forms often necessitate treatment.

For localized skin lesions, skin-directed therapies are typically the first line of treatment. These can include topical corticosteroids, phototherapy modalities like narrow-band UVB and PUVA, and in some instances, superficial radiation therapy delivered in doses of 10–20 Gy [2, 5]. For lesions that are ulcerated, disfiguring, or refractory to other modalities, surgical intervention may be contemplated.

In instances where multiple skin lesions are present, systemic methotrexate, often administered in doses of 20 mg weekly, can be an effective option.

For patients with systemic manifestations of LCH, a more aggressive treatment regimen is usually warranted, following established guidelines (e.g., [6]). This may entail chemotherapy combinations that include agents like vinblastine, methotrexate, and cytarabine. Moreover, targeted therapies like imatinib and BRAF inhibitors may also be indicated in specific instances where molecular alterations are identified in LCH cells.

12.2 Erdheim-Chester Disease (ECD)

12.2.1 Practice Essentials

- ECD is a rare, potentially lethal histiocytosis with frequent multiorgan involvement, especially the bone
- Peak occurrence in middle-aged males
- Eyelid xanthelasma is the major cutaneous manifestation

Although ECD may coexist with LCH, belonging to the same family of L-group histiocytoses, and though, in general, it shares with LCH a spectrum of clonal MAPK pathway activating mutations (also identified in both instances in the $CD34^+$ hematopoietic progenitors), they are very distinct clinically and histopathologically. We still do not understand the mechanisms that explain the various clinical presentations and the histopathological variance for either LCH or ECD as they develop in individual patients [4]. The identification of a pathogenic mutation in the MAPK or PI3K pathways is paramount in establishing a diagnosis of ECD, given the rather nonspecific histopathological features.

12.2.2 Clinical Manifestations

The average age at which ECD is diagnosed falls between 55 and 60 years, with males being disproportionately affected—exhibiting a threefold higher incidence compared to females. The disease is multisystemic, most frequently affecting the skeletal system—osteosclerosis is observed in over 90% of patients. In addition, cardiovascular involvement is noted in approximately half of the patients, while retroperitoneal fibrosis occurs in around 30%.

Dermatological manifestations are comparatively less frequent, occurring in fewer than 20% of ECD patients. However, it's important to note that skin involvement can sometimes be the predominant clinical feature leading to an eventual diagnosis of the disease. The most frequent cutaneous presentation is xanthelasma of the eyelids in approximately 25% of patients with cutaneous ECD. These eyelid xanthelasmas can often be quite pronounced, extending into the deeper orbital (intraconal) soft tissues and resulting in exophthalmos [7]. While extraorbital xanthelasmas are relatively rare, they have nonetheless been reported in the medical literature. Otherwise, the lesions may be relatively unspecific, such as ulcerated papules and nodules (Fig. 12.2).

12.2.3 Workup and Diagnosis

12.2.3.1 Histopathology and Molecular Diagnosis

Biopsy is necessary for the diagnosis of ECD. Skin biopsy shows foamy mononucleated histiocytes, multinucleated histiocytes, and Touton cells. ECD histiocytes are positive for CD68, CD163, and factor XIIIa, but negative for CD1a and CD207 (Table 12.2). Approximately 20% of patients with ECD also have LCH lesions, and the histopathological features of LCH and ECD may coexist in the same biopsy (ECD/LCH overlap). Unfortunately, neither the morphological features nor the IHC profile are entirely specific for ECD and will be observed in other cutaneous xanthogranulomatous lesions, although certainly, they help in distinguishing ECD from LCH and RDD. Besides histopathology, the diagnosis rests on typical clinical features and molecular profiles.

Molecular testing for BRAF (as a first initial step) is required in cases of suspected ECD. Approximately 50–55% of ECD patients have *BRAF* V600E mutations, but V600E mutations are more frequent in patients with cutaneous involvement (76%), and almost always found in xanthelasma-like lesions [8]. Patients who are V600E negative may have mutations in *MAP2K1*, *NRAS*, *KRAS*, and *ARAF* which require NGS sequencing. A minority of patients may have ALK translocation reminiscent of anaplastic lymphomas, and therefore ALK immunohistochemistry has been suggested as a part of the standard workup in patients with ECD or other progressive histiocytoses who are *BRAF* V600E and *MAP2K1* negative [1].

12.2.3.2 Imaging

PET with 18F-fluorodeoxyglucose (FDG) combined with CT has been shown to have high specificity for detecting skeletal changes and retroperitoneal fibrosis. FDG-PET scanning is more useful in follow-up than in the initial assessment of patients with ECD [9]. Heart MRI has been suggested in all patients to rule out cardiac involvement [10, 11]. Brain MRI is indicated in patients with neurological symptoms.

In patients with eyelid xanthelasmas, a CT scan of the face is recommended to assess the involvement of the orbit.

12.2.4 Differential Diagnosis

Eyelid xanthelasmas are often benign and commonly encountered in individuals suffering from hypercholesterolemia, diabetes, or thyroid dysfunction. They are seldom subjected to biopsy. When examined pathologically, these lesions are characterized by large, benign histiocytes loaded with lipids in the dermal layer. These histiocytes typically stain positive for CD68 but are negative for S100. Notably, Touton cells are absent, and there is a lack of an inflammatory infiltrate. However, biopsy should be considered in cases

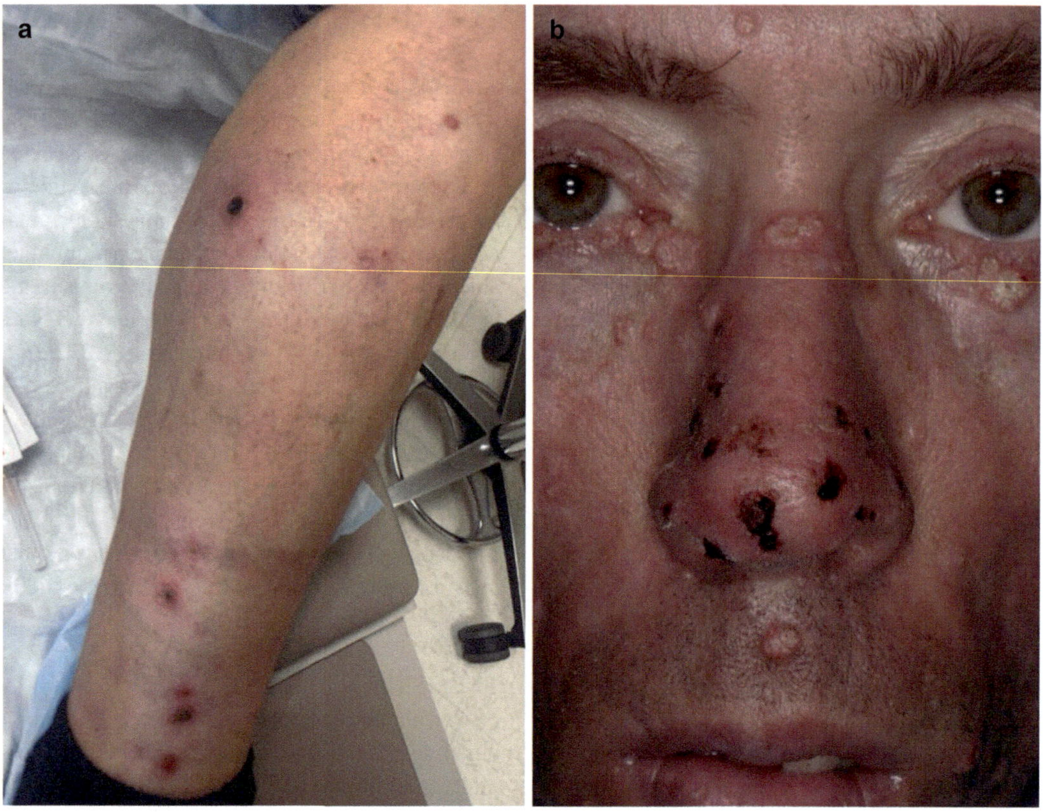

Fig. 12.2 Erdheim-Chester disease. (**a**) Ulcerated papules on the lower extremities. (**b**) Ulcerated lesions on the nose and yellowish papules on the face

Table 12.4 Differential diagnosis of eyelid xanthomas

Disease type	Clinical features
Erdheim-Chester disease	Thick, edematous plaques. Frequent involvement of the orbit. Ulceration is rare. Poor prognosis
Benign eyelid xanthoma	Thin plaques without infiltration in the deeper tissues. No functional impairment
Orbital xanthogranuloma	Clinically similar to ECD. Good prognosis
Necrobiotic xanthogranuloma	Involvement of anterior orbit, often fibrotic and ulcerated lesions. Poor prognosis due to frequent association with hematological cancers (lymphoma, multiple myeloma), and with paraproteinemia
Asthma-associated xanthogranuloma	Anterior orbit, association with asthma, frequent cervical lymphadenopathy. Good prognosis
IgG4 disease	Plaques resembling xanthomas or xanthogranulomas. Retroperitoneal fibrosis

where middle-aged or older individuals suddenly develop prominent xanthelasma, especially when accompanied by additional ophthalmological signs.

Eyelid xanthelasmas can also be observed in other types of histiocytic disorders. These include adult-onset xanthogranuloma, adult-onset asthma accompanied by periocular xanthogranuloma, and necrobiotic xanthogranuloma (Table 12.4) [12]. Therefore, a thorough histopathological differential diagnosis is crucial, particularly when these lesions present in an unusual manner or unexpected patient demographics.

12.2.5 Therapy

There is no consensus regarding the treatment of eyelid lesions. Intralesional corticosteroids, surgical excision, evaporation with CO_2 laser, and radiotherapy have been described as successful in case series. For edematous, bulky lesions, systemic prednisone in combination with methotrexate as a steroid-sparing agent was shown to be effective, although relapses after cessation of therapy are frequent.

Systemic treatment of patients with ECD should follow the current therapeutic guidelines.

12.3 C-Group Histiocytoses Primarily Affecting the Skin: AXG, GEH, PNH

Xanthogranulomas, the most common diseases within the C-group, comprise the histiocytoses with the primary cutaneous manifestations. The three main disease entities are adult xanthogranuloma (AXG), generalized eruptive histiocytosis (GEH), and progressive nodular histiocytosis (PNH).

12.3.1 Practice Essentials

- AXG, GEH, and PNH are non-Langerhans cell histiocytoses, mainly localized in the skin.
- Cutaneous manifestations include papules and nodules with yellow to brown hue.
- Good prognosis, rare extracutaneous dissemination.

12.3.2 Clinical and Histopathological Features

AXG typically manifests as an isolated nodule with flesh-colored, yellow, or brownish hues. Clinically, these lesions are rather nondescript, which frequently necessitates their biopsy or surgical removal for definitive diagnosis. This diagnosis is ultimately confirmed by histopathological examination. Histopathologically, the lesions are characterized by a unique cellular composition that includes foamy cells, giant cells, and Touton cells, along with a mixture of macrophages, lymphocytes, and eosinophils. In more chronic or older lesions, fibrotic changes may also be evident.

GEH, on the other hand, shares histological similarities with AXG but sets itself apart clinically. Specifically, GEH presents with multiple macules and papules, displaying a range of colors from skin-toned to red and even brown.

PNH is another distinct entity, primarily affecting individuals in their 60s. Similar to GEH patients, those with PNH also develop a multitude of skin lesions. However, PNH lesions are generally deeper and exhibit a more fibrous texture. It is worth noting that these lesions can also occasionally extend to involve the oral and conjunctival mucosal surfaces. Remarkably, spontaneous regression of skin lesions can occur after years, contributing to the complexity of managing this condition.

12.3.3 Clinical Differential Diagnosis

Solitary lesions characteristic of AXG may be mistaken for dermatofibromas or other benign connective tissue tumors, which sometimes results in them not being biopsied for further evaluation. In terms of histopathological differential diagnosis, these lesions could also be confused with Spitz nevi. Fortunately, the distinction is readily made by histopathological examination and associated phenotype.

For GEH and PNH, a definitive diagnosis is typically secured through biopsy findings. Further differentiation from other forms of non-Langerhans cell histiocytoses is achieved through meticulous clinicopathological correlation and by ruling out systemic involvement. It is crucial to differentiate GEH from eruptive xanthoma which is associated with hyperlipidemia. Additionally, infections caused by atypical mycobacteria, *Leishmania*, and *Mycobacterium leprae* should also be excluded from the list of potential diagnoses.

12.3.4 Workup and Diagnosis

For patients who are asymptomatic and present with a solitary AXG lesion, additional investigations are generally not necessary.

When dealing with multiple lesions in cases of GEH and PNH, distinguishing these conditions from other types of histiocytoses like xanthoma disseminatum (XD), as well as from secondary infectious granulomas, can be particularly challenging. As part of the diagnostic workup, it is advisable to order blood tests, including a lipid profile, to rule out any underlying hyperlipidemia. Age-appropriate cancer screening, which includes serum electrophoresis, should also be conducted to exclude the possibility of monoclonal gammopathies.

If the diagnosis remains uncertain, a skin biopsy should be examined and cultured for the presence of infectious agents such as mycobacteria and Leishmania. The need for any further investigations would then be determined based on the individual patient's presenting symptoms and clinical signs.

12.3.5 Treatment

There is no consensus regarding the therapy of C-group histiocytoses. Solitary lesions of AXG are usually surgically removed. The disseminated forms, GEH and PHN are therapeutically challenging. Case reports suggest evidence of phototherapy and prednisone with methotrexate. Kinase inhibitors (cobimetinib, regorafenib) may be spectacularly successful in patients with *BRAF* or *MAPK* mutations [13–15].

12.4 C-Group Histiocytoses with Frequent Systemic Involvement: Xanthoma Disseminatum (XD), Necrobiotic Xanthogranuloma (NXG), and Multicentric Reticulohistiocytosis (MRH)

12.4.1 Practice Essentials

- XD and NXG are cutaneous C-group histiocytoses, frequently affecting other organs.
- XD presents as disseminated skin papules and nodules and is associated with diabetes insipidus in 40% of cases.
- NXG manifests as an ulcerated plaque and is co-morbid with monoclonal gammopathies and multiple myeloma.
- MRH displays "coral bead" periungual plaques and is associated with destructive arthritis.

12.4.2 Clinical Features

Even though XD, NXG, and MRH are collectively categorized as C-group histiocytoses, their clinical presentations can be markedly different (Table 12.1, Fig. 12.3).

XD commonly affects young men and presents with multiple yellow or brown papules and nodules. These lesions are typically situated in the flexor regions of the extremities as well as in the periocular area of the face. In approximately 50% of cases, mucosal involvement is also observed. A noteworthy complication is the frequent involvement of the pituitary gland, leading to diabetes insipidus in as many as 40% of affected individuals [1].

NXG lesions are most often seen in the periocular region and display a range of characteris-

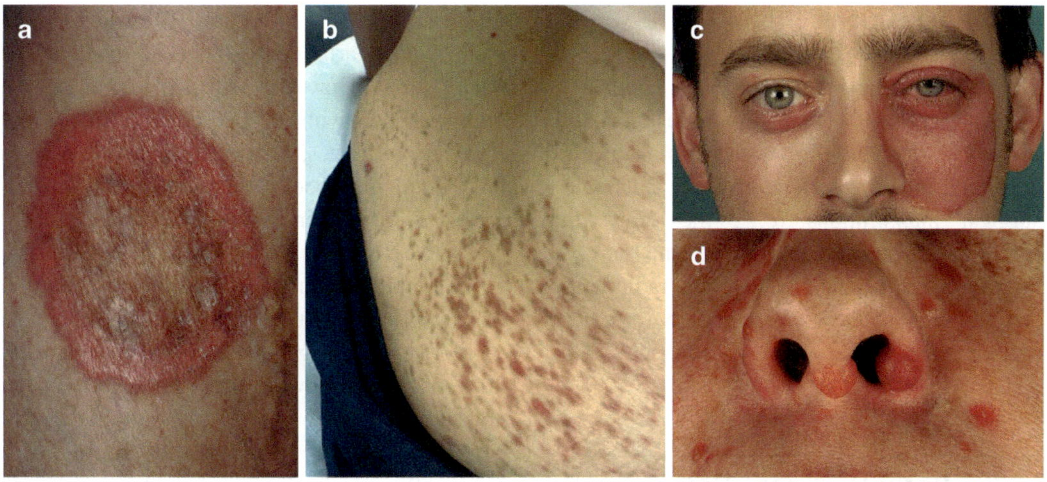

Fig. 12.3 Clinical spectrum of C-group histiocytosis. (**a**) Adult xanthogranuloma (AXG) presenting as a plaque on the arm. (**b**) Generalized eruptive histiocytosis (GEH) with multiple papules on the trunk. (**c**) Necrobiotic xanthogranulonma in the periorbital area. (**d**) Xanthoma disseminatum (XD) presenting as polymorphic yellow papules on the face

tics, from fibrotic and ulcerated to edematous plaques. Their color can vary from yellowish hues to purplish tones. Frequently, NXG lesions are accompanied by scarring and telangiectasias, adding complexity to their clinical presentation.

The patient demographic for MRH skews toward middle-aged and elderly women. The skin manifestations are widespread, but a key diagnostic indicator is the occurrence of destructive arthritis, predominantly affecting the distal joints of the fingers. Skin lesions manifest as papules and nodules, often concentrated around the nails on the distal fingers, creating a distinctive "coral bead" sign. Oral or nasal mucosa involvement is reported in approximately 50% of the cases. Furthermore, individuals with MRH exhibit a heightened incidence of both cancer and autoimmune diseases.

12.4.3 Workup and Diagnosis

The diagnosis of XD, NXG, and MRH is primarily established through a blend of clinical observations and pathological findings.

In MRH, the histopathological examination reveals oncocytic histiocytes and multinucleated giant cells featuring eosinophilic, ground-glass-like cytoplasm, with scant Touton giants. These cells are typically PAS positive and immunoreactive for CD68, CD163, and lysozyme, and Factor XIIIa may be positive in multiple lesions. They do not usually show positivity for S100 or Langerhans cell markers such as CD207 and CD1a. On the other hand, XD and NXG histopathology often shows the presence of Touton giant cells, accompanied by a more prominent lymphocytic and plasmacytic inflammatory infiltrate. Notably, necrosis and ulceration are especially more frequent in NXG cases.

Differentiating these entities from GEH and PNH can be challenging and is often feasible only after systemic involvement has been ruled out.

The following investigations should be considered:

- Blood work, including lipid profile, electrolytes, plasma, and urine osmolarity
- Antinuclear antibodies, rheumatoid factor to rule out autoimmunity
- Serum and urine electrophoresis to rule out monoclonal gammopathy
- Age-appropriate cancer screening
- X-ray of the hands and any symptomatic joint to rule out bone lesions

12.4.4 Treatment

Therapeutic options depend on the number and localization of the lesions. Single lesions can be excised or treated with intradermal injections of corticosteroids. Lesions in areas not amenable to surgical interventions (e.g., the orbit) may respond to systemic therapy with methotrexate, interferon α, plasmapheresis, or radiotherapy [16]. MRH has been described to respond to methotrexate, JAK inhibitors, and anti-TNF-α agents [17–19].

12.5 Rosai-Dorfman(-Destombes) Disease (RDD)

12.5.1 Practice Essentials

- Non-LCH ($S100^+$, $CD68^+$, $CD1a^-$, $CD207^-$) involving often skin and the lymph nodes, and associated with signs of systemic inflammation.
- There are five major clinical forms: familial, classical (nodal), skin only, extranodal, and RDD associated with another inflammatory or neoplastic disease.
- Cutaneous manifestations are painless nodules with a predilection to the torso and the head and neck region.

12.5.2 Clinical Features

The clinical presentation of RDD varies depending on its form. In its classic manifestation, RDD is typified by painless cervical lymphadenopathy, often accompanied by systemic inflammatory signs such as fever, weight loss, fatigue, elevated erythrocyte sedimentation rate (ESR), polyclonal hypergammaglobulinemia, and elevated ferritin levels. Though cervical lymph nodes are the primary site of involvement, other lymph node groups like axillary and inguinal nodes can also be affected, albeit less commonly.

Skin involvement occurs in approximately 50% of patients. The cutaneous lesions are diverse but generally manifest as painless nodules or non-ulcerated tumors. These tend to be localized primarily on the torso and the head and neck regions. However, virtually any part of the body can be involved. The coloration of these skin lesions varies, ranging from violaceous to the natural skin tone, particularly when the infiltration is situated in the deeper skin layers [20] (Fig. 12.4).

Extranodal, extracutaneous involvement is observed in about 40% of RDD cases, affecting a wide range of organ systems. Approximately 20% of cases show multisystem involvement, and the number of affected sites has a negative correlation with the patient's prognosis. Frequently involved sites outside the lymph nodes include the upper respiratory tract, manifesting as rhinosinusitis, and the orbit, where symptoms like proptosis and periorbital edema may occur. Osteolytic lesions can also be present in the bones.

RDD has been associated with other medical conditions, both inflammatory and neoplastic. Some of the most commonly associated conditions include:

- IgG4-related disease
- Hematological malignancies like various forms of leukemias, lymphomas, and myelodysplastic syndromes
- Other histiocytic disorders, such as LCH or ECD
- Systemic lupus erythematosus
- Autoimmune hemolytic anemia
- HIV infection

12.5.3 Workup and Diagnosis

12.5.3.1 Skin Biopsy

The histopathology of RDD) is distinct and can offer a definitive diagnosis in many cases. Histiocytes in RDD usually have enlarged hyperchromatic nuclei and abundant eosinophilic cytoplasm. One of the hallmark features is emperipolesis, a phenomenon where histiocytes engulf intact inflammatory cells like lymphocytes, without destroying them. The biopsy may also show associated fibrosis and a prominent inflammatory infiltrate that typically includes

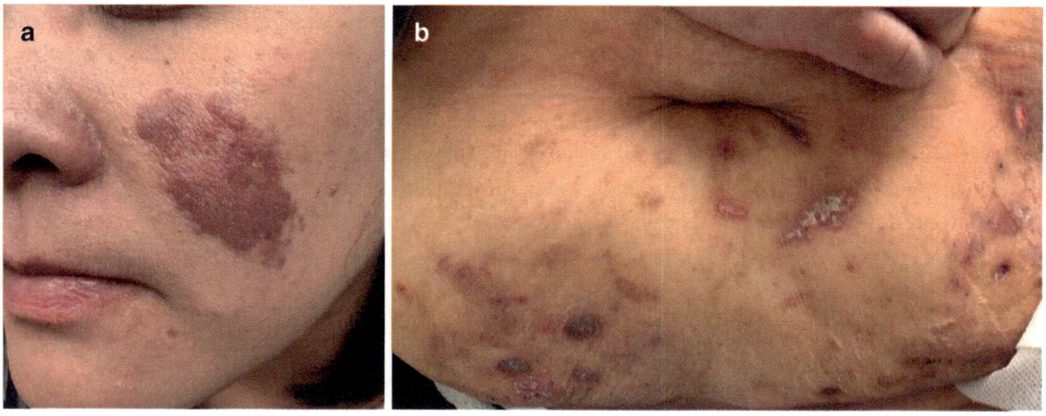

Fig. 12.4 Skin lesions in Rosai-Dorfman disease. (**a**) A well-demarcated, purple, infiltrated plaque on the cheek. (**b**) Relative nonspecific, polymorphic papular, and ulcerative lesions on the abdomen

plasma cells and lymphocytes. IHC studies, in typical cases with no overlap with ECD or LCH, confirm expression of CD68, CD163, S100, OCT2 and no expression of CD1a (in most), CD207, CD21, CD23, or CD35. Of note, CD30 may be focally positive in a subset of cases.

Interestingly, the plasma cells often test positive for IgG4; if they are abundant, this should prompt further evaluation to rule out IgG4-related disease (see below, [21]).

Molecularly, while the *BRAF* V600E mutation is quite rare in RDD, mutations in genes like *KRAS*, *NRAS*, and *MAP2K1* have been reported in approximately a third of cases, especially noncutaneous, head and neck cases. NGS is considered for cases that are refractory to standard therapy or in those involving multiple organs to provide further diagnostic and therapeutic guidance [22].

RDD can have clinical and histopathological features overlapping with other histiocytic disorders, particularly LCH and ECD. Detailed differentiation between these diseases often requires a comprehensive approach, incorporating clinical presentation, imaging studies, and histopathological findings (Table 12.2).

12.5.3.2 Laboratory Investigations and Imaging

Imaging and systemic evaluations are indispensable for formulating an accurate prognosis and determining the appropriate therapeutic approach in RDD. RDD confined to the skin is generally considered benign and often classified as a C-group histiocytosis. Nevertheless, the risk for complications and a less favorable prognosis escalates considerably when there is extranodal or multiorgan involvement. For these more complex cases, a diagnostic workup akin to that recommended for LCH may be employed.

The presence of IgG4-positive plasma cells in the biopsy tissue may raise concerns for a potential underlying IgG4-related disease (IgG4-RD), especially given that the pathogenesis of RDD remains somewhat elusive. At this point, there is no conclusive evidence that the two disorders are pathogenetically related. It is a confounding issue, as numerous classic or cutaneous-only RDD patients display IgG4 positivity on histological examination and IgG4-positive plasma cells are especially abundant in cases involving the liver, lungs, or colon. However, for most of these patients, blood IgG4 levels are not concurrently elevated [21]. Therefore, the IgG4/IgG ratio should be evaluated in all cases with significant IgG4 expression, and most clinical centers will opt to meticulously scrutinize IgG4-positive cases when this ratio exceeds expected values to decisively rule out or confirm IgG4-RD [22].

Although elevated serum levels of IgG4 bolster the diagnosis of IgG4-RD, normal levels do not definitively exclude the disease. Additional clinical parameters such as eosinophilia, as well as biochemical and radiological indicators of liver, kidney, and pancreatic dysfunction, may corroborate a diagnosis of systemic involvement. As part of the comprehensive workup, imaging studies frequently include CT scans, MRI, and PET/CT scans aimed at assessing various organs like the pancreas, bile ducts, salivary glands, kidneys, retroperitoneum, and lungs.

12.5.4 Therapy

Asymptomatic patients with skin-only or classic nodal RDD have a good prognosis, and the purpose of the symptomatic treatment can be sufficient. Options include intralesional corticosteroid injections, low-dose prednisone (0.5–1 mg/kg for 2–3 weeks followed by gradual taper over 2 months) and/or low-dose methotrexate. Other therapies to consider are rituximab and cobimetinib in RDD with mutations of MAPK-ERK pathway [5].

12.6 Malignant Histiocytoses (M-Group)

12.6.1 Practice Essentials

- Malignant histiocytosis is a rare, aggressive cancer derived from the histiocytes.
- Secondary malignant histiocytoses are associated with other hematopoietic malignancies, such as lymphomas and leukemias.
- Skin involvement is rare and clinical features are uncharacteristic, ranging from solitary tumors to disseminated, infiltrative lesions.

12.6.2 Clinical and Histopathological Features

Malignant histiocytosis typically affects the parenchymatous organs (liver, spleen), lymph nodes, and bone marrow and may, in rare cases, involve the skin secondarily. There are case reports of the primary skin malignant histiocytosis (histiocytic sarcoma), but due to the paucity of cases, this entity has not been well defined [23]. Clinically, the skin lesions present as solitary or multiple nodules or tumors, often with ulceration, with a predilection to the head and neck region. Prognosis is unfavorable. The diagnosis relies on immunohistochemistry and is made by excluding other skin tumors with anaplastic morphology, such as lymphoma, malignant melanoma, Merkel cell carcinoma or blastic plasmacytoid dendritic cell tumor.

12.6.3 Therapy

Malignant histiocytosis are aggressive tumors and the optimal treatment is not established.

12.7 HLH

12.7.1 Practice Essentials

- Hemophagocytic lymphohistiocytosis (HLH) is a multiorgan, hyperinflammatory syndrome driven by T-cells and activated macrophages, and develops secondary to cancers, infections, or autoimmune diseases.
- Cardinal manifestations are: fever, cytopenias, hepatosplenomegaly, and hyperferritinemia.
- Skin manifestations are uncharacteristic and comprise morbilliform exanthem, panniculitis, purpuric lesions, or erythroderma.

12.7.2 Clinical Manifestations

Patients with hemophagocytic lymphohistiocytosis (HLH) often present with a clinical picture that closely mimics sepsis. The array of symptoms and signs is extensive and includes persistent fever exceeding 38 °C, hepatosplenomegaly, cytopenias affecting multiple blood cell lines, hypertriglyceridemia, hypofibrinogenemia, and elevated levels of soluble interleukin-2 receptor (sCD25). The complexity of these manifestations often renders the diagnosis of HLH challenging, necessitating a high index of clinical suspicion.

In pediatric populations, HLH can be primary and is frequently attributable to monogenic mutations in genes that regulate cytotoxic T-cell activation (such as FHL2-5, XLP1, RAB27A, LYST), aberrant inflammasome activation (like XLP2, NLRC4), or result from various immunodeficiencies (MAGT1, ITK, CD27, CTPS1, MST1, Dock 8, Dock 2, ORAI1, STIM1, Coroinin1A). Although primary HLH is predominantly observed in pediatric patients, it is worth noting that manifestations can sometimes extend into early adulthood.

On the other hand, in adult patients, HLH is more commonly secondary in nature, arising as a complication of an underlying disease. The most frequent triggers include hematological malignancies, infections (such as HIV, EBV, or even COVID-19), specific immunotherapeutic interventions, and complications post-allogeneic bone marrow transplantation [5].

Cutaneous manifestations are fairly common in HLH but tend to be nonspecific. The skin symptoms can sometimes mimic those observed in infectious diseases and may range from morbilliform exanthems and vasculitic rashes to erythroderma [24, 25]. In some instances, patients might develop more severe skin lesions that resemble panniculitis (Fig. 12.5).

12.7.3 Diagnosis and Treatment

In patients with skin rash, the biopsy is often performed, but its utility is limited. HLH is diagnosed based on the totality of clinical and laboratory findings. Several diagnostic criteria have been proposed [5, 26, 27] but are not properly validated in adult patients. Treatment is a medical emergency and there are several therapeutic protocols available [5].

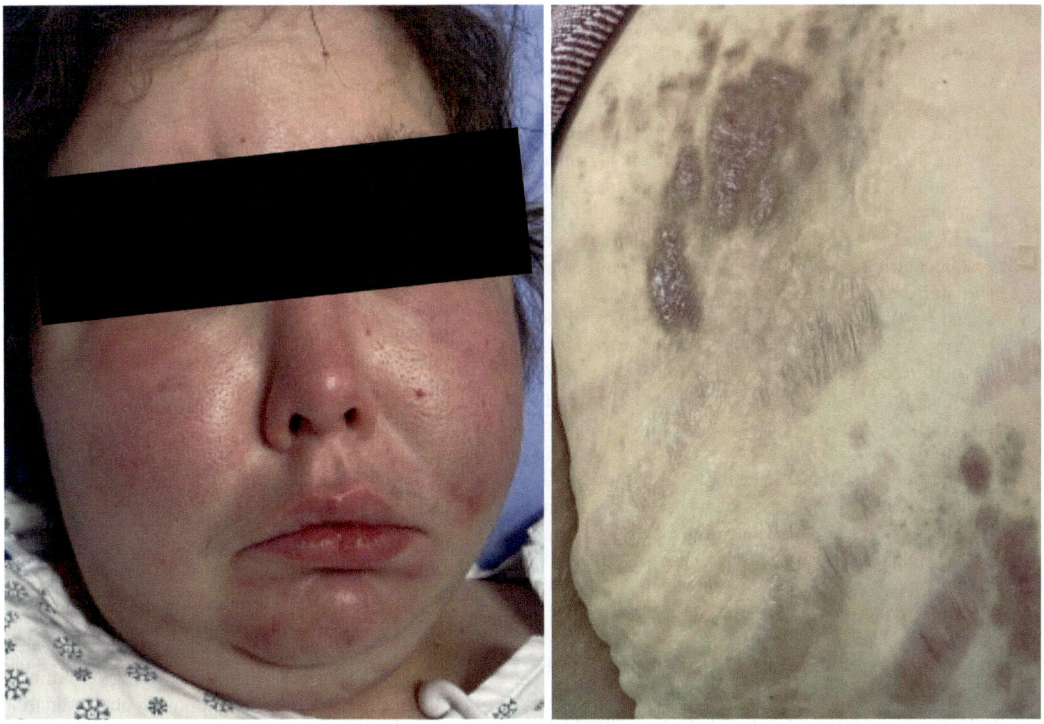

Fig. 12.5 Hemophagocytic lymphohistiocytosis (HLH) in a 31-year-old female with FHL3 gene mutation manifesting as panniculitis on the face and the upper legs. The biopsy from the lesions was consistent with subcutaneous panniculitic T-cell lymphoma (CD3$^+$ CD5$^+$ CD7$^+$ CD2$^+$ CD4$^+$ CD8$^+$, granzyme and TIA-1$^+$. EBER negative, Ki67 positivity in 70% CD8$^+$ cells). Six months after the initial diagnosis, the patient developed fever, hepatosplenomegaly, and hyperferritinemia, which led to the diagnosis of HLH

References

1. Emile J-F, Abla O, Fraitag S, Horne A, Haroche J, Donadieu J, et al. Revised classification of histiocytoses and neoplasms of the macrophage-dendritic cell lineages. Blood. 2016;127:2672–81.
2. Goyal G, Tazi A, Go RS, Rech KL, Picarsic JL, Vassallo R, et al. International expert consensus recommendations for the diagnosis and treatment of Langerhans cell histiocytosis in adults. Blood. 2022;139:2601–21.
3. Figueras-Nart I, Vicente A, Sánchez-Schmidt J, Jou-Muñoz C, Bordas-Orpinell X, Celis-Passini VP, et al. Langerhans cell histiocytosis presenting as fingernail changes. JAAD Case Rep. 2016;2:485–7.
4. McClain KL, Bigenwald C, Collin M, Haroche J, Marsh RA, Merad M, et al. Histiocytic disorders. Nat Rev Dis Primers. 2021;7:73.
5. Salama HA, Jazieh AR, Alhejazi AY, Absi A, Alshieban S, Alzahrani M, et al. Highlights of the management of adult histiocytic disorders: Langerhans cell histiocytosis, Erdheim-Chester disease, Rosai-Dorfman disease, and hemophagocytic lymphohistiocytosis. Clin Lymphoma Myeloma Leuk. 2021;21:e66–75.
6. Girschikofsky M, Arico M, Castillo D, Chu A, Doberauer C, Fichter J, et al. Management of adult patients with Langerhans cell histiocytosis: recommendations from an expert panel on behalf of Euro-Histio-Net. Orphanet J Rare Dis. 2013;8:72.
7. Watermann DF, Kiesewetter F, Frosch PJ. [Skin manifestations of Erdheim-Chester disease. Case report and review of the literature]. Hautarzt. 2001;52:510–7.
8. Chasset F, Barete S, Charlotte F, Cohen-Aubart F, Arnaud L, Le Pelletier F, et al. Cutaneous manifestations of Erdheim-Chester disease (ECD): clinical, pathological, and molecular features in a monocentric series of 40 patients. J Am Acad Dermatol. 2016;74:513–20.
9. Arnaud L, Malek Z, Archambaud F, Kas A, Toledano D, Drier A, et al. 18F-fluorodeoxyglucose-positron emission tomography scanning is more useful in follow-up than in the initial assessment of patients with Erdheim-Chester disease. Arthritis Rheum. 2009;60:3128–38.
10. Haroche J, Cluzel P, Toledano D, Montalescot G, Touitou D, Grenier PA, et al. Images in cardiovascular medicine. Cardiac involvement in Erdheim-Chester disease: magnetic resonance and computed tomographic scan imaging in a monocentric series of 37 patients. Circulation. 2009;119:e597–8.
11. Masci PG, Zampa V, Barison A, Lombardi M. Cardiovascular involvement in Erdheim-Chester disease. Int J Cardiol. 2012;154:e24–6.
12. Kanakis M, Petrou P, Lourida G, Georgalas I. Erdheim-Chester disease: a comprehensive review from the ophthalmologic perspective. Surv Ophthalmol. 2022;67:388–410.
13. Diamond EL, Durham BH, Ulaner GA, Drill E, Buthorn J, Ki M, et al. Efficacy of MEK inhibition in patients with histiocytic neoplasms. Nature. 2019;567:521–4.
14. Hua M, Jiang T, Cheng J, Fu J, Dun X, Taibo A, et al. Treatment of progressive nodular histiocytosis: a case report. Ann Transl Med. 2022;10:1143.
15. Berce PC, Cardwell L, Essenmacher AN, Michaelis LC, Wanat KA. Progressive nodular histiocytosis with dramatic response to cobimetinib. JAAD Case Rep. 2022;22:110–3.
16. Nockowski P, Woźniak Z, Reich A, Maj J. Xanthoma-like skin changes in an elderly woman with a normal lipid profile. Acta Dermatovenerol Croat. 2017;25:167–9.
17. Trotta F, Castellino G, Lo Monaco A. Multicentric reticulohistiocytosis. Best Pract Res Clin Rheumatol. 2004;18:759–72.
18. Niaki OZ, Penn E, Scott DA, Cobos G, Vleugels RA, Weinblatt ME. Treatment of severe multicentric reticulohistiocytosis with upadacitinib. JAMA Dermatol. 2021;157:735–7.
19. Macía-Villa CC, Zea-Mendoza A. Multicentric reticulohistiocytosis: case report with response to infliximab and review of treatment options. Clin Rheumatol. 2016;35:527–34.
20. Landim FM, Rios HO, Costa CO, Feitosa RGF, Rocha Filho FD, Costa AAA. Cutaneous Rosai-Dorfman disease. An Bras Dermatol. 2009;84:275–8.
21. Bruce-Brand C, Schneider JW, Schubert P. Rosai-Dorfman disease: an overview. J Clin Pathol. 2020;73:697–705.
22. Abla O, Jacobsen E, Picarsic J, Krenova Z, Jaffe R, Emile J-F, et al. Consensus recommendations for the diagnosis and clinical management of Rosai-Dorfman-Destombes disease. Blood. 2018;131:2877–90.
23. Magro CM, Kazi N, Sisinger AE. Primary cutaneous histiocytic sarcoma: a report of five cases with primary cutaneous involvement and review of the literature. Ann Diagn Pathol. 2018;32:56–62.
24. Dourra M, Mussad S, Singer R. Cutaneous manifestations in a patient with reactive hemophagocytic lymphohistiocytosis. Cureus. 2020;12:e10089.
25. Morrell DS, Pepping MA, Scott JP, Esterly NB, Drolet BA. Cutaneous manifestations of hemophagocytic lymphohistiocytosis. Arch Dermatol. 2002;138:1208–12.
26. Debaugnies F, Mahadeb B, Ferster A, Meuleman N, Rozen L, Demulder A, et al. Performances of the H-score for diagnosis of hemophagocytic lymphohistiocytosis in adult and pediatric patients. Am J Clin Pathol. 2016;145:862–70.
27. Fardet L, Galicier L, Lambotte O, Marzac C, Aumont C, Chahwan D, et al. Development and validation of the HScore, a score for the diagnosis of reactive hemophagocytic syndrome. Arthritis Rheumatol. 2014;66:2613–20.

13 Hypereosinophilic Syndrome

Robert Gniadecki, Minakshi Taparia, Jean Deschenes, Jori Hardin, and Etienne Mahe

13.1 Practice Essentials

- Hypereosinophilic syndrome (HES) is a heterogeneous group of diseases characterized by peripheral eosinophilia (defined as >1.5 × 10^9/L) and/or tissue eosinophilia and with signs of tissue damage related to the excessive eosinophils.
- Skin rash is present at the disease onset in up to 25% of patients.
- Lymphocyte variant HES (L-HES) is associated with the highest risk of skin involvement.
- HES may be very difficult to differentiate from secondary hypereosinophilia and patients are best managed in a multidisciplinary team.

Hypereosinophilia is related to a diverse collection of disorders characterized by varying degrees of peripheral blood eosinophilia above 1.5 × 10^9/L and/or tissue hypereosinophilia. Hypereosinophilic syndrome (HES) is the term used when hypereosinophilia is associated with tissue/organ damage that represents the direct effect of cytokines and other products released by the eosinophils. The diverse causes of eosinophilia range from reactive, inflammatory conditions (majority) to idiopathic. Amid that spectrum, there is a complex array of clonal proliferations due either to hematopoietic neoplasms or to abnormal clonal lymphoid populations that produce eosinophilia through an interleukin-mediated mechanism. The latter is represented by the lymphocyte variant of HES, and the former includes entities such as myeloid/lymphoid neoplasms with eosinophilia and tyrosine kinase gene fusion, eosinophilia associated with another well-characterized myeloid neo-

R. Gniadecki (✉)
Division of Dermatology, University of Alberta, Edmonton, AB, Canada
e-mail: gniadeck@ualberta.ca

M. Taparia
Division of Hematology, University of Alberta Hospital, Edmonton, AB, Canada

J. Deschenes
Department of Pathology and Laboratory Medicine, Cross Cancer Institute, Edmonton, AB, Canada
e-mail: Jean.Deschenes@albertaprecisionlabs.ca

J. Hardin
Division of Dermatology, University of Calgary, Calgary, AB, Canada
e-mail: Jori.hardin@albertahealthservices.ca

E. Mahe
Department of Pathology & Laboratory Medicine, and Hematology & Hematological Malignancies, University of Calgary, Calgary, AB, Canada
e-mail: etienne.mahe@albertaprecisionlabs.ca

R. Gniadecki et al. (eds.), *Diseases of Blood and Skin*, https://doi.org/10.1007/978-3-031-65292-9_13

plasm, such as CML or some types of AML and chronic eosinophilic leukemia. The unifying feature across these disparate categories of HES is peripheral blood eosinophilia, which has traditionally been defined as a count exceeding 1.5×10^9/L, measured in the peripheral blood (PB) on two different occasions, at least 4 weeks apart, and theoretically lasting at least 6 months. This conventional definition, however, has come under scrutiny as potentially being too stringent when it comes to blood eosinophilia. There are documented cases where HES has been diagnosed with lower levels of peripheral blood eosinophilia. For patients with leukopenias, the relative percentage of eosinophils in relation to total leukocytes—often exceeding 3–5%—might serve as a more clinically relevant indicator. A careful review of tissue samples, such as the bone marrow, may reveal tissue hypereosinophilia and related damage in some of these cases to help confirm the diagnosis, but this is a rare circumstance.

Idiopathic HES is a type of HES where one fails to reveal any potential cause or etiology for tissue-damaging hypereosinophilia. By definition, when organ damage is absent and blood eosinophilia is present in isolation for more than 6 months, with no detected cause (after a thorough clinical investigation), idiopathic hypereosinophilia or hypereosinophilia of unknown significance is the preferred term.

To offer clarity amidst this complexity, several classification systems for HES exist. In this text, we adopt a simplified approach to classification, which aligns with the upcoming WHO-HAEM 2022 and with the International Consensus Classification (2022) for eosinophilic disorders and systemic mastocytosis, as delineated in Table 13.1 [1, 2].

13.2 Clinical Manifestations

The typical age of onset for hypereosinophilic syndrome (HES) lies between 40 and 50 years, with a noticeable male predominance [3]. Patients commonly present with a constellation of non-specific but distressing signs and symptoms, including weakness and fatigue, fever, cough, dyspnea, joint pain, and rhinitis [2]. The mean eosinophil count across these cases is 6.6×10^9/L in one large retrospective study [4].

Cutaneous manifestations are relatively frequent but are often non-specific, occurring in about 15% of HES patients overall. This rate seems to be highest in lymphocytic variant HES (L-HES or LV-HES), where up to 25% of patients can present with various forms of skin rash right at the inception of the disease. The most prevalent symptom of skin involvement is pruritus. While the cutaneous manifestations in HES can be indistinct, they often mimic conditions like atopic dermatitis, eczema, or urticaria. In L-HES, more severe skin conditions like angioedema, anasarca (generalized skin edema), and erythroderma have been primarily reported. Interestingly, the incidence of skin involvement appears to escalate as the disease advances, reaching up to 70% in cases of L-HES (LV-HES) and around 30% in other types of HES [3] (Table 13.2). This increasing prevalence of cutaneous involvement correlates with the progression of the disease.

Dermatologic manifestations emerge as the most frequently encountered clinical feature of HES (Fig. 13.1). These are followed closely by pulmonary symptoms, which commonly include cough, dyspnea, and asthma, and gastrointestinal symptoms like diarrhea and abdominal pain. Overall, more than 80% of HES patients who initially present with skin-related symptoms will exhibit pathological changes in at least one extra-

Table 13.1 Classification of hypereosinophilias/hypereosinophilic syndromes (HE/HES). Modified from [1, 2]

Hypereosinophilia/HES type	Defining features
Myeloid-lymphoid neoplasms with eosinophilia and tyrosine kinase gene fusion (MLN-TK or MLN-eo-TK)	Approximately 25% of HES
	Hypereosinophilia due to neoplastic expansion of eosinophils based on various tyrosine kinase fusions.
	Specific genetic alterations: *PDGFRA* rearrangement, *PDGFRB* rearrangement, *FGFR1* rearrangement, *JAK2* rearrangement, *FLT3* rearrangement, *ETV6::ABL1* fusion
	Other defined tyrosine kinase fusions: *ETV6::FGFR2; ETV6::LYN; ETV6::NTRK3; RANBP2::ALK; BCR::RET; FGFR1OP::RET*
Chronic eosinophilic leukemia (CEL)	10% of HES cases
	Presence of clonal cytogenetic and/or molecular genetic abnormality, or blast cells are ≥2% in the peripheral blood or >5% in the bone marrow[a]
	No rearrangement of *PDGFRA, PDGFRB*, or *FGFR1*; no *PCM1-JAK2, ETV6-JAK2*, or *BCR-JAK2* fusion gene
	Not meeting criteria for *BCR-ABL1*-positive chronic myeloid leukemia, PV, ET, PMF, CNL, CMML, AML or atypical CML
	Blast cell count in the peripheral blood and BM < 20%
Idiopathic hyperosinophilia/HES (I-HE/HES)	Most common variant (>60% of HES cases)
	Diagnosis of exclusion. Rule out other forms of HES and secondary reactive hypereosinophilia
	I-HE is used when there is no organ/tissue damage secondary to the effect of the eosinophils-associated cytokines and enzymatic products
	I-HES is used when there is hypereosinophilia-related tissue or organ damage
Lymphocyte-variant HES (L-HES, also known as LV-HES)	Least common (<5% of HES). HE driven by cytokine-producing, immunophenotypically-aberrant clonal T-cell population

[a]For the ICC, in the absence of a clonal cytogenetic abnormality and/or somatic mutation(s) or increased blasts, typical bone marrow findings supportive of the diagnosis will suffice (in the presence of persistent eosinophilia, provided other causes of eosinophilia having been excluded). These include increased cellularity with dysplastic meg also known as ryocytes with or without dysplastic features in other lineages, including eosinophils and often significant fibrosis, associated with an eosinophilic infiltrate

Table 13.2 Skin manifestations of HES [3, 5, 6]

Pruritus
Nonspecific, eczematous rash
Eczema mimicking atopic dermatitis
Eczema mimicking nummular dermatitis
Urticaria
Angioedema
Skin edema (anasarca)
Eosinophilic fasciitis
Skin ulcers

cutaneous organ at some point or another. The lungs are most often implicated in this multi-organ involvement [5]. This high rate of extracutaneous organ pathology in patients with skin manifestations likely reflects an overrepresentation of the L-HES within this specific patient subset.

Given the multi-systemic nature of HES, a comprehensive organ-specific workup is required for accurate diagnosis and treatment planning. The specific organ manifestations of HES are methodically outlined in Table 13.3.

Prognosis in untreated HES is poor. With appropriate management, 5-year survival rate is approximately 80%. Negative predictive factors are M-HES, presence of another malignancy, lack of response to systemic corticosteroids, cardiac involvement, and the height of eosinophilia.

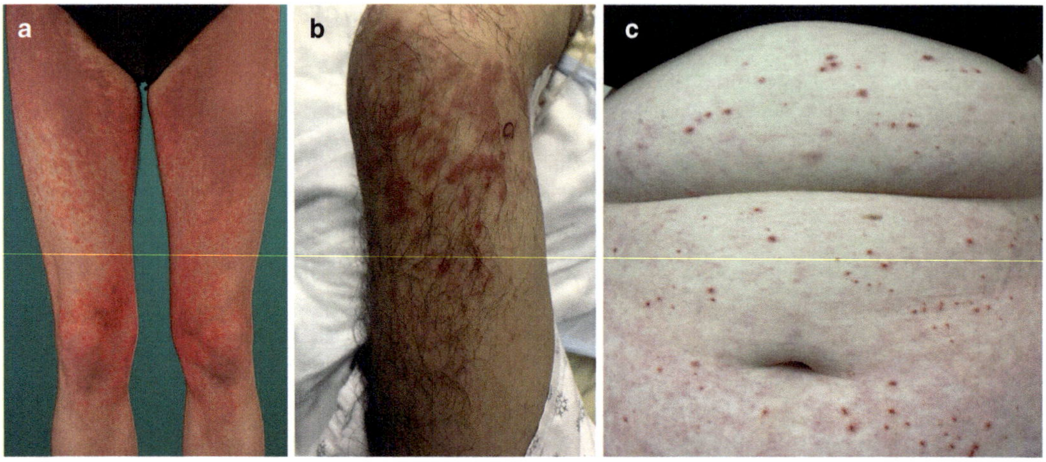

Fig. 13.1 Clinical spectrum of skin findings in hypereosinophilic syndrome (HES). (**a**) Confluent, urticarial rash on both lower extremities extending to the abdomen in a patient with idiopathic HES. (**b**) Itchy, bilateral popular eruption on lower legs in lymphocyte-variant HES. (**c**) Papular, intensely pruritic rash in a 34-year-old female with lymphocyte-variant HES

Table 13.3 Non-dermatological manifestations of HES [3]

Pulmonary	Cough, dyspnea, asthma, rhinitis, pleural effusions
Gastrointestinal	Diarrhea, abdominal pain
Organ enlargement	Splenomegaly, hepatomegaly
Hematological	Anemia, thrombocytopenia, lymphadenopathy
Rheumatological	Joint pain, arthritis, myalgia
Neurological	Neuropathy, paresthesia, stroke
Cardiac	Heart failure, myocarditis, pericarditis, mitral insufficiency, peripheral vascular disease, ischemia
Constitutional	Fatigue, fever, weight loss, night sweats

13.3 Diagnosis

13.3.1 Diagnostic Approach

13.3.1.1 Scenario 1: Hypereosinophilia

A common diagnostic scenario is a referral from a dermatologist who is managing a patient with persistent eosinophilia and a chronic skin rash, who wishes to consider HES as an underlying disease. Such situations are not uncommon as the dermatologist may be the initial point of contact due to the high incidence of skin rashes in HES and the difficulties in the early diagnosis of organ manifestations.

Hypereosinophilia accompanies numerous skin diseases, and the differentiation from HES may be very challenging for a dermatologist. Thus, diagnosis of HES should ideally take place in a multidisciplinary team [7]. Several algorithms have been published [2, 7], and the simplified approach is proposed in Table 13.4. Note that the diagnosis of I-HE is a diagnosis of exclusion in patients in whom Steps 1–3 ruled out MLN-eo-TK (myeloid/lymphoid neoplasms with eosinophilia and tyrosine kinase fusion genes), an underlying myeloid neoplasm, and L-HES, and secondary causes of hypereosinophilia, and in whom there is no evidence of tissue damage.

13.3.1.2 Scenario 2: Skin Biopsy

Another clinical scenario is when a hematologist or clinical immunologist refers a patient with difficult-to-diagnose eosinophilia to biopsy skin rash to help with the diagnosis. There exists a common but misplaced belief that the histopathological evaluation of skin lesions might offer definitive clues for diagnosing underlying hypereosinophilia. However, the reality is that the histopathological findings in skin lesions associated

Table 13.4 Diagnostic algorithm for patients with persistent eosinophilia and skin rash

Step 1	Screen for secondary causes of hypereosinophilia	Screen for infection, drug-induced eosinophilia, atopic dermatitis, lupus erythematosus and other collagen vascular disease, underlying malignancy, solid tumor or lymphoma-related hypereosinophilia, metabolic cause (adrenal insufficiency)
		Skin biopsy
	Assess tissue damage	Blood: complete blood count, electrolytes, renal and hepatic function tests, metabolic screen, IgE levels
		CT chest & abdomen, abdomen ultrasound
		Pulmonary function test
		ECG, Echocardiogram
		Additional tests depend on clinical findings. Consider sinus imaging, nerve conduction studies/EMG and/or biopsy of affected tissues (e.g., gastrointestinal tract, lungs, heart, nerves, etc.)
Step 2	Rule out MLN-eo-TK or an underlying recognized myeloid/mast cell neoplasm	Combined blood and bone marrow assessment
		Blood: Serum B12, IgE, tryptase level, peripheral blood smear: abnormal myeloid population, blast percentage
		Blood and/or marrow: FIP1L1-PDGFRA fusion by FISH or RT-PCR, TCR by PCR, Lymphocyte immunophenotyping by flow cytometry (abnormal T cells), NGS myeloid gene panel
		Bone marrow: Dysplasia and abnormal maturation; fibrosis, blast percentage, look for mast cell disease (including mast cell IHC, if serum tryptase is abnormal), standard karyotyping
Step 3	Rule out L-HES	Typical phenotypic changes in T cells in L-HES are: loss of CD3, double negative cells ($CD4^-CD8^-CD3^+$), elevated expression of CD5, loss of CD7, and loss of CD27

with HES are often as variable and nonspecific as the clinical manifestations themselves, as outlined in the table above. The skin manifestations in HES are likely more a result of the release of proinflammatory mediators from activated eosinophils than of a mechanism intrinsic to HES. It is worth emphasizing that eosinophilic infiltration in the skin can be conspicuously absent or merely scant in a significant proportion of patients. Furthermore, in the case of lymphocytic variant HES (L-HES), abnormal lymphocytes are often not detectable in skin biopsies.

The histopathological findings are generally reflective of the clinical presentation of the skin lesions. For example, eczematous rashes typically display spongiotic dermatitis, while urticarial lesions are consistent with what one would expect to find in chronic spontaneous urticaria [5, 6]. Therefore, the primary utility of skin biopsy in this context is to exclude other hypereosinophilic skin conditions, such as scabies or bullous pemphigoid. In these cases, identifying the causative parasite or demonstrating a positive pattern of immunofluorescence can swiftly lead to a more accurate diagnosis.

13.3.2 Differential Diagnosis

Differentiating true HES from hypereosinophilia stemming from an as-yet-undiagnosed underlying condition poses a major diagnostic challenge. Often, the clinician faces a complex interplay of symptoms and laboratory findings that may be misleading or nonspecific. The dermatologist, who frequently serves as the initial point of clinical contact due to the high prevalence of skin manifestations in hypereosinophilic conditions, is particularly positioned to grapple with this diagnostic complexity.

Several diseases are known to result in persistent eosinophilia and may also present with skin

Table 13.5 Differential diagnosis of HES in a patient presenting with concurrent skin rash

Malignant diseases	Solid tumors
	Cutaneous T-cell lymphomas, in particular, Sézary syndrome (Chap. 7)
	Chronic lymphocytic leukemia (Chap. 3)
Inflammatory diseases	Scabies
	Papuloerythroderma Ofuji
	Bullous pemphigoid (pre-bullous stage)
	Atopic dermatitis
	Drug-induced eosinophilia, including DRESS (drug reaction with eosinophilia and systemic symptoms) syndrome
	Eosinophilic granulomatosis with polyangiitis
	Eosinophilic fasciitis
	IgG4-related disease (see Chap. 15)
	Systemic mastocytosis (see Chap. 14)
	Graft versus Host (GvHD, see Chap. 17)
	Kimura disease (see Chap. 15)
	Rosai-Dorfman disease (see Chap. 15)
	Systemic lupus erythematosus

rashes, thereby complicating the diagnostic landscape. The comprehensive list of these conditions, along with their distinguishing characteristics, is delineated in Table 13.5 [7].

It is imperative to exercise caution and avoid prematurely labeling a patient as having an idiopathic condition until other potential etiologies for hypereosinophilia have been exhaustively ruled out. This is especially true given that treatment approaches can vary significantly depending on the underlying cause of eosinophilia.

Scabies can be quite difficult to diagnose and may be associated with severe eosinophilia, and relatively nonspecific skin rash. Papuloerythroderma has a characteristic morphology with a confluent, papular rash that on the abdomen produces a "deck-chair" sign (sparing of the folds) and peripheral hypereosinophilia. Papuloerythroderma is not a specific disease and may be a morphological representation of several skin diseases of diverse pathogenesis, such as Sézary syndrome, bullous pemphigoid in its prebullous stage, or adult-onset atopic dermatitis. Some patients with papuloerythroderma may fulfill the criteria of I-HES.

Particular difficulties may be encountered in differentiating between L-HES and early Sézary syndrome. In early phases, patients with SS often present with skin lesions resembling atopic dermatitis or other forms of eczema [8]. In those patients, eosinophilia may reach the levels seen in HES. Flow cytometry of peripheral blood reveals a clonal population of T-cells which, unlike L-HES, have a phenotype of normal, mature T-helper cells ($CD3^+CD4^+CD8^-$) and loss of CD5, CD7, and CD27 (Chap. 7). However, uncommonly, Sézary syndrome may present with the aberrant double negative phenotype ($CD4^-CD8^-$) or have a decrease in CD3 expression mimicking L-HES.

Adverse drug reactions are another confounding factor and are particularly prevalent among elderly patients on numerous medications, making it exceedingly difficult to establish a causative relationship between a particular medication and the skin condition. Additionally, eosinophilia often accompanies the exanthematous or eczematous rashes seen in drug reactions, and abnormal peripheral blood T-cell populations have been detected in patients with drug reactions, leading to an incorrect diagnosis of L-HES [9, 10].

13.3.3 Treatment

Therapy should be tailored to the type of HES [2, 7]. Systemic corticosteroids are particularly useful in L-HES and I-HES but have been used in any other type of HES symptomatically to reduce eosinophilia, pruritus, and eczematous skin rashes.

Patients with genetic mutations are treated with targeted therapy, including Imatinib for *PDGFRA/PDGFRB* rearranged disease, or JAK2 inhibitors (e.g., ruxolitinib). Patients with CEL-NOS and L-HES are treated with hydroxyurea, interferon, or imatinib. Anti-interleukin-5 (IL-5) targeted therapies such as mepolizumab, benralizumab, or depemokimab are effective, especially in I-HES.

Patients with widespread, pruritic skin lesions can often be helped with topical emollients, topical steroids, and narrow-band UVB phototherapy.

References

1. Wang SA, Orazi A, Gotlib J, Reiter A, Tzankov A, Hasserjian RP, et al. The international consensus classification of eosinophilic disorders and systemic mastocytosis. Am J Hematol. 2023;98:1286–306.
2. Shomali W, Gotlib J. World Health Organization-defined eosinophilic disorders: 2022 update on diagnosis, risk stratification, and management. Am J Hematol. 2022;97:129–48.
3. Requena G, van den Bosch J, Akuthota P, Kovalszki A, Steinfeld J, Kwon N, et al. Clinical profile and treatment in hypereosinophilic syndrome variants: a pragmatic review. J Allergy Clin Immunol Pract. 2022;10:2125–34.
4. Ogbogu PU, Bochner BS, Butterfield JH, Gleich GJ, Huss-Marp J, Kahn JE, et al. Hypereosinophilic syndrome: a multicenter, retrospective analysis of clinical characteristics and response to therapy. J Allergy Clin Immunol. 2009;124:1319–25.e3.
5. Zayas J, Peters MS, Butterfield JH, Pongdee T, Sokumbi O. Clinical and histopathological features of hypereosinophilic syndrome with cutaneous involvement: The Mayo Clinic Experience. J Cutan Pathol. 2023;50:455–65.
6. Khoury P, Lee C-CR, Abiodun AO, Klion AD. Skin histopathology in patients with dermatologic manifestations of hypereosinophilic syndrome. J Allergy Clin Immunol. 2015;135:AB266.
7. Thomsen GN, Christoffersen MN, Lindegaard HM, Davidsen JR, Hartmeyer GN, Assing K, et al. The multidisciplinary approach to eosinophilia. Front Oncol. 2023;13:1193730.
8. Mangold AR, Thompson AK, Davis MD, Saulite I, Cozzio A, Guenova E, et al. Early clinical manifestations of Sézary syndrome: a multicenter retrospective cohort study. J Am Acad Dermatol. 2017;77:719–27.
9. Weingertner N, Mitcov M, Chenard M-P, Cribier B. Intralymphatic CD30+ T-cell proliferation during DRESS: a mimic of intravascular lymphoma. J Cutan Pathol. 2016;43:1036–40.
10. Magro C, Guo R, Nguyen GH, Tsang H, Momtahen S. Pityriasis lichenoides-like drug reaction: a clinical histopathologic study of 10 cases. Dermatol Online J. 2017;23:13030/qt7xd8j71z.

Mastocytosis and Mast Cell Activation Disorders

14

Robert Gniadecki, Minakshi Taparia, Jean Deschenes, Jori Hardin, and Etienne Mahe

Mastocytosis represents a group of rare and diverse neoplasms characterized by the abnormal accumulation of mast cells in various organs or tissues. This condition is typically driven by the constitutive activation of the KIT receptor. The established classification recognizes three distinct disease types: systemic mastocytosis (SM), cutaneous mastocytosis (CM), and mast cell sarcoma (MCS) [1] (Table 14.1).

The clinical presentation of mastocytosis is heterogeneous, spanning from skin-limited disease, particularly evident in pediatric cases of CM, where onset commonly occurs within the first 2 years of life. Notably, many pediatric cases experience spontaneous regression of skin lesions during puberty [1]. In contrast, adult patients often present with sysmetic mastocytosis (SM), a more aggressive variant with extracutaneous involvement, potentially associated with multi-organ dysfunction/failure and shortened survival.

It is crucial to distinguish SM from nonclonal mast cell activation syndrome (MCAS, see below), wherein patients manifest recurrent symptoms of systemic mast cell activation with varying severity, accompanied by an increase in

Table 14.1 Classification of mast cell disorders

Cutaneous mastocytosis
Urticaria pigmentosa/Maculopapular cutaneous mastocytosis: Monomorphic and polymorphic forms
Diffuse cutaneous mastocytosis
Cutaneous mastocytoma
Systemic mastocytosis
Bone marrow mastocytosis
Indolent systemic mastocytosis (ISM)
Smoldering systemic mastocytosis (SSM)
Aggressive systemic mastocytosis (ASM)
Systemic mastocytosis with an associated hematologic neoplasm (SM-AHN)
Mast cell leukemia (MCL)
Mast cell sarcoma
Mast cell activation disorders (MCAD)
Mast cell activation syndrome (MCAS)
Other mast cell activation disorders

R. Gniadecki (✉)
Division of Dermatology, University of Alberta, Edmonton, AB, Canada
e-mail: r.gniadecki@ualberta.ca

M. Taparia
Division of Hematology, University of Alberta Hospital, Edmonton, AB, Canada
e-mail: mtaparia@ualberta.ca

J. Deschenes
Department of Pathology and Laboratory Medicine, Cross Cancer Institute, Edmonton, AB, Canada
e-mail: Jean.Deschenes@albertaprecisionlabs.ca

J. Hardin
Division of Dermatology, University of Calgary, Calgary, AB, Canada
e-mail: Jori.hardin@albertahealthservices.ca

E. Mahe
Department of Pathology & Laboratory Medicine, and Hematology & Hematological Malignancies, University of Calgary, Calgary, AB, Canada
e-mail: etienne.mahe@albertaprecisionlabs.ca

R. Gniadecki et al. (eds.), *Diseases of Blood and Skin*, https://doi.org/10.1007/978-3-031-65292-9_14

mast cell mediator release. Additionally, there is an elevated frequency of hereditary α-tryptasemia (HαT), a condition linked to an increased copy number of the *TPSAB1* gene and elevated baseline serum tryptase levels, observed in both MCAS and SM patients.

In more than 90% of SM cases, a somatic point mutation in the *KIT* gene at codon 816 is detected. Other rare activating *KIT* alterations include mutations in the extracellular (e.g., deletion of codon 419 on exon 8 or A502_Y503dup in exon 9), transmembrane (e.g., NM_000222:KIT p.F522C), or juxtamembrane (e.g., NM_000222:KIT p.V560G) domains. These are detected in less than 1% of advanced SM cases but are enriched in cases of indolent SM. Most patients with advanced SM and *KIT* p.D816V mutation exhibit additional somatic mutations, frequently involving *TET2, SRSF2, ASXL1, RUNX1, and JAK2.* Associated hematologic (usually myeloid) neoplasms may be detected in these patients [1] (Table 14.2).

Indolent SM stands out as the most prevalent subtype (Table 14.1), characterized by the absence of comorbid hematologic neoplasms, none or very few B findings, and absence of C findings (refer to Tables 14.2 and 14.3). Conversely, smoldering SM manifests with two or more B findings but lacks C findings. Notably, indolent SM carries a more favorable prognosis compared to the smoldering variant.

Table 14.2 Diagnostic criteria for systemic mastocytosis. At least one major and one minor or three minor criteria should be fulfilled for the diagnosis of SM.

Major Criterion:
Multifocal dense infiltrates of mast cells (15 mast cells in aggregates) in BM biopsies and/or in sections of other extracutaneous organs
Minor Criteria:
>25% of all mast cells are atypical cells (type I or type II) in bone marrow smears or are spindle-shaped in dense and diffuse mast cell infiltrates in sections of BM or other extracutaneous organ(s). In tissue sections, an abnormal mast cell morphology counts in both a dense infiltrate and a diffuse mast cell infiltrate. In the bone marrow smear, an atypical morphology of mast cells does not count as an SM criterion when mast cells are located within or adjacent to bone marrow particles. Morphologic criteria of atypical mast cells have been described
Activating KIT point mutation(s) at codon 816 or in other critical regions of KIT in BM or another extracutaneous organ(s)
Mast cells in bone marrow, blood, or another extracutaneous organ(s) aberrantly express 1 or more of the following antigens: CD2, CD25, and CD30
Baseline serum tryptase concentration > 20 ng/mL in the absence of an associated hematologic neoplasm. In the case of hereditary alpha-tryptasemia (HαT), the tryptase level should be adjusted

Table 14.3 B ("burden of disease") and C ("cytoreduction-requiring") findings of systemic mastocytosis (based on [2] reproduced with permission)

B-findings	C-findings
Mast cells infiltration in BM > 30% and/or serum tryptase level > 200 ng/mL	Cytopenias: Absolute neutrophil count <1000 g/dL, hemoglobin <10 g/dL, platelet <100,000 μL
Dysmyelopoiesis with normal or slightly abnormal blood cell count	Organomegaly (hepatomegaly with ascites, splenomegaly with hypersplenism)
KIT p.D816V mutation with variant allele frequency (VAF) ≥ 10% in bone marrow cells or peripheral blood leukocytes	Malabsorption resulting in weight loss and low albumin level
Organomegaly (without impaired organ function) as the following:	Osteolysis that may be associated with osteoporosis and pathologic fractures
Palpable hepatomegaly without liver impairment	
Palpable lymphadenopathy or size of the visceral lymph nodes >2 cm on CT scan	
Palpable splenomegaly	

The second most common variant of SM is characterized by its association with a hematologic neoplasm. This subtype fulfills the diagnostic criteria for SM while concurrently presenting with a non-mast cell disorder, such as myeloproliferative neoplasm, myelodysplastic syndrome, or acute myeloid leukemia. Chronic myelomonocytic leukemia (CMML) is the most frequently observed neoplasm associated with this subtype.

In rare instances, SM takes on an aggressive form, presenting with C finding(s). Despite having fewer mast cells in the bone marrow and lacking an association with any hematologic neoplasm, this aggressive variant results in substantial infiltration of mast cells in various organs (Table 14.3).

14.1 Adult-Onset Mastocytosis

14.1.1 Practice Essentials

- Adult-onset CM is associated with SM in >90% of cases.
- The most common type of mastocytosis in adults is indolent SM, whereas pediatric mastocytosis is usually confined to the skin.
- It is not possible to distinguish between normal and clonally expanded mast cells in skin biopsies, and therefore confirmatory biopsies have to be obtained from bone marrow or other affected organs.

14.1.2 Clinical Manifestations [3]

The organs most frequently affected in mastocytosis include the skin and bone marrow. Skin involvement is observed in more than 80% of all patients with mastocytosis. While the majority of adult-onset mastocytosis cases develop between 20 and 35 years of age, later onset is also noted. Maculopapular CM, specifically urticaria pigmentosa, is the predominant type in adults. The appearance of skin lesions becomes a significant indicator of SM since CM is rare in adults, in contrast to pediatric cases where the majority are confined to the skin.

14.1.2.1 Maculopapular Cutaneous Mastocytosis—Urticaria Pigmentosa

Characteristic features of small, round, brown, or red monomorphic lesions are commonly observed in adult-onset mastocytosis with cutaneous involvement (Figs. 14.1 and 14.2). The number of lesions varies widely among patients, ranging from fewer than ten to nearly universal. Lesions typically initiate on the thigh, axilla, or lower trunk, gradually spreading over several years to the upper trunk, distal extremities, and lateral neck. Facial skin, however, is typically spared.

The frequency of skin involvement differs across various types of SM. Over 95% of patients with indolent SM exhibit maculopapular skin mastocytosis, while the frequency decreases in advanced SM. Additionally, skin lesions may exhibit regression as systemic involvement increases.

An important clinical feature of CM is Darier's sign. This sign is elicited by gently stroking a lesion around five times using moderate pressure with a tongue spatula. Within a few minutes, a wheal-and-flare reaction occurs on the lesion, distinct from the surrounding skin. Darier's sign is crucial in the diagnosis of mastocytosis, although its absence in adult patients does not exclude the diagnosis. Hence, the term "urticaria pigmentosa" has been replaced in favor of maculopapular CM.

14.1.2.2 Other Morphological Types of Cutaneous Mastocytosis in Adults

Telangiectasia macularis eruptiva perstans (TMEP) presents as telangiectatic macular lesions, predominantly found on the chest, shoulders, neck, and upper back. Historically, these lesions have been considered a distinct form of CM due to an increased number of mast cells observed in biopsies from the affected skin. However, individuals with TMEP-like lesions, lacking evidence of maculopapular mastocytosis, do not exhibit signs of systemic involvement. Consequently, in expert opinion, TMEP is no longer regarded as a reliable manifestation of mastocytosis.

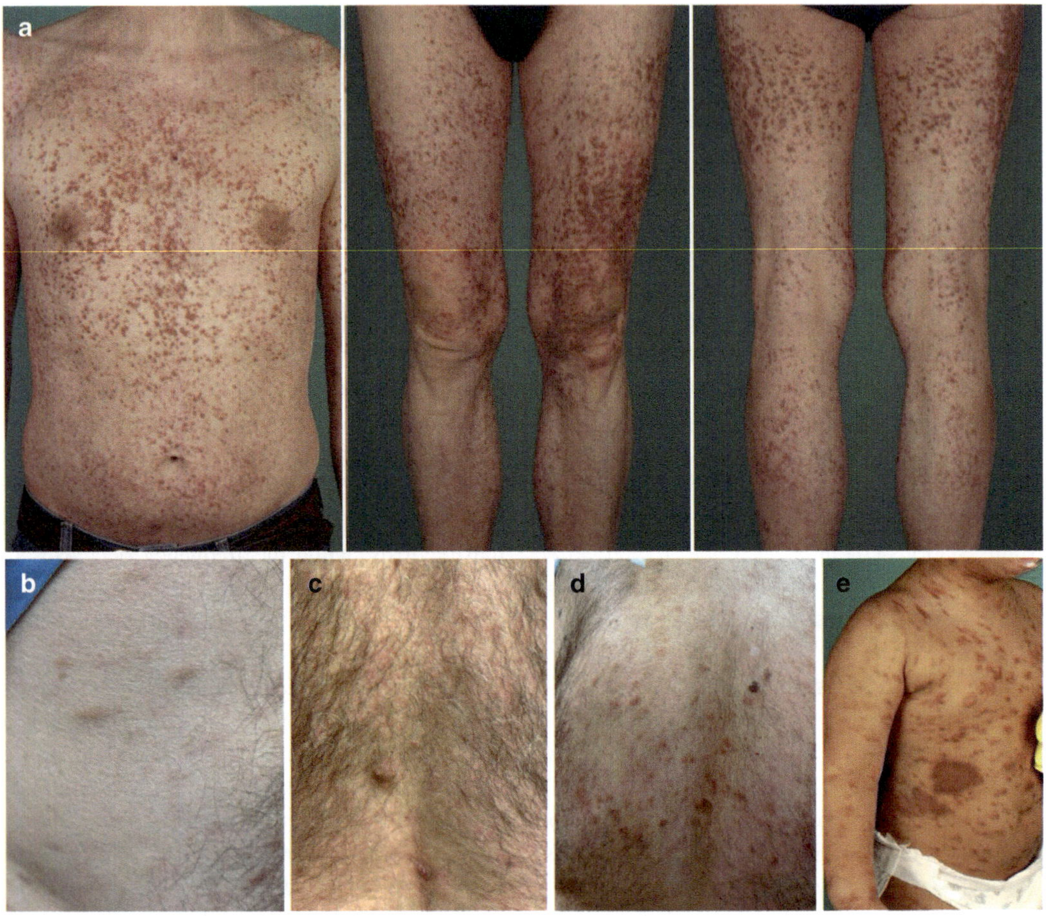

Fig. 14.1 Urticaria pigmentosa/maculopapular cutaneous mastocytosis. (**a**) Monomorphic form manifesting with a widespread maculopapular rash with a characteristic purple-brown color. Many patients present with a milder disease with only a few lesions (**b–d**). Compare the relative uniformity of the lesions in adults to the more polymorphic urticaria pigmentosa in a child (**d**)

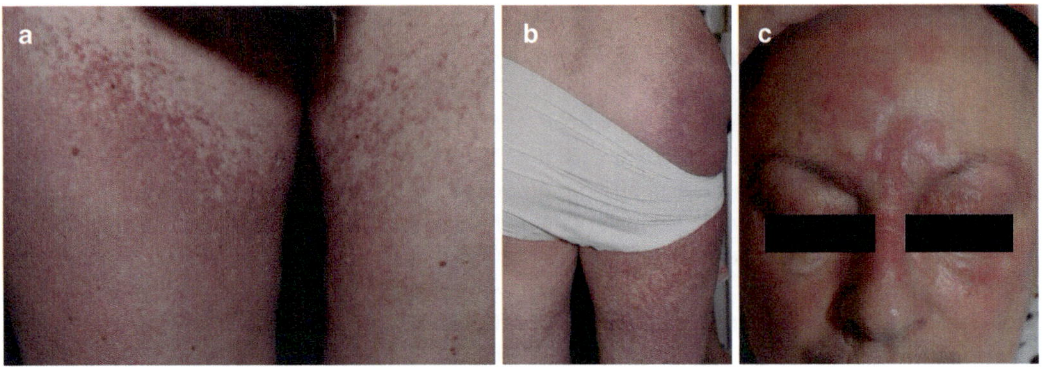

Fig. 14.2 Systemic mastocytosis with an associated hematologic neoplasm (SM-AHN). (**a, b**) Characteristic maculopapular cutaneous mastocytosis on the skin of lower legs extending to the trunk. Several years after the debut of cutaneous mastocytosis, this patient developed infiltrative facial lesions diagnosed as folliculotropic mycosis fungoides

Table 14.4 Differences in skin manifestations in adult and pediatric mastocytosis

Feature	Adult-onset	Pediatric
Most common mastocytosis	Indolent SM	Cutaneous mastocytosis
Skin lesions	Maculopapular, monomorphic (urticaria pigmentosa)	Urticaria pigmentosa, polymorphic lesions, mastocytoma, diffuse CM
Distribution of skin lesions	Trunk, thighs	Trunk, head, extremities
Spontaneous regression	No	Yes
Frequency of anaphylaxis	50%	10%
Laboratory findings	Tryptase levels >20 μg/L Frequent KIT^{D816V} mutations	Tryptase levels <20 μg/L Rare KIT^{D816V} mutations

Other clinical forms of CM have been described, primarily in pediatric-onset disease but occasionally appearing in adults (Table 14.4). Diffuse CM is exceptionally rare in adults, predominantly described in pediatric patients. Manifestations include generalized erythema, often accompanied by pachydermia (thickened skin), occasional papules, or verrucous, darker surfaces. Dermographism, marked by pronounced and persistent skin reactions to minimal mechanical irritation, is commonly observed. Some cases of diffuse CM may initially present with large blisters, elicited by rubbing or scratching, and prolonged bleeding from skin wounds, likely due to local release of heparin. Mastocytoma is almost exclusively found in children, presenting as a single elevated brown or yellow lesion, occasionally with blistering and a prominent Darier's sign. Mastocytomas typically do not persist into adulthood. They may undergo fibrous changes and appear yellow, resembling xanthelasma, termed xanthelasmoid CM.

14.1.3 Diagnosis and Risk Stratification

14.1.3.1 Histopathology

In clinical practice, the contemporary diagnostic approach for SM initiates with a bone marrow examination [4]. This preference stems from the near-universal involvement of the bone marrow in adult mastocytosis. Notably, histological diagnostic criteria for non-bone marrow and extracutaneous organ involvement in SM lack standardization. Additionally, a bone marrow examination enables the identification of a second hematologic neoplasm, if present.

Neoplastic mast cells typically express CD25 and/or CD2. The abnormal expression of CD25 with or without CD2, along with CD30 expression, is considered a minor criterion contributing to the diagnosis of SM. This approach ensures a comprehensive assessment of mastocytosis, emphasizing the importance of bone marrow examination as a pivotal step in confirming the diagnosis and evaluating potential secondary hematologic neoplasms.

14.1.3.2 Skin Biopsy

Mast cells exhibit a significant increase, several-fold in number, within the lesional dermis. For optimal detection, the preferred staining method for mast cells is immunohistochemical, with a focus on tryptase. This preference arises from the fact that degranulated mast cells may be overlooked in sections stained with Giemsa or toluidine blue.

Unlike bone marrow infiltrates in SM, no specific aberrantly expressed marker of clonal cutaneous mast cells has been identified thus far. Specifically, staining cutaneous mast cells for CD25 often yields negative results. It's noteworthy that mast cells in skin lesions may also show negative staining for CD25 or CD2 in patients with SM, even when bone marrow mast cells in the same individuals exhibit positive staining for CD25 or CD2. This highlights the complexity and variability in the expression of these markers in different tissue compartments.

14.1.3.3 Laboratory Tests

Serum tryptase levels play a pivotal role in the diagnosis of SM, serving as an obligatory parameter. Beyond tryptase, a comprehensive diagnostic assessment involves additional laboratory parameters. Complete blood counts, liver enzymes, creatinine, and albumin levels prove helpful in evaluating organ involvement and contribute to risk stratification.

Molecular testing is a crucial component of the diagnostic process. The presence of the *KIT* p. D816V mutation is identified in over 90% of patients with adult-onset mastocytosis and serves as one of the minor diagnostic criteria. The preferred screening tests include allele-specific quantitative PCR or droplet digital PCR. Notably, the presence of *KIT* p. D816V in other blood cells, in addition to mast cells, holds prognostic significance. Multilineage involvement is associated with a worse prognosis.

In cases presenting with blood eosinophilia and bone marrow mast cell proliferation, screening for *FIP1L1-PDGFRA*, using either fluorescence in situ hybridization (FISH) or reverse transcription-polymerase chain reaction (RT-PCR), is recommended. These instances, characterized by *PDGFRA/PDGFRB*-rearranged neoplasms with bone marrow mast cell proliferation and blood eosinophilia, are distinct from SM. They are appropriately classified as "Myeloid or lymphoid neoplasms with eosinophilia and tyrosine kinase gene fusions" according to both the International Council for Standardization in Haematology (ICSH) and World Health Organization (WHO) classifications. This nuanced approach ensures a thorough and accurate diagnosis in the context of diverse mastocytosis presentations.

14.1.3.4 Imaging

Imaging plays a crucial role in the diagnostic and prognostic evaluation of SM. CT or MRI of the skeleton is a primary focus due to the common involvement of the skeletal system, which serves as a prognostic factor. Up to 90% of SM patients exhibit osseous involvement, making MRI and CT the preferred modalities for assessing osseous lesions and bone marrow. While FDG-PET can demonstrate SM activity, its exact role in the context of SM is still evolving.

Abdominal CT and chest CT are essential for gastrointestinal (GI) imaging in SM. Thickened walls of the small intestine, large intestine, and stomach are common radiological features, often exhibiting a nodular appearance due to lamina propria infiltration. Bowel wall thickening, seen on CT scans, can be associated with strictures and lymph node enlargement. The liver is affected in 61% of SM cases, particularly in aggressive variants, with common imaging findings including hepatomegaly, ascites, and periportal adenopathy. Lymphadenopathy is a frequent occurrence, with periportal, retroperitoneal, mesenteric, and axillary regions being commonly affected.

Brain MRI is essential for evaluating neuropsychiatric abnormalities reported in select cases of mastocytosis. MRI typically reveals punctuate asymmetric homogeneously enhancing lesions in the cortical, subcortical, or deep brain regions. According to studies, white matter abnormalities and increased perfusion to the basal ganglia are detected in a significant percentage of cases. However, it is crucial to note that MRI findings are non-specific, and their appearance is believed to be linked to an inflammatory reaction in patients with mastocytosis.

14.1.3.5 Risk Stratification

Patients with SM are further subclassified into subtypes based on the histopathological features and the presence of B- and C-symptoms (Tables 14.1, 14.2, and 14.3; Fig. 14.3).

14.1.4 Differential Diagnosis

In the process of diagnosing SM, it is important to consider and rule out other hematologic malignancies that may accompany this condition. Additionally, HαT, characterized by an increased copy number of the TPSAB1 gene and elevated baseline serum tryptase levels, should be considered in both MCAS and SM patients.

Mast cell activation disorder, as discussed in the following chapter, also presents a differential diagnosis to be taken into account.

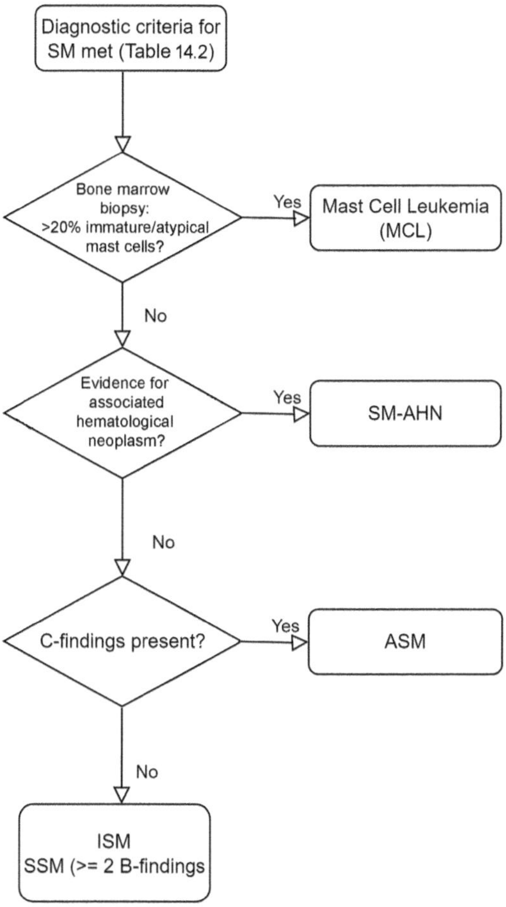

Fig. 14.3 Diagnosis and risk stratification of patients with SM. For abbreviations, see Table 14.1

14.1.5 Treatment

The treatment approach for mastocytosis is diverse, ranging from observation with preventive measures to manage mast cell degranulation triggers, and symptomatic relief, to more targeted and cytoreductive therapies aimed at neoplastic mast cells.

Patients are advised to avoid triggers of degranulation, aspirin, opioids, and alcohol. For skin pruritus and flushing, H1 antagonists (at doses used for chronic spontaneous urticaria) can be beneficial. Leukotriene antagonists (montelukast, zafirlukast) and sodium cromolyn are sometimes used, although their effectiveness for skin symptoms is limited. Systemic steroids are considered second-line therapy, but their use is restricted due to associated toxicities, particularly the heightened risk of osteoporosis in mastocytosis patients. Prophylactic prescription of bisphosphonates, vitamin D supplementation, and calcium is often recommended.

Maculopapular CM may respond to PUVA (psoralen plus ultraviolet A) therapy and improvement was seen in 70% of patients with disease-free periods ranging from weeks to years [5, 6]. In one study 25% of the patients showed an improvement for more than 5 years [5]. The efficacy of narrow-band UVB therapy is probably lower than seen in PUVA, but some patients achieve good responses [7].

Anaphylaxis is more prevalent in mastocytosis patients (in some studies between 25% and 50% of patients), particularly those with indolent SM. Omalizumab, an anti-IgE monoclonal antibody, has shown efficacy in treating recurrent, treatment-refractory anaphylaxis in both atopic and non-atopic mastocytosis patients. Patients with a history of anaphylaxis are often prescribed self-injectable epinephrine (Epi-Pen) and are trained, along with their caregivers, in its use. Wearing a medical identification bracelet and having access to self-injectable epinephrine is recommended for patients with a history of anaphylaxis. Perioperative management is crucial for mastocytosis patients undergoing surgery to prevent severe cardiovascular shock. Adequate premedication is essential in such cases.

Systemic treatment is individualized and varies based on disease risk. Cytoreductive therapy, such as cladribine-based chemotherapy or potent tyrosine kinase inhibitors (e.g., avapritinib and midostaurin), is used in cases of aggressive, advanced, or treatment-refractory disease. Recent data suggests promising results with these tyrosine kinase inhibitors, demonstrating a marked decrease in bone marrow mast cell burden and the potential for molecular remissions.

For select cases, allogeneic stem cell transplant (ASCT) has shown the potential to prolong overall and progression-free survival in SM patients. However, the choice of treatment is highly individualized, taking into account the specific characteristics and risk profile of each patient.

14.2 Mast Cell Activation Disorders (MCAD)

14.2.1 Practice Essentials

- Mast cell activation disorders (MCAD) are a heterogeneous group of disorders characterized by symptoms and signs attributed to excessive release of mast cell mediators.
- MCAS is a subtype of MCAD which may be related to mastocytosis (primary), to pre-existing allergic disease (secondary MCAS), associated with HαT, or idiopathic.
- Patients with MACS are at risk of developing anaphylactic shock.

MCAD are defined as pathological and excessive release of mast cell mediators leading to cutaneous and systemic symptoms and signs of hypersensitivity. The classification of mast cell activation disorders is summarized in Table 14.5.

MCAS is suspected when the following criteria are satisfied (Table 14.6):

- Clinical symptoms are severe, involving at least two organs
- There is biochemical evidence of mast cell activation
- There is clinical response to drugs targeting mast cells

MCAS manifests in four clinical variants (Table 14.5), with primary (monoclonal) MCAS being the most significant hematologically, as it coexists with an underlying proliferative mast cell disease that fully or partially meets the criteria for SM. Secondary MCAS is associated with IgE-mediated allergy, unrelated to a proliferative mast cell disorder. Additionally, MCAS can be linked to HαT, an autosomal dominant genetic condition present in up to 5% of the general population, characterized by elevated tryptase synthesis leading to a baseline serum elevation exceeding 8 ng/mL. Finally, idiopathic MCAS is diagnosed in patients meeting the disease's diagnostic criteria but lacking an underlying proliferative, allergic, or genetic condition [8].

MCAS is often associated with various comorbidities that exacerbate symptoms and signs. These comorbidities include atopy (such as atopic dermatitis and asthma), CM, other autoimmune diseases with a T helper type 2 (Th2) acti-

Table 14.5 Classification of MCAD

Mast cell activation syndrome (MCAS)	
Monoclonal MCAS	The *KIT* p.D816V mutation is detected and MCs may display CD25 and/or CD30 (a) with confirmed mastocytosis (CM or SM) (b) only two minor SM criteria are met
Secondary MCAS	An IgE-mediated allergy, another hypersensitivity reaction, or another immunologic disease that can induce MCA and thus MCAS is diagnosed, but no neoplastic MCs or *KIT* p.D816V is found
HαT-associated MCAS	Hereditary alpha-tryptasemia (HαT) is detected and all diagnostic MCAS criteria are fulfilled
Idiopathic MCAS	Criteria to diagnose MCAS are met, and primary, secondary, or HαT-related MACS are ruled out. May be accompanied by comorbidities, such as atopy, autoimmune disease, or infections
MCAD, unspecified	Criteria of MACS are not fulfilled, but patients present with symptoms and signs suggestive of mast cell activation

Table 14.6 Diagnostic criteria for mast cell activation syndrome (MCAS) (based on [8], reproduced with permission)

Clinical symptoms	Typical clinical signs of severe, recurrent (episodic) systemic mast cell activation are present (often in the form of anaphylaxis) (definition of systemic: involving at least two organ systems)
Biochemical evidence of mast cell activation	Increase in serum tryptase level from the individual's baseline to 120% + 2 ng/mL. Other mast cell-derived biomarkers of mast cell activation may also be used but are less specific compared with the increase in serum tryptase level
Response to therapy	Response of symptoms to therapy with antihistamines or other mast cell stabilizing agents

vation profile (like bullous pemphigoid, graft versus host disease, and rheumatoid arthritis), as well as infections, both viral and parasitic.

In some cases, patients may present with symptoms and signs that only partially fulfill the criteria for MCAS. For such individuals, the appropriate diagnosis is MCAD-NOS (not otherwise specified).

Conceptually, the relationship between MCAD, MCAS, and mastocytosis is visualized in the figure below, providing a comprehensive overview of their interconnections [9]. This conceptual framework helps in understanding the complex landscape of mast cell disorders and their varying clinical presentations (Fig. 14.4).

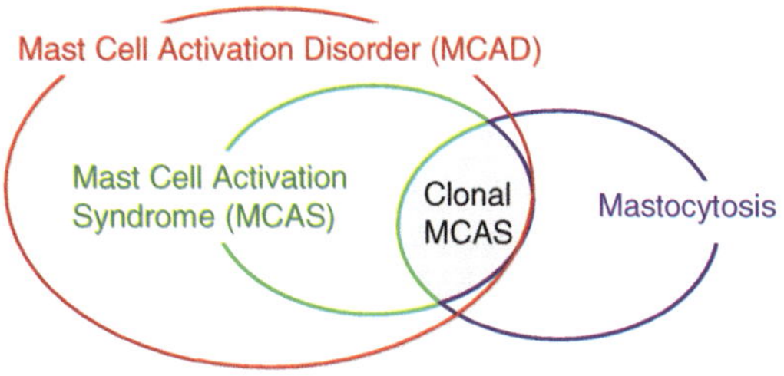

Fig. 14.4 Relationship between different mast cell disorders (modified from [9]). Mastocytosis is a clonal proliferative disorder that may be associated with MCAD and REMA score (see Sect. 14.2.3) may be helpful in determining the indication for bone marrow biopsy

Table 14.7 Clinical manifestations of mast cell activation disorders (MCAD)

Anaphylaxis	
Skin	Pruritus, flushing, urticaria, angioedema, dermatographism, anal pruritus
Gastro-intestinal	Diarrhea, abdominal bloating, abdominal pain, vomiting, gastroesophageal reflux
Cardiovascular	Hypotension, hypertension, syncope, tachycardia
Pulmonary	Shortness of breath, wheezing, throat swelling
Skeletal	Bone fractures, osteoporosis, osteopenia
Psychiatric	Brain fog, poor concentration, memory loss, anxiety, depression, headaches

14.2.2 Clinical Manifestations

Symptoms of MCAD are diverse, encompassing various organ systems, including gastrointestinal, dermatologic, orthopedic, cardiovascular, respiratory, neuromuscular, and psychiatric manifestations (Table 14.7). MCAD symptoms can manifest spontaneously or be triggered by various factors such as surgical procedures, infections, ingestion of certain foods (especially histamine-rich foods), or medications.

Dermatologic symptoms are typical and common in MCAD, including flushing, anal pruritus, urticaria, and angioedema. Numerous other skin manifestations have been reported, such as migratory pruritus or rash, cellulitis, xerostomia, telangiectasias, eczema, Raynaud's syndrome, increased sweating, alopecia, poor wound healing, and onychodystrophy [10]. Interestingly, studies have also reported clotting disorders in MCAD patients, presenting as bruising, purpura, or small vessel vasculitis.

Despite these dermatologic manifestations, it is crucial to note that skin signs in MCAD are not specific and require careful consideration in the context of a broad differential diagnosis. Differential diagnosis should account for various primary cutaneous diseases, including atopic eczema, contact dermatitis, spontaneous urticaria, or psychodermatoses.

14.2.3 Diagnosis

Patients exhibiting clinical signs suggestive of mast cell activation disorder should undergo a comprehensive diagnostic workup to confirm or rule out the presence of a mast cell disorder and further classify it based on Table 14.5. Alongside documenting anaphylaxis and organ involvement, the following diagnostic panel is recommended:

- Routine blood work including hematology panel, blood chemistry (liver enzymes, kidney function tests, CRP, electrolytes, calcium, thyroid hormones).
- Serum tryptase, baseline, and during MCAD episode. The normal tryptase range in adults is

1 to 15 ng/mL, average 5 ng/mL, and levels greater than 11.5 ng/mL (the 95th percentile) are considered to be elevated [11]. Diagnosis of MCAS requires a symptom-related increase above the baseline of 20% plus 2 ng/mL. Patients with elevated baseline should be further evaluated for possible HαT, which should be differentiated from secondary causes of histamine elevation such as myeloid neoplasm or chronic renal failure. High baseline tryptase levels (>20 ng/mL) may be a sign of SM even in the absence of other symptoms and for those patients, REMA score was proposed as a useful tool to determine the need for bone marrow biopsy and KIT mutation screen [9]. The score is computed based on the known risk factors (male sex, absence of urticaria/angioedema—1 point each, serum tryptase >25 ng/mL—2 points, history of pre-syncope/syncope—3 points, subtract 1 point for female patients and those with tryptas levels <15 ng/mL, subtract 2 points for patients with a history of urticaria and/or angioedema). Score ≥2 is highly predictive of clonal mast cell disease in a patient with MCAD.

- Other mast cell mediators. In patients with normal levels of tryptase, some authors advocated for testing for other mast cell mediators to conclusively rule out MCAD. The tests that might be useful are: urinary N-MH (N-methylhistamine) levels (reflecting total histamine production), urinary prostaglandin PGD2 metabolites, urinary leukotriene LTE4, and interleukin-6 (IL-6) [11]. Unfortunately, those tests are not readily available in all centers.
- Testing for HαT (*TPSAB1* gene copy number) can be considered in patients with elevated basal tryptase levels to rule out HαT.

14.2.4 Management

The management of patients with MCAS may necessitate multidisciplinary care, contingent on the symptoms and their severity. Referral to an allergist can be beneficial for ruling out other allergic diseases, assisting with the management of anaphylactic episodes, and educating patients on identifying and avoiding specific triggers of histamine release and mast cell activation. These triggers may include vigorous exercise, stress, sleep deprivation, surgical procedures, medications (especially opiates, NSAIDs, quinolones), alcohol, or histamine-rich foods (fermented products, cured pork meat, etc.).

Patients with elevated basal tryptase levels may be at risk for anaphylaxis provoked by factors such as arthropod bites, NSAIDs, radiological contrast media, and agents used in general anesthesia [9, 11].

Although data are limited, monitoring bone marrow density and recommending supplementation with calcium and vitamin D is advised, as mast cell mediators may induce excessive bone resorption and osteoporosis in MCAD patients.

Pharmacological treatment of MCAD primarily relies on antihistamines, with a preference for non-sedating antihistamines (cetirizine, fexofenadine, loratadine, desloratadine, levocetirizine) at doses up to fourfold higher than the FDA-recommended doses. Blocking both H1 and H2 receptors is usually recommended. Leukotriene blockers (montelukast, zafirlukast) can enhance therapeutic benefits. Sodium cromolyn, at doses starting from 100 mg daily with subsequent titration up to 1000 mg in four divided doses daily, may improve skin, gastrointestinal, and neuropsychiatric symptoms [9, 11].

In cases resistant to conventional treatment, there may be potential benefits from interferon -α-2b, omalizumab, or imatinib mesylate, as suggested by current medical literature [11]. The management approach should be tailored to the individual patient's symptoms, response to treatment, and overall clinical profile. Regular follow-up and close collaboration among healthcare providers are essential for optimizing the care and well-being of individuals with MCAS.

References

1. Khoury JD, Solary E, Abla O, Akkari Y, Alaggio R, Apperley JF, et al. The 5th edition of the World Health Organization Classification of Haematolymphoid Tumours: myeloid and histiocytic/dendritic neoplasms. Leukemia. 2022;36:1703–19.
2. Elsaiey A, Mahmoud HS, Jensen CT, Klimkowski S, Taher A, Chaudhry H, et al. Mastocytosis—a review of disease spectrum with imaging correlation. Cancers. 2021;13:5102.
3. Hartmann K, Escribano L, Grattan C, Brockow K, Carter MC, Alvarez-Twose I, et al. Cutaneous manifestations in patients with mastocytosis: consensus report of the European Competence Network on Mastocytosis; the American Academy of Allergy, Asthma & Immunology; and the European Academy of Allergology and Clinical Immunology. J Allergy Clin Immunol. 2016;137:35–45.
4. Pardanani A. Systemic mastocytosis in adults: 2023 update on diagnosis, risk stratification and management. Am J Hematol. 2023;98:1097–116.
5. Godt O, Proksch E, Streit V, Christophers E. Short- and long-term effectiveness of oral and bath PUVA therapy in urticaria pigmentosa and systemic mastocytosis. Dermatology. 1997;195:35–9.
6. Vella Briffa D, Eady RA, James MP, Gatti S, Bleehen SS. Photochemotherapy (PUVA) in the treatment of urticaria pigmentosa. Br J Dermatol. 1983;109:67–75.
7. Brazzelli V, Grassi S, Merante S, Grasso V, Ciccocioppo R, Bossi G, et al. Narrow-band UVB phototherapy and psoralen-ultraviolet A photochemotherapy in the treatment of cutaneous mastocytosis: a study in 20 patients. Photodermatol Photoimmunol Photomed. 2016;32:238–46.
8. Valent P, Hartmann K, Bonadonna P, Gülen T, Brockow K, Alvarez-Twose I, et al. Global classification of mast cell activation disorders: an ICD-10-CM-adjusted proposal of the ECNM-AIM consortium. J Allergy Clin Immunol Pract. 2022;10:1941–50.
9. Akin C. How to evaluate the patient with a suspected mast cell disorder and how/when to manage symptoms. Hematology Am Soc Hematol Educ Program. 2022;2022:55–63.
10. Mihele DM, Nistor PA, Bruma G, Mitran CI, Mitran MI, Condrat CE, et al. Mast cell activation syndrome update—a dermatological perspective. J Pers Med. 2023;13:1116.
11. Castells M, Butterfield J. Mast cell activation syndrome and mastocytosis: initial treatment options and long-term management. J Allergy Clin Immunol Pract. 2019;7:1097–106.

15 Inflammatory Lymphadenopathies with Skin Involvement

Robert Gniadecki, Minakshi Taparia,
Jean Deschenes, Jori Hardin, and Etienne Mahe

Patients frequently present in clinical settings with both skin rash and lymphadenopathy, a combination that poses diagnostic challenges. Although these symptoms often lead clinicians to suspect malignancies like lymphoma, many non-malignant conditions can present similarly. This chapter aims to clarify this complex area, which sits at the intersection of multiple medical specialties, including dermatology, rheumatology, clinical immunology, and hematology.

The conditions covered in this chapter are listed in Table 15.1.

Table 15.1 Syndromes of reactive lymphadenopathies with skin involvement

Disease	Typical skin involvement
Kikuchi disease	Rash on the face and upper trunk in 25% of patients
Kimura disease	Deep nodules and tumors on the head and neck area, including the orbits
Castleman disease	Paraneoplastic pemphigus
Unicentric CD (uCD)	Kaposi sarcoma
Idiopathic multicentric CD (mCD)	Nonspecific exanthems
Human herpesvirus-8 (HHV8)-associated mCD	
POEMS-associated mCD	
IgG4-related disease	Skin nodules and plaques in the head and neck area
	Subcutaneous tumors originating from inflamed salivary or lacrimal glands

R. Gniadecki (✉)
Division of Dermatology, University of Alberta, Edmonton, AB, Canada
e-mail: r.gniadecki@ualberta.ca

M. Taparia
Division of Hematology, University of Alberta Hospital, Edmonton, AB, Canada
e-mail: mtaparia@ualberta.ca

J. Deschenes
Department of Pathology and Laboratory Medicine, Cross Cancer Institute, Edmonton, AB, Canada
e-mail: Jean.Deschenes@albertaprecisionlabs.ca

J. Hardin
Division of Dermatology, University of Calgary, Calgary, AB, Canada
e-mail: Jori.hardin@albertahealthservices.ca

E. Mahe
Department of Pathology & Laboratory Medicine, and Hematology & Hematological Malignancies, University of Calgary, Calgary, AB, Canada
e-mail: etienne.mahe@albertaprecisionlabs.ca

R. Gniadecki et al. (eds.), *Diseases of Blood and Skin*, https://doi.org/10.1007/978-3-031-65292-9_15

15.1 Kikuchi Disease

15.1.1 Practice Essentials

- A rare, self-limited, benign condition characterized by painful lymphadenopathy, primarily affecting cervical lymph nodes which may be accompanied by fever, abnormal white blood cell counts, and a variety of systemic symptoms.
- Highest prevalence in younger women of Asian origin.
- The course is subacute with spontaneous resolution within 3–4 months.

15.1.2 Clinical Manifestations

Kikuchi disease, also known as Kikuchi-Fujimoto disease or histiocytic necrotizing lymphadenitis, is a rare, benign condition primarily observed in East Asian populations. The clinical presentation often includes painful cervical lymphadenopathy, fever, and variable white blood cell counts, such as leukocytosis or neutropenia [1].

Patients may also develop lymphadenopathy at other sites and experience a variety of systemic symptoms, including fatigue, night sweats, weight loss, headache, joint pain, upper respiratory tract, and gastrointestinal symptoms.

Antinuclear antibodies, anti-DNA antibodies, and rheumatoid factor are typically negative. Viral serologies are also negative.

Skin involvement is observed in approximately 25% of patients presenting as heterogeneous skin lesions. These may include papules, plaques, acneiform lesions, or erythema multiforme-like changes, typically localized on the face and upper trunk [1, 2]. The condition usually resolves spontaneously within 1–6 months, although recurrence has been documented in up to 20% of cases [3].

15.1.3 Diagnosis

The diagnosis of Kikuchi disease is predominantly made through excisional biopsy of an involved lymph node, in conjunction with clinical symptoms that align with the condition. Histopathologically, the disease evolves through distinct phases: proliferative, necrotic, and xanthogranulomatous [4]. In the proliferative phase, affected lymph nodes display preserved architecture with evidence of follicular hyperplasia and an expanded cortex, while notably lacking in neutrophils and eosinophils. The necrotic phase is defined by the development of circumscribed necrotic areas in the expanded paracortex, with prominent, characteristic apoptotic change. The final xanthogranulomatous phase is marked by the presence of foamy histiocytes on biopsy specimens.

Laboratory tests offer limited diagnostic utility but are essential for the exclusion of other conditions that may present with a similar clinical picture to Kikuchi disease (Table 15.2).

Of note, a Kikuchi-like clinical-pathological picture may occur with systemic lupus erythematosus (about 5–20% of patients) or another autoimmune condition (rheumatoid arthritis, Sjögren syndrome, etc.) or develop before a diagnosis of autoimmune disease is made. In instances where systemic lupus erythematosus is diagnosed concurrently, given the nonspecific features of the clinical and histopathological data, the lymph node changes are often considered to be part of the spectrum of lupus lymphadenitis.

15.1.4 Differential Diagnosis

See Table 15.2.

15.1.5 Treatment

No effective treatment is established. Corticosteroids, in combination with intravenous immunoglobulin, have been employed in the management of Kikuchi disease. Although the disease often demonstrates a predilection for spontaneous remission, it should be noted that recurrence occurs in approximately 20% of cases.

Table 15.2 Differential diagnosis of Kikuchi disease

Disease	Differentiating features
Lymphomas	Can be difficult to differentiate from Hodgkin and non-Hodgkin B- and T-cell lymphomas
	Aberrant immunohistochemical profiles or histological effacement by atypical lymphoid cells may help, but Kikuchi may at times stimulate T-cell lymphoma
	Molecular studies for T- and B-cell clonality may be useful; however, TCRγ will generate false positive results in a significant subset of cases [5]
Kimura disease	Different histopathology and clinical findings. Prominent peripheral eosinophilia
Systemic lupus erythematosus	No tendency for spontaneous remissions. Positive lupus serology, specific skin lesions for SLE (photosensitivity, butterfly rash, nail fold capillary changes). Histopathology may be indistinguishable, but $CD4^+$ tends to predominate over $CD8^+$ T-cells in SLE
Infections	The presence of specific pathogens detected either in lymph nodes or through clinical laboratory methods. Look for tuberculosis, histoplasmosis, cat-scratch disease (*Bartonella*), syphilis, infectious mononucleosis, and HIV
	Histopathology shows many differences depending on the specific agent (granulomas, neutrophils, viral cytopathic inclusions, geographic necrosis)

15.2 Kimura Disease

15.2.1 Practice Essentials

- A rare inflammatory disease, mostly in middle-aged Asian males involving lymph nodes and the skin of the head and neck.
- Systemic symptoms are uncommon; however, some patients have fever and/or renal impairment.
- Peripheral eosinophilia and elevated IgE.

15.2.2 Clinical Manifestations

Kimura disease primarily affects younger males of East Asian descent and manifests as a chronic, relapsing inflammatory disorder [6–8]. Clinically, the condition is often characterized by bilateral cervical lymphadenopathy. Additional features may include fever, elevated levels of peripheral blood eosinophilia, and increased IgE. Involvement of the nasal sinuses can result in symptoms resembling those of chronic sinusitis. Renal involvement is present in up to 15% of patients and poses a risk for progression to nephrotic syndrome if not managed timely [6, 8].

Dermatologically, Kimura disease frequently exhibits cutaneous features that include infiltrative papules, plaques, or nodules, most commonly on the head and neck area. These lesions tend to be localized in the deeper skin layers, leaving the overlying skin appearing unremarkable. The condition can also give rise to nonspecific skin manifestations, such as pruritus, urticaria, and chronic eczema [6, 8].

15.2.3 Diagnosis

15.2.3.1 Biopsy

A biopsy of the enlarged lymph nodes is required for diagnosis and for differentiating Kimura disease from other malignant or inflammatory conditions. Excisional lymph node biopsy is preferred.

Histopathological examination typically reveals preserved nodal architecture with follicular hyperplasia, reactive germinal centers, and a mixed paracortical infiltrate of plasma cells, lymphocytes, and macrophages. Eosinophilic infiltrates are prominent in interfollicular areas and are associated with necrosis, proteinaceous debris (often containing IgE), vascularization of germinal centers, eosinophilic folliculolysis, and micro-abscesses formation with frequent stromal sclerosis. Occasionally, eosinophils may coalesce to form small granulomas [9].

The skin's inflammatory infiltrate mirrors that of the lymph nodes, characterized by benign follicular hyperplasia, eosinophil presence, fibrosis, and the arborizing vascular proliferation of postcapillary venules [6].

15.2.3.2 Laboratory Investigations and Imaging

Diagnostic confirmation is often aided by laboratory findings of peripheral eosinophilia and elevated IgE levels. Additional blood tests, such as antinuclear antibodies, ANCA, and serum immunoglobulin fractions (including IgG4), as well as inflammatory markers, can help differentiate Kimura disease from other conditions with similar presentations (see Table 15.3). Ultrasonography and/or computed tomography (CT) are valuable tools for assessing lymph node involvement and may guide the selection of the most suitable biopsy site.

15.2.4 Differential Diagnosis

Kimura disease should be differentiated from other conditions that manifest with lymph node enlargement and infiltrative skin lesions. Notably, it shares clinical and histopathological similarities with IgG4-related disease (IgG4-RD), Castleman disease (CD), and, to a lesser extent, Kikuchi disease. These conditions often present with eosinophilic infiltrates and tissue fibrosis, complicating the diagnostic process (Table 15.3).

Another diagnostic challenge is differentiating cutaneous lesions of Kimura disease from cutaneous pseudolymphoma. Both conditions can display similar histological features, adding complexity to the diagnosis.

Moreover, cutaneous manifestations of Kimura disease must be differentiated from those seen in angiolymphoid hyperplasia with eosinophilia (ALHE). While both disorders show eosinophilic infiltrate and small-vessel hyperproliferation, their underlying pathology diverges significantly. ALHE represents a neoplastic process involving blood vessels, while Kimura disease is fundamentally an inflammatory condition [9, 11]. Unlike Kimura disease, which may manifest systemic symptoms and commonly exhibits abnormally enlarged lymph nodes, ALHE is primarily cutaneous in presentation, characterized by dome-shaped papules and nodules (typically on the scalp and ears), and practically never directly involves the lymph nodes.

Table 15.3 Differential diagnosis of Kimura disease

Disease	Differentiating features
Angiolymphoid hyperplasia with eosinophilia (ALHE)	Occurs in all racial groups. More superficial (dermal) lesions, often smaller in ALHE. Lack of systemic symptoms and lymphadenopathy. The biopsy shows lymphocyte- and eosinophil-rich hyperplasia of the vascular endothelium with hobnail cells but no germinal centers. Peripheral blood eosinophilia is less common, with an increase in IgE levels very rare [10]
IgG4-RD	Large amounts of scattered $IgG4^+$ plasma cells
Castleman disease	Hyperplastic germinal centers with plasma cells; only small numbers of eosinophils. Concomitant autoimmune phenomena
Kikuchi disease	Necrotizing features in lymph node biopsy, peripheral eosinophilia absent. No eosinophils in affected lymph nodes
Eosinophilic granulomatosis with polyangiitis (Churg-Strauss syndrome)	Asthma, involvement of paranasal sinuses, severe constitutional symptoms, presence of vasculitis and ANCA positivity, peripheral neuropathy
Hypereosinophilic syndrome (HES) (Chap. 13)	Persistent eosinophilia, organ damage, mutations in M-HES, abnormal peripheral lymphocytes in L-HES. Differentiation from I-HES may be problematic; however, Kimura disease has more prominent lymphadenopathy
Hyper IgE syndrome (Chap. 16)	High IgE, staphylococcal skin infections, no lymphadenopathy, frequent involvement of the lungs

15.2.5 Treatment

The primary treatment for Kimura disease includes surgical resection of the affected tissues or localized radiotherapy (20–45 Gray). Intralesional corticosteroids can be used for cutaneous lesions. Systemic therapy comprises systemic corticosteroids, cyclosporine, dupilumab, JAK inhibitors (tofacitinib, baracitinib), and low-dose imatinib mesylate [12–16].

15.3 Castleman Disease (CD)

15.3.1 Practice Essentials

- CD is a group of 4 related diseases of follicular dendritic cells in the lymph nodes, characterized by lymphadenopathy with associated systemic signs and symptoms.
- Histopathological examination of the lymph node is necessary for the diagnosis.
- Paraneoplastic pemphigus is the most severe skin disease associated with CD.

15.3.2 Clinical Manifestations

CD typically emerges in patients during their 4th or 5th decade, presenting a spectrum of clinical manifestations that vary considerably in terms of symptom severity and prognosis.

Unicentric Castleman disease (uCD) is the milder clinical variant, characteristically involving a single lymph node or occasionally a few lymph nodes in the same anatomical region. These patients often exhibit minimal systemic manifestations and the likelihood of organ involvement remains low.

On the other hand, multicentric CD (mCD) extends its involvement to multiple nodal regions. This form can be further distinguished into idiopathic mCD and those associated with human herpesvirus HHV8 infection or the rare POEMS syndrome (discussed in Chap. 4). The onset of mCD invariably brings along pronounced systemic symptoms such as fever, weight loss, malaise, and fatigue. Furthermore, these patients confront a heightened risk of developing secondary autoimmune complications and extensive organ involvement. Notably, all CD variants carry a potential risk of malignant lymphoma transformation, with the risk particularly accentuated in HHV8-associated mCD. The primary clinical features of CD are delineated in Table 15.4 [17].

15.3.3 Skin Signs

CD does not have specific cutaneous manifestations and skin signs in patients with CD reflect the concurrent autoimmune and neoplastic pathologies [18, 19]. Paraneoplastic pemphigus stands out as a particularly aggressive dermal manifestation, characterized by erosive lesions on both the skin and mucosal surfaces, with severe involvement of the vermillion lip often being a helpful clue. Those with HHV8-associated mCD may display cutaneous manifestations of Kaposi sarcoma. The mCD variant linked to POEMS syndrome often showcases dermatological signs typical of monoclonal gammopathies (refer to Chap. 4). Additionally, patients might manifest with lesions reminiscent of lichen planus, purpuric eruptions (particularly in the backdrop of thrombocytopenia), or nonspecific maculopapular inflammatory lesions. It is worth noting that these cutaneous symptoms can manifest several years after the disease onset [20, 21].

15.3.4 Diagnosis

15.3.4.1 Lymph Node Biopsy

Acquiring a biopsy from the enlarged lymph node remains a pivotal step in the diagnostic process of CD. Histopathological examination delineates three distinct variants: the hyaline vascular variant, which reveals regressed germinal centers; the plasma cell variant, character-

Table 15.4 Clinical features of different types of CD (from [17], reproduced with permission)

		mCD		
Feature	uCD	Idiopathic mCD	POEMS-associated mCD	HHV8-associated mCD
Clinical course	Benign	Aggressive		
Systemic symptoms	+/–	+		
		Elevated markers of systemic inflammation: ESR, CRP, ferritin		
Lymphadenopathy	One station, often central	Several lymph node stations, both central and peripheral		
Organ and blood involvement	+/–	Common: Organomegaly, renal dysfunction, anemia, thrombocytopenia, elevated liver enzymes		
Hypergammaglobulinemia	+/–	+	+ (monoclonal)	+
Autoimmunity	Rare	Autoimmune hemolytic anemia, immune thrombocytopenia, interstitial lung disease		
Risk of paraneoplastic pemphigus (PNP)	+/–	+	+/–	+
Risk of malignancy	Lymphoma		Myeloma	Lymphoma and Kaposi sarcoma

ized by hyperplastic germinal centers coupled with increased polytypic plasmacytosis; and the mixed variant. Notably, the plasma cell variant predominates in HHV8-associated mCD. In that subtype, besides abundant polytypic plasma cells, limited numbers of HHV8-infected atypical large cells with plasmablastic or immunoblastic morphology are found in the mantle zones of reactive secondary follicles, with a restricted monotypic expression of IgM λ[17]. This is related to the effect of HHV8, which has been shown to induce and upregulate RAG-mediated B-cell receptor rearrangement revision, resulting in the biased expression of λ light chain and loss of κ-positive cells among the infected plasmablasts [22].

15.3.4.2 Skin Biopsy

A skin biopsy does not provide significant diagnostic value in CD. This is primarily because the skin pathology does not mirror the characteristic histopathology observed in lymph nodes in the context of CD. Nevertheless, a skin biopsy becomes essential when dealing with ulcerative or lichenoid mucosal lesions, assisting in discerning the onset of paraneoplastic pemphigus. Any violaceous or pigmented papules or plaques should be biopsied to exclude Kaposi sarcoma or cutaneous lymphoma. Additionally, purpuric lesions merit a biopsy to evaluate the presence of vasculitis. In several instances, biopsies may merely demonstrate nonspecific lymphocytic infiltrates, underscoring a generalized systemic inflammatory response.

15.3.4.3 Laboratory Investigations

A thorough laboratory workup should encompass a complete blood count, evaluation of inflammatory markers like ESR, CRP, and ferritin, and an autoimmune screen, which includes antinuclear antibodies, direct antiglobulin test, and ANCA. Additionally, liver and kidney function tests, serum and urine protein electrophoresis, and serological testing for HIV, CMV, and EBV should be part of the routine diagnostic investigations.

15.3.4.4 Imaging

Positron emission tomography-computed tomography (PET/CT) is typically recommended to gauge the extent of lymph node and systemic organ involvement and also to aid in choosing the optimal site for biopsy. In particular, a high-resolution chest CT emerges as the imaging modality of choice for ruling out pulmonary involvement. Pulmonary involvement (bronchiolitis obliterans) is a negative prognostic feature in patients with paraneoplastic pemphigus.

15.3.5 Diagnostic Criteria

Table 15.5 summarizes consensus diagnostic criteria for idiopathic CD (from [17], reproduced with permission).

15.3.6 Differential Diagnosis

Distinguishing CD from other pathologies is crucial given the overlap in clinical presentation. Patients manifesting with lymphadenopathy, cutaneous rashes, and systemic manifestations present a diagnostic challenge. Prime among the differentials are Kikuchi disease, IgG4-related disease, and malignant lymphomas with skin involvement, each with its unique histopathological and clinical features (see Tables 15.2 and 15.3). Additionally, when confronted with non-specific skin eruptions and associated autoimmune manifestations, differential diagnosis can extend to primary autoimmune entities such as lupus erythematosus or adult-onset Still's disease. In such intricate cases, a lymph node biopsy (preferably excisional) can provide invaluable insights, steering the diagnostic process toward a conclusion.

15.3.7 Treatment

Treatment of uCD is usually surgical (excision of the involved lymph nodes) or using radiotherapy. For mCD, there is evidence for the beneficial effect of systemic corticosteroids, tocilizumab (anti-IL6 antibody), and rituximab. Management of paraneoplastic pemphigus is described in Chap. 18, Sect. 18.1.

Table 15.5 Diagnostic criteria for CD

Inclusion criteria	Exclusion criteria
I. Major criteria (need both)	**Infection-related disorders**
Histopathologic lymph node	HHV8
Enlarged lymph nodes in ≥2 lymph node stations	EBV LPD
II. Minor criteria (need ≥2 of 11 with ≥1 laboratory criterion)	Inflammation and adenopathy by other infection
Laboratory	**Autoimmune/inflammatory disease**
Elevated ESR or CRP	SLE
Anemia	Rheumatoid arthritis
Thrombocytopenia/tosis	Adult-onset Still disease
Renal dysfunction or proteinuria	Juvenile idiopathic arthritis
Polyclonal hypergammaglobulinemia	Autoimmune LPS
Hypoalbuminemia	**Malignant LPD**
Clinical	Lymphoma
Constitutional symptoms	Multiple myeloma
Large spleen and/or liver	Primary lymph node plasmacytoma
Fluid accumulation	FDC sarcoma
Eruptive cherry angiomata or violaceous papules	POEMS syndrome
Lymphocytic interstitial pneumonitis	

Features supportive of, but not required for, diagnosis include: elevated IL-6, soluble IL-2 receptor (sIL-2R), VEGF, immunoglobulin A (IgA), IgE, lactate dehydrogenase (LDH), and/or β2-microglobulin (B2M); reticulin fibrosis of bone marrow (particularly in patients with TAFRO syndrome); paraneoplastic pemphigus, bronchiolitis obliterans–organizing pneumonia, autoimmune cytopenias, polyneuropathy (without diagnosing POEMS), glomerular nephropathy, inflammatory myofibroblastic tumor

CRP C-reactive protein, *EBV LPD* Epstein-Barr virus lymphoproliferative disease, *ESR* erythrocyte sedimentation rate, *FDC* follicular dendritic cell, *LPD* lymphoproliferative disorder, *LPS* lymphoproliferative syndrome, *SLE* systemic lupus erythematosus

15.4 IgG4-Related Disease (IgG4-RD)

15.4.1 Practice Essentials

- IgG4-RD is an inflammatory, fibrotic, multiorgan disease that occasionally may manifest with lymphadenitis and infiltrative skin lesions. It can clinically simulate malignancy.
- Increased numbers of $IgG4^+$ plasma cells in lesional tissue, combined with key histopathological findings and appropriate clinical and laboratory data (including serum levels of IgG4), at times supplemented by imaging studies, are required for the diagnosis.
- Treatment comprises systemic corticosteroids and rituximab. The prognosis is grave in patients who do not receive timely systemic therapy.

15.4.2 Clinical Manifestations

IgG4-RD is a systemic disease affecting several organs [23–26]. The symptomatology is rich and summarized in Table 15.6.

Table 15.6 The main clinical features of IgG4-RD

Organ/system	Main features
Gastrointestinal	Pancreatitis, diabetes, malabsorption, hepatic failure and cirrhosis, cholangitis, icterus
Cardiovascular	Aorta aneurysm, pericarditis, stroke, peripheral vascular ischemia, Raynaud phenomenon
Neurologic	Ophthalmic nerve involvement, ocular motor nerve and muscle involvement (diplopia, ptosis), cranial nerve palsy
Soft tissue	Retroperitoneal fibrosis, exophthalmos
Other organ involvement	Lung (pulmonary fibrosis, bronchial asthma), kidneys (tubulointerstitial nephritis, membranous glomerulonephritis, kidney failure), glandular organs (salivary gland and lacrimal gland involvement, Küttner's tumor [unilateral sclerosing sialadenitis]), endocrine organs (mostly thyroid), sinusitis

The constellation of organ involvement in IgG4-RD may vary vastly from patient to patient, but the symptomatology tends to follow four main phenotypic patterns: gastrointestinal (hepatic and pancreatic involvement), fibrotic (retroperitoneal fibrosis, cardiovascular involvement), head and neck dominant (neurologic, ophthalmic and thyroid involvement), and the systemic (Mikulicz-type: organ and glandular involvement; kidneys, lungs, salivary and lacrimal glands) [24]. Accompanying these patterns, constitutional symptoms frequently manifest, with patients reporting weight loss, low-grade fevers, fatigue, and arthralgias, all hinting at the systemic nature of the disease.

Skin and lymph node involvement are hallmark features of systemic IgG4-RD. Patients often exhibit lymphadenopathy, predominantly cervical or axillary, although a generalized spread can sometimes be noted. These enlarged lymph nodes are typically non-tender upon palpation. Intriguingly, in certain cases, the lymphadenopathy is confined to nodes proximate to other affected body regions, offering a hint into the focal nature of the disease's pathology.

Skin manifestations in IgG4-RD are prevalent in about half of the patients. These dermatological changes are twofold. Firstly, there are primary skin lesions directly resulting from the skin's infiltration by $IgG4^+$ plasma cells. The frequency of these primary lesions is relatively low (about 5–6% of patients). Secondly, secondary lesions arise as a consequence of the inflammation associated with IgG4-RD [27]. The features of primary and secondary lesions are shown in Table 15.7.

15.4.3 Diagnosis and Staging

15.4.3.1 Tissue Diagnosis

Characteristic histopathological findings observed in abnormal tissues remain very important for the diagnosis of IgG4-RD but should be interpreted in the appropriate clinical context.

Classic histological features include a triad of marked lymphoplasmacytic T-cell-rich infiltrate, fibrosis with a "storiform" pattern, and

Table 15.7 Skin lesions in IgG4-RD

Type of lesion	Characteristics
Primary lesions	
Cutaneous plasma cell infiltration	Red-brown, sometimes pigmented papules and nodules, mostly on the trunk. IgG4⁺ plasma cells in the biopsy.
Secondary lesions	
Pseudolymphoma-like lymphocytic infiltrates	Papules, nodules, and plaques on the trunk, head, and neck. Often, the dominance of B-cells that may be monotypic.
Lesions resembling angiolymphoid hyperplasia with eosinophilia (ALHE)	Papules and plaques with predilection to the face. Biopsy resembling ALHE or Kimura disease.
Papulosquamous skin eruptions	Scaly plaques resembling clinical psoriasis. Should be differentiated from the psoriasiform lesions of secondary syphilis, as numerous plasma cells may be present in the biopsy.
Purpura	Petechiae. Biopsy may show features of leukocytoclastic vasculitis.

obliterative phlebitis. Often, eosinophils can be readily identified within these infiltrates. They are accompanied by a significant number of polytypic $IgG4^{+}$ plasma cells, which have to be enumerated to exceed strict, pre-defined diagnostic threshold determined based on the type of sample and the tissue of origin. The characteristic features might not uniformly manifest in all biopsied tissues, and their presence can vary depending on the affected organ. For example, the classic histological triad may lack one or two of its components in lymph nodes (except in the inflammatory pseudo-tumor pattern), in the lung, in lacrimal glands, and minor salivary glands.

Paradoxically, while biopsies from enlarged lymph nodes are less likely to show archetypal storiform fibrosis or obliterative phlebitis, they are also prone to show an excess of $IgG4^{+}$ plasma cells for unrelated reasons, such as chronic inflammatory conditions or malignancy, also highlighting that IgG4 enumeration alone is not sufficient to secure the diagnosis. The same observation is valid, to a lesser extent for some other anatomical sites [28, 29].

Of note, skin biopsies, when they contain the primary lesions, tend to more consistently reflect the classic pattern of IgG4-RD. A note of caution, however: the presence of $IgG4^{+}$ cells is not exclusively indicative of IgG4-RD, as they can be identified in other dermatological conditions (as shown in Table 15.9). Moreover, several plasma cell-rich skin lesions, such as primary cutaneous marginal zone lymphoma (pcMZL/LPD), can express IgG4, further complicating the differential diagnosis; however, in the case of pcMZL/LPD, these plasma cells are generally (but not invariably) monotypic (showing light chain restriction) and are accompanied by sheets of B cells, as opposed to the predominant T-cells observed in IgG4 disease.

Table 15.8 Proposed workup for IgG4-RD

Investigation	Comment
Serum IgG4	Elevated above 1.4 g/L in >70% of patients. Correlates with disease burden. Normal values do not exclude diagnosis of IgG4-RD and low or moderate elevations lack specificity[a]
Serum IgG4/IgG ratio	Values >0.1 have higher diagnostic specificity than absolute values of IgG4
Serum IgE	Elevated in 30% of patients, mainly systemic type IgG4-RD
Peripheral eosinophils	
Serum complement C3, C4	Low values indicate kidney disease
CRP	Correlates with disease activity and the risk of retroperitoneal fibrosis
Histopathology	
Biopsy from the skin and other affected sites	A biopsy is required for the definitive diagnosis. Biopsies from some sites may not show typical findings, e.g., lymph node, lacrimal gland, submandibular salivary gland
Other investigations	
Liver function tests, kidney function tests, pancreatic enzymes, TSH, and thyroid hormones	Screen for involvement of parenchymatous organs
Chest CT	Identifies lung involvement
FDG-PET/CT	Identifies involved organs. Useful for selecting sites for biopsy

[a]5–10% of patients with other conditions and systemic inflammation will show elevated levels [25, 30]

15.4.3.2 Laboratory Investigations and Imaging

To gauge the disease's spread and activity, specific laboratory and imaging modalities are employed as outlined in Table 15.8 [24, 31]. Furthermore, based on the clinical presentation, tailored imaging, and additional tests can be employed to further elucidate the disease's involvement and severity.

Several diagnostic criteria are available (the Mayo Clinic criteria and the Japanese Comprehensive Clinical Diagnostic criteria), but they are not universally adopted [25]. Histopathology is the current gold standard for diagnosis.

15.4.4 Differential Diagnosis

IgG4-RD has a wide differential diagnosis, depending on the spectrum of organ involvement. In the hematology-dermatology clinic, the most common differential diagnoses are from other diseases that produce a constellation of lymphadenopathy and skin rash and from those that may occasionally express $IgG4^+$ plasma cells in the infiltrate (Table 15.9).

15.4.5 Treatment

Many patients have an indolent course for years. However, IgG4 RD poses a significant risk of fatal complications related to the involvement of the aorta, retroperitoneal fibrosis, or pachymeningitis. All patients are treated systemically with glucocorticosteroids. Typically, patients are started on Prednisone at dosages ranging from 0.5–1 mg/kg. After an initial phase of 2–4 weeks, the dose is then gradually tapered. Given the side-effect profile of long-term corticosteroid use, especially a 40% risk of diabetes in IgG4 RD, a steroid-sparing agent is often added to the regimen [32]. Common choices include azathioprine, mycophenolate mofetil, or methotrexate.

In situations where the disease is more aggressive or unresponsive to the standard regimen, intravenous rituximab has demonstrated efficacy [23, 24, 31].

Table 15.9 Differential diagnosis of IgG4-RD

Disease	Similarities	Differentiating features
Inflammatory diseases		
Kimura disease		Lack of organ involvement
Rosai–Dorfman disease	Increased IgG^+ plasma cells	Overall histiocytic process, low number of $IgG4^+$ plasma cells, systemic investigation recommended if $IgG4^+$ plasma cells are markedly increased
Kikuchi disease		Lack of organ involvement
Castleman disease	Plasma cell infiltrate	Typical morphology of CD; low number of $IgG4^+$ plasma cells
Cutaneous lesions of lupus erythematosus	Cutaneous infiltrates may show a mixture of lymphocytes and $IgG4^+$ plasma cells. Involvement of internal organs	Presence of antinuclear antibodies and other lupus-specific antibodies
Sarcoidosis	Affects many organs	Granulomas are not a feature of IgG4-RD; sarcoid has no increase in $IgG4^+$ plasma cells
Malignancies, histiocytic and lymphoid proliferations		
Primary cutaneous marginal zone B-cell lymphoma	Presence of plasma cells expressing IgG4 in lesional skin	Features of B-cell lymphoma are noted
Primary cutaneous small-medium cell $CD4^+$ lymphoproliferative disease		Plasma cells are very often monotypic and do not achieve the numbers typical for IgG4-RD. lymphadenopathy is usually absent in primary cutaneous lymphomas
Lymphoid hyperplasias	Nodules or infiltrated plaques, preferentially on the face, polyclonal lymphocytic infiltrate with admixture of plasma cells	Lack of fibrosis and infiltration of blood vessels in the skin. Small number of $IgG4^+$ plasma cells
Xanthogranulomas	Eyelid swelling and exophthalmos may clinically resemble lacrimal gland inflammation in IgG-RD	Inflammatory infiltrate in IgG4-RD is dominated by plasma cells and T-cells rather than histiocytes
Hypereosinophilic syndrome	Peripheral eosinophilia may be prominent, especially in systemic type IgG4-RD	Lack of IgG4 cells in skin lesions
Infectious diseases		
Syphilis Borreliosis	Plasma cells in skin lesions may express IgG4	Positive syphilis or *Borrelia* serology. Response to antibiotics

For localized, therapy-resistant skin manifestations, there are potential therapeutic measures that can be employed, such as topical corticosteroids or intralesional corticosteroid injections. However, it's important to note that current evidence supporting the effectiveness of these local treatments remains limited.

References

1. Perry AM, Choi SM. Kikuchi-Fujimoto disease: a review. Arch Pathol Lab Med. 2018;142:1341–6.
2. Seno A, Torigoe R, Shimoe K, Tada J, Arata J, Suwaki M. Kikuchi's disease (histiocytic necrotizing lymphadenitis) with cutaneous involvement. J Am Acad Dermatol. 1994;30:504–6.
3. Park HS, Sung MJ, Park SE, Lim YT. Kikuchi-Fujimoto disease of 16 children in a single center of Korea. Pediatr Allergy Immunol. 2007;18:174–8.
4. Kuo TT. Kikuchi's disease (histiocytic necrotizing lymphadenitis). A clinicopathologic study of 79 cases with an analysis of histologic subtypes, immunohistology, and DNA ploidy. Am J Surg Pathol. 1995;19:798–809.
5. Hartmann S, Melle F, Motta G, Agostinelli C, Sabattini E, Pileri S, et al. Clonal T-cell proliferations occasionally occur in Kikuchi-Fujimoto disease. Hum Pathol. 2023;138:103–11.
6. Chen H, Thompson LDR, Aguilera NSI, Abbondanzo SL. Kimura disease: a clinicopathologic study of 21 cases. Am J Surg Pathol. 2004;28:505–13.

7. Kim WJ, Kim HK. Current concepts of Kimura disease: pathophysiology and evolution of treatment. Arch Craniofac Surg. 2022;23:249–55.
8. Sun Q-F, Xu D-Z, Pan S-H, Ding J-G, Xue Z-Q, Miao C-S, et al. Kimura disease: review of the literature. Intern Med J. 2008;38:668–72.
9. Abuel-Haija M, Hurford MT. Kimura disease. Arch Pathol Lab Med. 2007;131:650–1.
10. Zou A, Hu M, Niu B. Comparison between Kimura's disease and angiolymphoid hyperplasia with eosinophilia: case reports and literature review. J Int Med Res. 2021;49:3000605211040976.
11. Adler BL, Krausz AE, Minuti A, Silverberg JI, Lev-Tov H. Epidemiology and treatment of angiolymphoid hyperplasia with eosinophilia (ALHE): a systematic review. J Am Acad Dermatol. 2016;74:506–12.e11.
12. Teraki Y, Terao A. Treatment of Kimura disease with dupilumab. JAMA Dermatol. 2022;158:329–30.
13. Bellinato F, Mastrosimini MG, Querzoli G, Gisondi P, Girolomoni G. Dupilumab for recalcitrant Kimura disease. Dermatol Ther. 2022;35:e15674.
14. Sun Q, Fu B, Li S, Fang H, Qiao J. Efficacy of tofacitinib in Kimura's disease in a patient with concomitant atopic dermatitis. Clin Exp Dermatol. 2021;46:1336–8.
15. Ueda M, Kogame T, Egawa G, Kambe N, Kabashima K. A case of Kimura disease with atopic dermatitis successfully treated with baricitinib. J Dermatol. 2023;50:e196–7.
16. O'Malley DP, Grimm KE. Reactive lymphadenopathies that mimic lymphoma: entities of unknown etiology. Semin Diagn Pathol. 2013;30:137–45.
17. Dispenzieri A, Fajgenbaum DC. Overview of Castleman disease. Blood. 2020;135:1353–64.
18. Wu D, Lim MS, Jaffe ES. Pathology of Castleman disease. Hematol Oncol Clin North Am. 2018;32:37–52.
19. Chavez-Alvarez S, Villarreal-Martinez A, Ocampo-Candiani J, Gomez-Flores M, Vazquez-Martinez O, Gonzalez-Saldivar G, et al. Cutaneous manifestations of Castleman disease. Int J Dermatol. 2020;59:1226–40.
20. Nakamura Y, Mori N, Yamazaki M, Yamakawa T. Different types of skin lesions in multicentric Castleman disease. Intern Med. 2022;61:2395–6.
21. Sato K, Shinkuma S, Fujimoto K, Hatanaka KC, Ujiie H, Nomura T, et al. Late-onset skin involvement on the forehead in multicentric Castleman disease. Int J Dermatol. 2017;56:e152–3.
22. Totonchy J, Osborn JM, Chadburn A, Nabiee R, Argueta L, Mikita G, et al. KSHV induces immunoglobulin rearrangements in mature B lymphocytes. PLoS Pathog. 2018;14:e1006967.
23. Kamisawa T, Zen Y, Pillai S, Stone JH. IgG4-related disease. Lancet. 2015;385:1460–71.
24. Lanzillotta M, Mancuso G, Della-Torre E. Advances in the diagnosis and management of IgG4 related disease. BMJ. 2020;369:m1067.
25. Nambiar S, Oliver TI. IgG4-related disease. In: StatPearls. StatPearls Publishing; 2023.
26. Miyabe K, Zen Y, Cornell LD, Rajagopalan G, Chowdhary VR, Roberts LR, et al. Gastrointestinal and extra-intestinal manifestations of IgG4-related disease. Gastroenterology. 2018;155:990–1003.e1.
27. Tokura Y, Yagi H, Yanaguchi H, Majima Y, Kasuya A, Ito T, et al. IgG4-related skin disease. Br J Dermatol. 2014;171:959–67.
28. Strehl JD, Hartmann A, Agaimy A. Numerous IgG4-positive plasma cells are ubiquitous in diverse localised nonspecific chronic inflammatory conditions and need to be distinguished from IgG4-related systemic disorders. J Clin Pathol. 2011;64:237–43.
29. Cheuk W, Chan JKC. Lymphadenopathy of IgG4-related disease: an underdiagnosed and overdiagnosed entity. Semin Diagn Pathol. 2012;29:226–34.
30. Ghazale A, Chari ST, Smyrk TC, Levy MJ, Topazian MD, Takahashi N, et al. Value of serum IgG4 in the diagnosis of autoimmune pancreatitis and in distinguishing it from pancreatic cancer. Am J Gastroenterol. 2007;102:1646–53.
31. Stone JH, Zen Y, Deshpande V. IgG4-related disease. N Engl J Med. 2012;366:539–51.
32. Chen LYC, Mattman A, Seidman MA, Carruthers MN. IgG4-related disease: what a hematologist needs to know. Haematologica. 2019;104:444–55.

16 Skin Manifestations of Adult-Onset Immunodeficiencies

Sandrine Menard, Robert Gniadecki, and Mohammed Osman

16.1 Practice Essentials

- Immunodeficiencies with adult-onset are rare and often unrecognized causes of diseases of skin and blood.
- Chronic variable immunodeficiency and selective IgA deficiency are the most common immunodeficiencies with adult onset.
- Skin is commonly affected in adult-onset immunodeficiencies. Typical infectious manifestations are mucocutaneous candidiasis, therapy-resistant warts, severe herpetic infections, and abscesses.
- Immunodeficiencies leading to immune dysregulation often manifest as skin eczemas or autoimmune diseases.
- Other important clinical warning signs are chronic and recurrent infection of the sinuses, recurrent pneumonia, and chronic diarrhea with weight loss.

Immunodeficiency disorders encompass an expanding array of conditions characterized by impaired immune system development or function. The etiology can be traced to genetic mutations (giving rise to primary immunodeficiency disorders), occur secondarily due to antibodies targeting various components of the immune system, or iatrogenic as a side effect of various medications [1, 2]. Notably, while a significant portion of these disorders makes their debut during childhood, some patients manifest symptoms later in life. This timeline distinction is pivotal, as disease management, including diagnosis, monitoring, and treatment strategies, must be tailored to the age group in question, taking into account the inherent differences between pediatric and adult presentations [3]. Whereas most pediatric-onset immunodeficiencies have a genetic cause, the root cause of adult-onset immune defects is often multifactorial.

In this chapter, we will focus on immunodeficiencies with an onset in adults, which typically have manifestations in the skin and may be associated with other hematological problems (Table 16.1).

Immunodeficiencies are quite rare and often remain undiagnosed. It is reasonable to consider immunodeficiency in patients presenting with the following signs and symptoms:

S. Menard
University of Montreal, Montreal, QC, Canada
e-mail: sandrine.menard.1@umontreal.ca

R. Gniadecki (✉)
Division of Dermatology, University of Alberta, Edmonton, AB, Canada
e-mail: r.gniadecki@ualberta.ca

M. Osman
Department of Medicine, University of Alberta, Edmonton, AB, Canada
e-mail: mosman@ualberta.ca

R. Gniadecki et al. (eds.), *Diseases of Blood and Skin*, https://doi.org/10.1007/978-3-031-65292-9_16

Table 16.1 Adult-onset immunodeficiencies with skin involvement

Disease	Typical skin manifestations	Associated hematological diseases
Antibody defects		
Common variable immunodeficiency	Bacterial skin infections	CLL
	Severe rosacea	Risk of lymphoma
	Seborrheic dermatitis	
Selective IgA deficiency (SIgAD)	Skin abscesses	Transfusion reactions
Lymphocyte defects		
Idiopathic CD4+ lymphocytopenia	Warts	Risk of lymphoma
Immune dysregulation syndromes		
Hyper IgE syndrome (HIES)	Eczema	Risk of lymphoma
	Staphylococcal infections	
Autoimmune polyendocrinopathy with candidiasis and ectodermal dystrophy (APECED)	Mucocutaneous candidiasis	Pernicious anemia
	Nail dystrophy	
Good syndrome	Lichen planus	Thymoma
VEXAS (vacuoles, E1 enzyme, X-linked autoinflammatory, somatic syndrome)	Herpes reactivation	Myelodysplastic syndrome
	Chondritis	Hemophagocytic lymphohistiocytosis (HLH)
	Vasculitis	
LRBA deficiency	Atopic dermatitis-like eczema	Lymphadenopathy
	Vitiligo	
Innate immune deficiencies		
GATA2 deficiency	Warts	Myelodysplastic syndrome
WHIM syndrome	Warts	Leukopenia
Chronic granulomatous disease (CGD)	Severe bacterial and fungal infections	Hemophagocytic lymphohistiocytosis (HLH)

- Recurrent, treatment-resistant infection of the sinuses, ears, nose, or throat
- Recurrent pneumonias
- Chronic diarrhea with weight loss
- Unusual infections not commonly seen in healthy individuals
- Suspicious skin manifestations (infections, eczemas, autoimmune conditions; see below)

Thus, in adults, skin manifestations are considered to be common warning signs of immunodeficiency.

16.2 Skin Manifestations of Adult-Onset Immunodeficiencies

Clinically, immunodeficiency disorders predispose patients to a myriad of complications such as frequent or severe infections, autoimmune reactions, inflammatory responses, malignancies, and allergic manifestations. From a dermatological perspective, the array of potential presentations is diverse. Most commonly, the patient will either present with cutaneous infection reflecting deficiencies in antimicrobial defense or with a non-infectious, inflammatory rash as a manifestation of immune dysregulation.

16.2.1 Skin Infections (Fig. 16.1)

Skin infections can be divided into four broad categories:

- "Normal" infections, which are commonly found in healthy individuals, have an unusual course in immunocompromised individuals, either because of resistance to treatment, high recurrence rate, or unusual severity. Examples are mucocutaneous candidiasis or recurrent

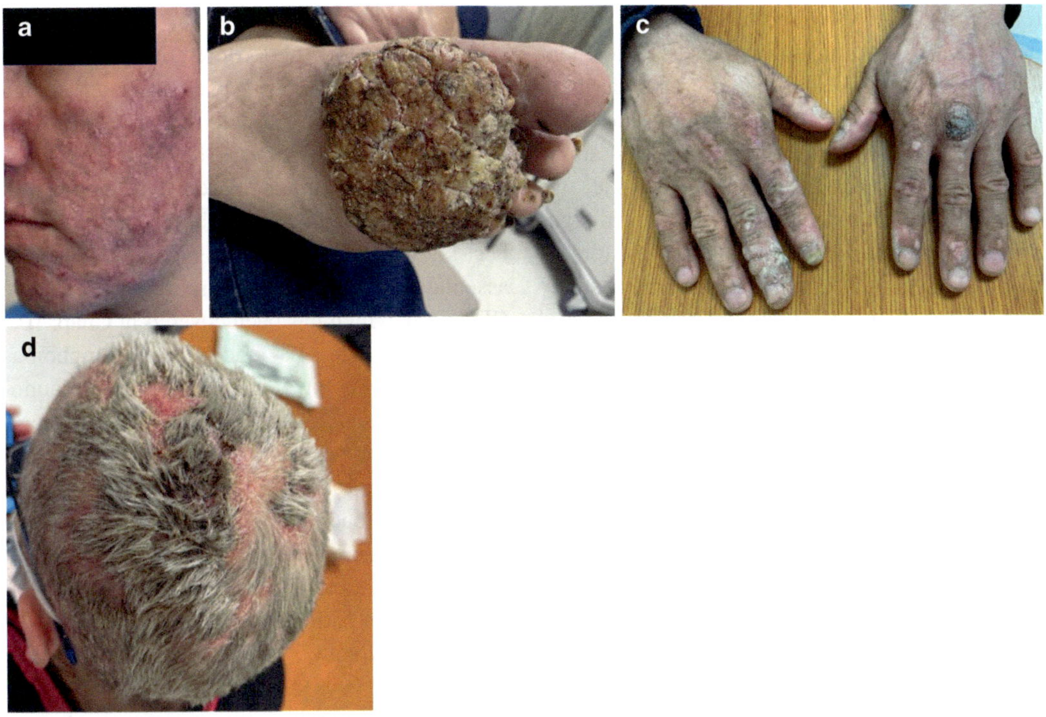

Fig. 16.1 Inflammatory and infectious diseases emerging in the context of underlying immunodeficiency. (**a**) Severe rosacea in a patient with common variable immunodeficiency (CVID). The lesions showed improvement following immunoglobulin replacement therapy. (**b, c**) Numerous hyperkeratotic, therapy-resistant warts in a patient with idiopathic CD4 lymphocytopenia (**b**) and in a patient with NK-cell deficiency (**c**). (**d**) Severe *Trichophyton mentagrophytes* fungal infection of the scalp (kerion) in a female patient with previously unrecognized CVID

and therapy-resistant staphylococcal abscesses.

- Reactivation of dormant infections. Viral reactivations are most commonly seen in this category. Human papillomavirus (HPV) is present in epidermal cells in most individuals, giving rise to warts. The control of HPV is achieved by the immune system, and decreased levels of immune surveillance lead to the emergence of florid warts, which may be extremely difficult, if not impossible to treat. Similar examples are severe reactivations of *Herpes simplex* and *Varicella zoster* virus (herpes zoster).
- Occurrence of skin disease in which infection plays a pathogenic role. Examples are very severe acne or rosacea (exacerbated by *Propionibacterium* [*Cutibacterium*] *acnes* or *Demodex* mites, respectively), seborrheic dermatitis (*Malassezia* spp.), or eczemas (*Staphylococcus aureus*).
- Atypical infections, not usually seen in immunocompetent individuals, such as *Bartonella*, or atypical *Mycobacteriae*. This type of infection is most common in iatrogenically immunosuppressed individuals.

16.2.2 Eczemas

Eczema (or dermatitis) are inflammatory skin diseases characterized by ill-defined erythematous patches or plaques accompanied by itch and secondary skin changes. Eczemas represent nonspecific inflammatory reactions of the skin to damage and thus may be classified as exogenous (caused by damage caused by external allergens and irritants) or endogenous, caused by the deficiencies in the skin barrier (e.g., atopic dermatitis). Dermatitis is a common manifestation of immunodeficiency and often resembles atopic dermatitis. Differentiation between those two conditions may be difficult, as the clinical signs may be identical. However, a lack of history of atopic dermatitis in childhood and an unusually high severity and treatment resistance should prompt consideration of immunodeficiency as an underlying cause.

16.2.3 Autoimmune and Autoinflammatory Skin Diseases

Immune dysregulation in immunodeficiencies may lead to the emergence of autoimmune skin diseases, such as vitiligo, alopecia areata, cutaneous lupus erythematosus, chondritis, vasculitis, or psoriasis. Those manifestations are quite rare.

16.2.4 Cutaneous Lymphomas and Lymphoproliferative Disorders

Systemic immunodeficiency-associated lymphoproliferative disorders constitute a diverse array of lesions characterized by varying clinicopathologic features and are usually grouped into four distinct types: posttransplant lymphoproliferative disorders (PTLDs), lymphomas linked to HIV infection, lymphoproliferations associated with primary immune disorders, and other iatrogenic immunodeficiency-associated lymphoproliferative disorders. The best characterized are those related to an infectious agent, Epstein-Barr virus (EBV) or Kaposi sarcoma–associated virus/human herpes virus 8 (HHV8) [4]. The EBV-related B-cell lymphoproliferations have been best studied. The severity may vary from benign B-cell hyperplasias, through indolent lymphomas (such as marginal zone B-cell lymphoma) to aggressive, high-grade B-cell lymphomas. In relation to cutaneous lymphoproliferation, the best-known type is cutaneous immunodeficiency-associated B-cell lymphoproliferative disease (ID-LPD), which has been covered in Chap. 10.

The incidence of T- and NK-cell lymphomas is comparatively lower in the context of immunodeficiency. In contrast to B-cell lymphoproliferations, it does not exhibit a robust association with EBV. Limited knowledge exists regarding immunodeficiency-associated T-cell lymphoproliferative disorders in the skin. We have observed the occurrence of rare primary cutaneous T-cell lymphomas in patients with underlying immunodeficiency. Notably, two patients with γδ MF were found to have common variable immunodeficiency. Intriguingly, immunosuppressed individuals appear to be at an elevated risk of another γδ T-cell lymphoma, specifically hepatosplenic γδ T-cell lymphoma. This risk has been documented in young patients with Crohn's disease undergoing immunosuppressive therapy with thiopurines and anti-tumor necrosis factor-α agents. We have documented the development of two cutaneous malignancies in a patient with recessive hyper IgE syndrome (DOCK8 mutation): Langerhans cell histiocytosis and aggressive epidermotropic CD8 T-cell lymphoma. Additionally, we have observed cutaneous $CD8^+$ T-cell lymphoproliferative diseases in two patients with idiopathic CD4 lymphocytopenia, which, despite being resistant to therapy, exhibited a protracted, indolent course. A similar case has recently been reported in a teenage patient with homozygous RAG1 mutations [5] (Fig. 16.2).

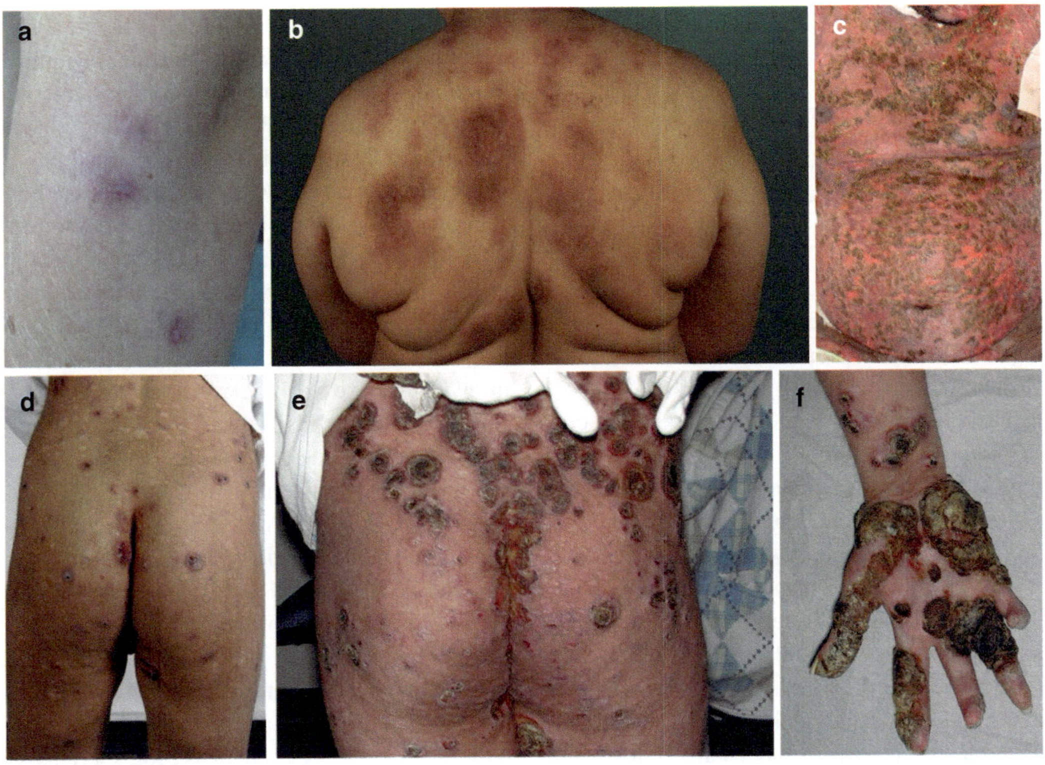

Fig. 16.2 Cutaneous T-cell lymphoproliferative diseases and lymphomas arising in patients with underlying immunodeficiency. (**a**) Skin nodules representing $CD8^+$ lymphoproliferative disease ($CD8^+$ $CD4^-$ $CD3^+$ TIA-1^+, granzyme-B^+ TCRγ polyclonal) in a 28-year-old female with idiopathic CD4 lymphocytopenia. The patient was monitored for 4 years, when she gradually developed additional lesions of the same morphology on the trunk and extremities. (**b**) Extensive $CD8^+$ lymphoproliferative disease in a patient with Common Variable Immunodeficiency (CVID). (**c**) γδ T-cell lymphoma manifesting as erythroderma and necrotic skin plaques in a patient with hypogammaglobulinemia (probably CVID). (**d–f**) A 14-year-old male patient with autosomal recessive hyper IgE syndrome who developed necrotic skin lesions. The photographs depict progression over 14 months. The initial biopsy from lesions in D showed Langerhans cell histiocytosis, whereas the biopsies taken from the more necrotic plaques revealed aggressive epidermotropic $CD8^+$ lymphoma

16.3 Common Variable Immunodeficiency (CVID)

Skin Manifestations

- Cutaneous abscesses
- Alopecia areata
- Vitiligo
- Granulomas

Hematological Comorbidities

- Lymphadenopathy, splenomegaly
- Increased risk of non-Hodgkin lymphoma, including cutaneous lymphomas
- Decreased numbers of naive B and T cells

Common variable immunodeficiency (CVID) stands out as the predominant symptomatic primary immunodeficiency, hallmarked by hypogammaglobulinemia and an impaired capability to produce specific immunoglobulins [6]. Its prevalence, hovering between 1:20,000 and 1:50,000, typically brings about a diagnosis in the second to fourth decade of life [7]. The primary diagnostic feature for CVID involves observing a decrease in serum IgG levels that fall two or more standard deviations below the mean for an age-specific normal range. This must also coincide with a similar drop in at least one of the other two isotypes, making it below the age-specific normal range. In adults, a significant reduction is typi-

Table 16.2 Secondary causes of hypogammaglobulinemia

Factor	IgG	IgA
Drugs: penicillamine, sulfasalazine, cyclosporine, NSAID, antiepileptics	+	+
Malignancies: chronic lymphocytic leukemia, lymphomas, thymoma	+	–
Another primary immunodeficiency	+	–

cally considered when IgG levels fall below 4 g/L, but some centers consider CVID already at the threshold of 6 g/L.

Clinically, CVID manifests as a kaleidoscope of presentations, ranging from recurrent infections, autoimmune reactions, and inflammatory disturbances to lymphoproliferative complications [8]. Approximately 40% of patients manifested skin-related symptoms, mainly skin infections of fungal, bacterial, and viral origins, notably abscesses and oral candidiasis.

In addition, patients may present with autoimmune and inflammatory skin conditions, such as alopecia areata, erythema nodosum, vitiligo, cutaneous granulomas reminiscent of sarcoidosis or granuloma annulare, or Sweet syndrome [9–11]. We have observed patients in whom CVID was diagnosed based on unusually severe or therapy resistant seborrheic dermatitis, acne or rosacea.

CVID should be differentiated from secondary causes of hypogammaglobulinemia (Table 16.2).

16.4 Selective IgA Deficiency (SIgAD)

Skin Manifestations

- Mostly asymptomatic
- Atopic dermatitis
- Urticaria
- Lupus erythematosus

Hematological Comorbidities

- Severe transfusion reactions (anaphylaxis with IVIg infusions)
- Not clear whether SIgAD is associated with malignancies

Selective immunoglobulin A deficiency (SIgAD) is the most common primary immune deficiency, with its prevalence ranging from 1:3000 to as high as 1:150, contingent on the studied population [12]. It is defined by a decrease in serum IgA levels below 0.07 g/L, with normal IgM and IgG levels in individuals >4 years of age. Most individuals are clinically asymptomatic. If symptoms occur, they become clinically evident during the second decade of life, but diagnoses in childhood are not uncommon [3]. These include recurrent pulmonary infections, predispositions to allergies, autoimmune diseases, gastrointestinal complications, and, on rarer occasions, malignancies. A noteworthy aspect of SIgAD is the heightened susceptibility to allergic conditions. In fact, between 25% and 50% of SIgAD patients come to medical attention primarily due to an allergic disease. Within this allergic spectrum, eczema, specifically atopic dermatitis, emerges as a frequently associated condition in SIgAD patients [12, 13]. As is the case for CVID, secondary causes of IgA deficiencies should be excluded, especially those related to the drugs (Table 16.2).

A significant proportion of SIgAD patients have anti-IgA antibodies in their serum and thus may develop severe transfusion reactions, especially when given intravenous immunoglobulins.

16.5 Idiopathic CD4 Lymphocytopenia

Skin Manifestations

- HPV infections: warts, genital condylomata
- Molluscum contagiosum
- Squamous cell carcinomas
- Mucocutaneous candidiasis
- Autoimmune conditions: psoriasis, lupus, vitiligo, vasculitis

Hematological Comorbidities

- EBV-related lymphomas
- Brain lymphomas

Idiopathic $CD4^+$ lymphocytopenia is a primary immune deficiency, predominantly diagnosed in adulthood, especially around the third decade of life [3]. The core feature of this condition is a diminished $CD4^+$ count below 300 cells/mm^3 without evidence of other causes of lymphopenia, such as HIV or immunosuppressive medications. Clinical manifestations encompass a spectrum from autoimmune disturbances and neoplasia to the more frequently seen opportunistic infections.

More than half (52%) of the patients exhibit cutaneous manifestations. The spectrum of reported infectious skin symptoms is related to persistent HPV infections (warts, condylomata) and fungal or bacterial infections (mycetoma, dermal abscesses). Additionally, patients report pruritus, erythroderma, and vesicular eruptions, probably related to immune dysregulation due to decreased activity of CD4 regulatory T cells [14].

16.6 Hyper IgE Syndrome

Skin Manifestations

- Atopic dermatitis-like eczema
- Staphylococcal infections
- Other infections: Molluscum contagiosum, Herpes simplex

Hematological Comorbidities

- Non-Hodgkin and Hodgkin lymphomas

Hyper IgE Syndrome (HIES) is a complex primary immunodeficiency disorder, hallmarked by significantly elevated serum IgE levels. The level of IgE is very high (>2000 IU/mL), but it may gradually decline in adulthood (inversely correlated with patients' age). Eosinophilia is present and is not correlated to IgE levels. The most frequently identified mutation is in the *STAT3* gene, leading to autosomal dominant HIES. Recessive forms of HIES due to *DOCK8* mutation are rare but have a more severe phenotype associated with profound immunodeficiency [15].

Clinically, patients with HIES are particularly susceptible to recurrent skin abscesses and pulmonary infections. *Staphylococcus aureus* is frequently the causative pathogen, although other bacteria and fungi can also be implicated. Cutaneous manifestations are prominent; patients often exhibit atopic dermatitis-like eczema, which can be severe and challenging to manage. Additionally, these individuals may develop other skin complications like molluscum contagiosum, herpes virus infections, and fungal infections. Mucocutaneous candidiasis is also common. Importantly, elevated IgE and eosinophilia do not correlate with the clinical severity of the disease [16].

Beyond its dermatological impact, HIES has notable systemic manifestations. Respiratory complications are prevalent, with patients commonly experiencing recurrent pneumonia, leading to the development of lung parenchymal damage over time. This damage can manifest as pneumatoceles or bronchiectasis, potentially resulting in chronic respiratory insufficiency.

Musculoskeletal anomalies further complicate the clinical picture. Patients may exhibit skeletal abnormalities such as scoliosis, craniosynostosis, and osteopenia. Dental and craniofacial anomalies, like retained primary teeth or a characteristic facial appearance, might also be observed.

Patients with HIES seem to have a predisposition to different lymphomas.

It is worth mentioning that with the advent of NGS a number of mutations in genes other than *STAT3* or *DOCK8* may result in clinical syndromes indistinguishable from HIES (e.g., *CARD11*, IL6 receptor, *ERBIN*, *PGM3*) [17].

16.7 Autoimmune Polyendocrinopathy with Candidiasis and Ectodermal Dystrophy (APECED)

Skin Manifestations

- Mucocutaneous candidiasis
- Vitiligo
- Nail pitting and nail dystrophy

Hematological Comorbidities

- Pernicious anemia

APECED is a distinct autosomal recessive immunodeficiency, hallmarked by a triad: chronic mucocutaneous candidiasis, persistent hypoparathyroidism, and Addison's disease. Additionally, the disorder presents with a spectrum of endocrine and non-endocrine features. The underlying etiology for APECED stems from mutations in the autoimmune regulator gene (AIRE), which is instrumental in fostering T-cell tolerance within the thymus. These patients develop antibodies against IL-17, which explains their susceptibility to fungal infections. Candidiasis is often the presenting sign and may manifest as chronic mucocutaneous candidiasis, persistent genital moniliasis, esophageal candidiasis and therapy-resistant angular cheilosis [10]. Other dermatological signs are nail pitting and nail dystrophy as a manifestation of ectodermal dystrophy, which are present in up to 50% of patients.

Although the disease typically debuts during childhood, APECED can be insidious, with some clinical manifestations presenting later in adulthood. In fact, novel disease components have been identified as late as the fifth decade [3, 18].

Patients with diagnoses of APECED develop several autoimmune diseases, including vitiligo and pernicious anemia. Major differential diagnoses are other immunodeficiencies associated with candidiasis, such as Dectin1 deficiency or mannan-binding lectin (MBL) deficiency, described in women with recurrent vulvovaginal candidiasis.

16.8 Good's Syndrome

Skin Manifestations

- Herpes reactivation
- Lichen planus
- Erythema multiforme

Hematological Comorbidities

- Thymoma
- Hypogammaglobulinemia
- Lymphopenia

Good's Syndrome, also known as thymoma with immunodeficiency, is a rare secondary immunodeficiency characterized by adult-onset combined B and T cell immunodeficiency in the setting of a thymoma [19]. The exact mechanism remains unclear but anti-cytokine autoantibodies arising in the context of thymoma autoimmunity play a role.

Clinical manifestations comprise a combination of infectious and autoimmune conditions with a predilection to the lung, where there is a high risk of *Pneumocystis jirovecii*, *Aspergillus*, *Candida*, and viral (HSV, VZV, CMV, HHV8) infections [19, 20]. Laboratory investigations reveal hypogammaglobulinemia affecting all immunoglobulin isotypes (IgG, IgA, IgM), lymphopenia particularly affecting $CD4^+$ T cells, and sometimes an absence of B cells.

In the skin the most commonly reported finding is oral lichen planus [21, 22]. Skin infections, particularly herpetic infections and bacterial abscesses, have also been described [23–25]). Patients seem to be at increased risk of developing erythema multiforme [26].

16.9 VEXAS (Vacuoles, E1 Enzyme, X-Linked Autoinflammatory, Somatic Syndrome)

Skin Manifestations

- Chondritis
- Neutrophilic dermatoses
- Vasculitis
- Herpes infections

Hematological Comorbidities

- Myelodysplastic syndrome
- HLH (hemophagocytic lymphohistiocytosis)

VEXAS syndrome is a monogenic autoinflammatory disorder afflicting adult males within the age bracket of 45–80 years. The condition's underpinnings lie in the somatic mutations affecting *UBA1* within hematopoietic cells [27, 28]. This genetic alteration results in a constellation of both inflammatory and hematological derangements. Patients often exhibit hematological anomalies, ranging from macrocytosis, cytopenias and myelodysplastic syndrome. The systemic inflammatory response encompasses multiple organs and tissues, including the skin, lungs, vasculature, and cartilage. Chondritis is the most common sign in patients with VEXAS and may precede other symptoms and signs. The disease has a severe course—patients develop neutrophilic dermatoses reminiscent of Sweet syndrome, cutaneous vasculitis and may develop HLH.

The diagnosis should be considered in patients with hematological abnormalities who develop severe inflammatory diseases in the skin and elsewhere. The presence of vacuoles in bone marrow cells and the *UBA1* mutation test are diagnostic (Fig. 16.3).

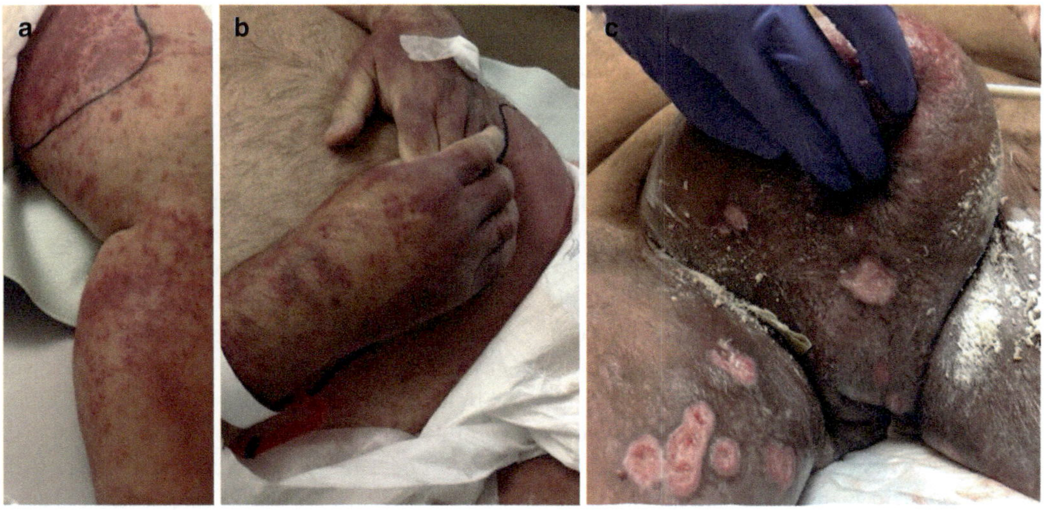

Fig. 16.3 VEXAS syndrome in a 64-year-old male. The patient presented with pancytopenia, fever, abdominal pain, peripheral edema, and diarrhea. Skin manifestations included a widespread purpuric and livedoid skin rash (**a, b**) and skin ulcers in the genital and gluteal area caused by HSV1 infection (**c**)

16.10 LRBA Deficiency

Skin Manifestations

- Atopic dermatitis
- Alopecia
- Vitiligo

Hematological Comorbidities

- Lymphadenopathy, splenomegaly
- Lymphopenia, thrombocytopenia
- Hypogammaglobulinemia

Lipopolysaccharide-responsive beige-like anchor protein (LRBA) deficiency is a rare autosomal recessive disorder caused by *LRBA* gene mutation [29]. The LRBA protein has a role in the endocytic pathway and in maintaining intracellular vesicle transport. When LRBA is deficient, there is an altered regulation of cytotoxic T lymphocyte antigen-4 (CTLA-4), a protein vital for immune tolerance. This results in cellular and humoral immune dysregulation.

The disease debuts before the age of 25. Clinical manifestations are numerous. Patients present with recurrent bacterial, viral, and fungal infections, mostly in the lungs. A significant proportion of patients with LRBA deficiency manifest with autoimmune and allergic complications such as autoimmune hemolytic anemia, immune thrombocytopenia, autoimmune neutropenia, asthma, and atopy. Hypothyroidism, diabetes mellitus, and growth hormone deficiency can occur. Gastrointestinal symptoms range from chronic diarrhea to more severe presentations such as inflammatory bowel disease-like symptoms. Hepatomegaly, splenomegaly, and lymphadenopathy are common and linked to autoimmunity.

The involvement of the skin reflects the autoimmune phenomena. Atopic dermatitis-like eczema, alopecia and vitiligo have been reported [30, 31].

16.11 GATA2 Deficiency

Skin Manifestations

- HPV-related infections (cutaneous warts, genital condylomata)
- Erythema nodosum
- Panniculitis
- Gingival hypertrophy
- Rosacea-like facial granulomas and lymphoedema

Hematological Comorbidities

- Myelodysplastic syndrome

GATA2 deficiency, a recently identified genetic immunodeficiency disorder, typically emerges around the median age of 20 years, although its onset spans a broad spectrum, from as early as 5 months to as late as 78 years. Notably, some carriers remain asymptomatic throughout life. Clinically, GATA2 deficiency exhibits diverse manifestations, with infections and hematological disturbances, such as myelodysplastic syndrome. Skin manifestations predominantly arise from complications related to chronic HPV infections. As a result, these patients face an elevated risk of HPV-related skin malignancies, encompassing squamous intraepithelial lesions, bowenoid papulosis, and invasive squamous cell carcinoma. Beyond these malignancies, Patients with GATA2 deficiency commonly exhibit other dermatological afflictions, such as warts, condylomata, lower extremity ulcers, distinct nodular skin lesions, cellulitis, and inflammatory conditions like erythema nodosum or panniculitis [10, 32, 33]. Facial lymphedema may mimic severe rosacea. Case reports indicated an association with cutaneous lymphomas [34].

16.12 WHIM Syndrome

Skin Manifestations

- HPV-related infections (warts, genital condylomata)

Hematological Comorbidities

- Panleukopenia
- Hypogammaglobulinemia

WHIM syndrome, an infrequent autosomal dominant immunodeficiency, is an acronym derived from its primary clinical manifestations: warts, hypogammaglobulinemia, infections, and myelokathexis. This syndrome stems from germline mutations, which result in an amplified function of the CXCR4 chemokine receptor. The perturbed function of CXCR4 disrupts the normal trafficking and homeostasis of immune cells, thereby making individuals susceptible to recurrent infections, especially those caused by HPV, leading to persistent and widespread warts. Furthermore, the unique feature of myelokathexis involves neutrophil retention in the bone marrow, which compounds the immunodeficient state [35]. WHIM syndrome typically emerges in late childhood, but its manifestation in adulthood is not uncommon [3]. A hallmark feature in these patients is the early and prolific development of skin warts, especially concentrated on the hands and feet. By their adolescent years, many affected individuals exhibit extensive warts, and those who become sexually active might subsequently develop genital warts. Beyond HPV-related warts, individuals with WHIM syndrome are intrinsically more susceptible to diverse soft-tissue infections. This augmented vulnerability often translates to recurrent episodes of cellulitis, persistent abscesses, and occasionally more invasive deep-tissue infections [35]. Patients are at risk of developing squamous cell carcinomas [36].

16.13 Chronic Granulomatous Disease (CGD)

Skin Manifestations

- Skin abscesses

Hematological Comorbidities

- HLH (hemophagocytic lymphohistiocytosis)

Chronic granulomatous disease (CGD) is a genetically inherited primary immunodeficiency. While it typically manifests during childhood, there are instances of onset in both early and later stages of adulthood [3]. Adult patients with CGD can be classified into three distinct groups: those initially diagnosed in infancy who have managed to reach adulthood, individuals who displayed symptoms during their childhood but only received a definitive diagnosis later in life, and those with a milder disease variant who experience symptom onset exclusively in their adult years. At its core, CGD arises from hereditary defects in one of the six components of the NADPH oxidase enzyme complex. This complex is pivotal in producing reactive oxygen species (ROS) during the respiratory burst of phagocytes, a crucial mechanism in neutralizing ingested pathogens [37]. The disease manifests through both infectious and inflammatory complications. Severe bacterial and fungal infections are seen in all patients.

Significantly, the skin emerges as one of the organs most frequently impacted by CGD [38]. Skin staphylococcal abscesses, cellulitis and lymphadenitis were described [39]. Atypical causes of abscesses such as *Serratia*, *Granulibacter*, and fungal or yeast infections can be present.

16.14 Diagnostic Approach

The most challenging part of the diagnostic process is to consider immunodeficiency as a possible cause of the disease. Classic presentations of immunodeficiencies, such as persistent, refractory infections, unexplained weight loss, or dermatological manifestations, can frequently be misattributed to coexisting hematological disorders or be perceived as adverse events related to therapeutic interventions. However, a deeper clinical insight may reveal that the immunodeficiency itself could underpin the pathophysiological cascade.

Once immunodeficiency is suspected, the usual initial screening panel aims at the assessment of the key components of the immune system: the immunoglobulins, complement, differential leukocyte counts, and T- and B-lymphocyte subsets (Table 16.3).

Further testing depends on clinical findings and the results of the screening tests. NGS sequencing is increasingly available and is being used to detect primary immunodeficiencies in complex cases.

Table 16.3 Screening panel in a patient with suspected immunodeficiency

Immunoglobulins	Quantitative immunoglobulins: IgG, IgM, IgA, IgE
	IgG subclasses: IgG1–4
Complement	C3
	C4
	CH50
Cells	Complete blood count with differential count
	Flow cytometry panel (T cells: CD3, CD4, CD8, CD45RA/RO, α/β, γ/δ; B cells: CD20, NK cells: CD56)
Autoimmunity	ANA (antinuclear antibody) screen
	ENA (extractable nuclear antigen)

16.15 Differential Diagnosis

Immunodeficiencies can mimic some blood diseases with skin manifestations. The most common differential diagnostic considerations are summarized in Table 16.4.

Table 16.4 Consideration for differential diagnoses of adult-onset immunodeficiencies

Immunodeficiency	Differential diagnoses
Common variable immunodeficiency	Secondary hypogammaglobulinemia due to comorbid CLL or lymphoma
Selective IgA deficiency (SIgAD)	Transfusion reactions
Hyper IgE syndrome (HIES)	In adult patients with HIES, IgE levels may be only moderately increased and accompanied by eosinophilia mimicking Kimura disease (Chap. 15) or hypereosinophilic syndrome (Chap. 13)
Good syndrome	Paraneoplastic pemphigus in Castleman's disease may mimic erosive oral lichen planus in Good's syndrome
VEXAS (vacuoles, E1 enzyme, X-linked autoinflammatory, somatic syndrome)	Hematophagocytic lymphohistiocytosis (HLH)
	Immunodeficiency secondary to myelodysplastic syndrome
GATA2 deficiency	Myelodysplastic syndrome
	Panniculitic inflammation in GATA2 deficiency may resemble subcutaneous panniculitic T-cell lymphoma (Chap. 9)
Chronic granulomatous disease (CGD)	Hemophagocytic lymphohistiocytosis (HLH)

References

1. Tangye SG, Al-Herz W, Bousfiha A, Cunningham-Rundles C, Franco JL, Holland SM, et al. Human inborn errors of immunity: 2022 update on the Classification from the International Union of Immunological Societies Expert Committee. J Clin Immunol. 2022;42:1473–507.
2. Staels F, Collignon T, Betrains A, Gerbaux M, Willemsen M, Humblet-Baron S, et al. Monogenic adult-onset inborn errors of immunity. Front Immunol. 2021;12:753978.
3. Rosenberg E, Dent PB, Denburg JA. Primary immune deficiencies in the adult: a previously underrecognized common condition. J Allergy Clin Immunol Pract. 2016;4:1101–7.
4. Natkunam Y, Gratzinger D, Chadburn A, Goodlad JR, Chan JKC, Said J, et al. Immunodeficiency-associated lymphoproliferative disorders: time for reappraisal? Blood. 2018;132:1871–8.
5. Avitan-Hersh E, Stepensky P, Zaidman I, Nevet MJ, Hanna S, Bergman R. Primary cutaneous clonal CD8+ T-cell lymphoproliferative disorder associated with immunodeficiency due to RAG1 mutation. Am J Dermatopathol. 2020;42:e11–5.
6. Yazdani R, Habibi S, Sharifi L, Azizi G, Abolhassani H, Olbrich P, et al. Common variable immunodeficiency: epidemiology, pathogenesis, clinical manifestations, diagnosis, classification, and management. J Investig Allergol Clin Immunol. 2020;30:14–34.
7. Westh L, Mogensen TH, Dalgaard LS, Bernth Jensen JM, Katzenstein T, Hansen A-BE, et al. Identification and characterization of a nationwide Danish adult common variable immunodeficiency cohort. Scand J Immunol. 2017;85:450–61.
8. Albin S, Cunningham-Rundles C. An update on the use of immunoglobulin for the treatment of immunodeficiency disorders. Immunotherapy. 2014;6:1113–26.
9. Zarezadeh Mehrabadi A, Aghamohamadi N, Abolhassani H, Aghamohammadi A, Rezaei N, Yazdani R. Comprehensive assessment of skin disorders in patients with common variable immunodeficiency (CVID). J Clin Immunol. 2022;42:653–64.
10. de Wit J, Brada RJK, van Veldhuizen J, Dalm VASH, Pasmans SGMA. Skin disorders are prominent features in primary immunodeficiency diseases: a systematic overview of current data. Allergy. 2019;74:464–82.
11. Cook QS, Zdanski CJ, Burkhart CN, Googe PB, Thompson P, Wu EY. Idiopathic, refractory sweet's syndrome associated with common variable immunodeficiency: a case report and literature review. Curr Allergy Asthma Rep. 2019;19:32.
12. Morawska I, Kurkowska S, Będnowska D, Hrynkiewicz R, Becht R, Michalski A, et al. The epidemiology and clinical presentations of atopic diseases in selective IgA deficiency. J Clin Med Res. 2021;10:3809.
13. Yazdani R, Azizi G, Abolhassani H, Aghamohammadi A. Selective IgA deficiency: epidemiology, pathogenesis, clinical phenotype, diagnosis, prognosis and management. Scand J Immunol. 2017;85:3–12.
14. Vijayakumar S, Viswanathan S, Aghoram R. Idiopathic CD4 lymphocytopenia: current insights. Immunotargets Ther. 2020;9:79–93.
15. Minegishi Y. Hyper-IgE syndrome, 2021 update. Allergol Int. 2021;70:407–14.
16. Buckley RH. The hyper-IgE syndrome. Clin Rev Allergy Immunol. 2001;20:139–54.
17. Gharehzadehshirazi A, Amini A, Rezaei N. Hyper IgE syndromes: a clinical approach. Clin Immunol. 2022;237:108988.
18. Capalbo D, De Martino L, Giardino G, Di Mase R, Di Donato I, Parenti G, et al. Autoimmune polyendocrinopathy candidiasis ectodermal dystrophy: insights into genotype-phenotype correlation. Int J Endocrinol. 2012;2012:353250.
19. Sipos F, Műzes G. Good's syndrome: brief overview of an enigmatic immune deficiency. APMIS. 2023;131(12):698–704.
20. Ni J, Zhang J, Chen Y, Wang W, Liu J. Variable clinical characteristics and laboratory results in five patients with Chinese Good's syndrome (thymoma and hypogammaglobulinemia): an 8-year retrospective analysis in a university hospital in China. BMC Immunol. 2021;22:50.
21. Fatrez B, Cuny J-F, Bursztejn A-C, Schmutz J-L, Moawad S. Good syndrome associated with lichen planus: a case report and review. Eur J Dermatol. 2020;30:756–7.
22. Macdonald JB, Mangold AR, Connolly SM. Good syndrome and lichen planus: case and review. J Eur Acad Dermatol Venereol. 2014;28:1828–30.
23. Shi Y, Wang C. When the good syndrome goes bad: a systematic literature review. Front Immunol. 2021;12:679556.
24. Fieschi C, Malphettes M, Galicier L, Oksenhendler E. [Adult-onset primary hypogammaglobulinemia]. Presse Med. 2006;35:887–94.
25. Hagiwara H, Iwata Y, Saito K, Watanabe S, Arima M, Ono Y, et al. Herpes vegetans accompanied by Good's syndrome. J Dermatol. 2018;45:e269–71.
26. Glick LR, Wilson WW, Fletcher M. A case of Good's syndrome complicated by erythema multiforme. BMJ Case Rep. 2019;12:e229999.

27. Grayson PC, Patel BA, Young NS. VEXAS syndrome. Blood. 2021;137:3591–4.
28. Beck DB, Ferrada MA, Sikora KA, Ombrello AK, Collins JC, Pei W, et al. Somatic mutations in and severe adult-onset autoinflammatory disease. N Engl J Med. 2020;383:2628–38.
29. Lopez-Herrera G, Tampella G, Pan-Hammarström Q, Herholz P, Trujillo-Vargas CM, Phadwal K, et al. Deleterious mutations in LRBA are associated with a syndrome of immune deficiency and autoimmunity. Am J Hum Genet. 2012;90:986–1001.
30. Tesch VK, Abolhassani H, Shadur B, Zobel J, Mareika Y, Sharapova S, et al. Long-term outcome of LRBA deficiency in 76 patients after various treatment modalities as evaluated by the immune deficiency and dysregulation activity (IDDA) score. J Allergy Clin Immunol. 2020;145:1452–63.
31. Kostel Bal S, Haskologlu S, Serwas NK, Islamoglu C, Aytekin C, Kendirli T, et al. Multiple presentations of LRBA deficiency: a single-center experience. J Clin Immunol. 2017;37:790–800.
32. Polat A, Dinulescu M, Fraitag S, Nimubona S, Toutain F, Jouneau S, et al. Skin manifestations among GATA2-deficient patients. Br J Dermatol. 2018;178:781–5.
33. Geier CB, Ellison M, Cruz R, Pawar S, Leiss-Piller A, Zmajkovicova K, et al. Disease progression of WHIM Syndrome in an International Cohort of 66 pediatric and adult patients. J Clin Immunol. 2022;42:1748–65.
34. Fertitta L, de Fontbrune FS, Battistella M, De Masson A, Bergeron A, Ranta D, et al. Folliculotropic mycosis fungoides associated with GATA2 deficiency: a new skin manifestation. Br J Dermatol. 2018;179:1420–1.
35. McDermott DH, Murphy PM. WHIM syndrome: immunopathogenesis, treatment and cure strategies. Immunol Rev. 2019;287:91–102.
36. Dotta L, Notarangelo LD, Moratto D, Kumar R, Porta F, Soresina A, et al. Long-term outcome of WHIM syndrome in 18 patients: high risk of lung disease and HPV-related malignancies. J Allergy Clin Immunol Pract. 2019;7:1568–77.
37. Gennery A. Recent advances in understanding and treating chronic granulomatous disease. F1000Res. 2017;6:1427.
38. Arnold DE, Heimall JR. A review of chronic granulomatous disease. Adv Ther. 2017;34:2543–57.
39. Roos D. Chronic granulomatous disease. Br Med Bull. 2016;118:50–63.

17 Cutaneous Manifestations of Graft Versus Host Disease (GvHD)

Robert Gniadecki, Minakshi Taparia, Jean Deschenes, Jori Hardin, and Etienne Mahe

17.1 Practice Essentials

- The most common cutaneous feature in acute graft-versus-host disease (aGvHD) is a maculopapular, morbilliform exanthem appearing 2–6 weeks after allogeneic hematopoietic stem cell transplant (HSCT).
- Skin involvement in chronic GVHD (cGvHD) is seen in 60–80% of allogeneic HSCT recipients and is comprised of poikiloderma, lichen-planus-like, or sclerodermoid skin morphology.
- Risk factors for GvHD include human leukocyte antigen (HLA) disparity between donor and recipient, higher age of the recipient and/or donor, female donor, and male recipient, use of peripheral G-CSF mobilized stem cells, increased number of allogeneic HSCT procedures, and the use of total body irradiation.
- cGvHD results in a 30–40% increased risk of non-relapse-related mortality and lower overall survival.
- Topical steroids and calcineurin inhibitors are first-line treatments in mild-to-moderate GvHD whereas systemic corticosteroids are effective in moderate-to-severe disease. Extracorporeal photopheresis is a therapy method with few side effects and achieves good results as a second-line therapy, especially in cutaneous manifestations.

17.2 Definition and Classification

Graft-versus-host disease (GvHD) presents as an intricate multi-organ disorder stemming from the introduction of immune-competent cells into the recipient's system. This phenomenon predominantly occurs within the context of allogeneic hematopoietic stem cell transplantation (HSCT), with rare instances linked to blood transfusion or solid organ transplantation [1].

R. Gniadecki (✉)
Division of Dermatology, University of Alberta, Edmonton, AB, Canada
e-mail: r.gniadecki@ualberta.ca

M. Taparia
Division of Hematology, University of Alberta Hospital, Edmonton, AB, Canada
e-mail: mtaparia@ualberta.ca

J. Deschenes
Department of Pathology and Laboratory Medicine, Cross Cancer Institute, Edmonton, AB, Canada
e-mail: Jean.Deschenes@albertaprecisionlabs.ca

J. Hardin
Division of Dermatology, University of Calgary, Calgary, AB, Canada
e-mail: Jori.hardin@albertahealthservices.ca

E. Mahe
Department of Pathology & Laboratory Medicine, and Hematology & Hematological Malignancies, University of Calgary, Calgary, AB, Canada
e-mail: etienne.mahe@albertaprecisionlabs.ca

R. Gniadecki et al. (eds.), *Diseases of Blood and Skin*, https://doi.org/10.1007/978-3-031-65292-9_17

For GvHD to manifest, the donor graft must encompass immunologically competent cells, while the host must lack the ability to mount an effective immune response to eradicate the transplanted cells. Recipients of HSCT undergo conditioning chemotherapy and/or radiotherapy to address an underlying malignancy. This dual-purpose treatment serves to both treat the malignancy and suppress the immune system, preventing the rejection of the donor graft. Subsequently, donor hematopoietic progenitor cells are introduced into the recipient. These donor cells may originate from an HLA-identical sibling, a matched but unrelated donor, or, less commonly, from an umbilical cord or a mismatched/haploidentical donor. The ensuing outcome is an immune-mediated response from the donor cells against the host malignancy, known as the graft-versus-tumor effect. GvHD ensues when immunocompetent donor cells recognize host tissues as foreign. Consequently, autologous transplants do not induce an immune response against the recipient but are also devoid of graft-versus-tumor effect [2].

The skin and mucosa are commonly affected by cGvHD, which constitutes the primary manifestations. However, the involvement of any organ is plausible, with a higher incidence observed in the liver, gastrointestinal tract, and lungs.

The classic categorization of GvHD divides it into two main groups: acute GvHD (aGvHD) encompasses manifestations within the initial 3 months (100 days) post-transplant, while chronic GvHD (cGvHD) refers to occurrences beyond day 100. Beyond the temporal distinction, aGvHD and cGvHD exhibit divergent immunological mechanisms and clinical presentations, allowing for an early diagnosis of cGvHD based on clinical features even before the 100-day mark [3]. The genesis of aGvHD unfolds through a three-phase process [2]:

1. Recipient tissue damage: The initial phase is characterized by recipient tissue damage resulting from the toxicity of the conditioning regimen. This damage triggers the release of inflammatory cytokines, creating an inflammatory milieu.
2. Donor lymphocyte activation: In the second phase, mature donor lymphocytes present within the graft enter this inflammatory environment. Upon contact with host and donor antigen-presenting cells expressing disparate host antigens, there is a subsequent expansion and activation of donor lymphocytes.
3. Expansion of alloreactive T-cells: The third and final phase involves the expansion of alloreactive T-cells derived from the donor. These cells transform into cytotoxic effector T-cells, instigating tissue injury and releasing additional inflammatory cytokines against the host.

The pathophysiology of cGvHD remains less comprehended, incorporating elements of allore-activity and autoimmunity. Notably, pathogenic T-cells emerge after the maturation of donor precursor cells within the recipient thymus, a process that is affected by aging, conditioning regimens, and acute graft-versus-host reactions [4]. Furthermore, cGvHD presents an imbalance between regulatory T cells (Tregs) and alloreactive effector T cells [2]. B cells also play a pivotal role in cGvHD. Host B cells activate alloreactive donor $CD4^+$ T cells, subsequently contributing to the activation and expansion of autoreactive B cells within the graft. These autoreactive donor B cells assume a central role in amplifying autoimmune responses and facilitating the epitope spreading of autoreactive T and B cells [5].

Advancements in stem cell transplantation protocols, such as reduced conditioning intensity pre-transplantation, donor lymphocyte infusion (DLI), and secondary allogeneic HSCT, have reshaped the onset timing of aGvHD and cGvHD symptoms. Recognizing this evolution, the GvHD working group of the US National Institutes of Health (NIH) has refined aGvHD further into classical (manifesting before 100 days) and persistent, recurrent, or delayed types (first aGvHD emerging after day 100) [2, 6]. Chronic GvHD is categorized into classic cGvHD (lacking signs of acute GvHD) and an overlap syndrome in which both aGvHD and cGvHD coexist (Table 17.1).

The development of aGvHD is significantly influenced by the mismatch of human leukocyte antigen (HLA) molecules, with an escalated risk correlating to a greater HLA disparity between the donor and recipient. However, even patients with matching HLA molecules can be susceptible to GvHD, emphasizing the intricate nature of this immunological phenomenon [8].

Several additional risk factors contribute to the likelihood of GvHD occurrence. These encompass the higher age of either the recipient or the donor, a scenario involving a female donor and a male recipient, the utilization of peripheral G-CSF mobilized stem cells, a diagnosis of chronic myeloid leukemia, an increased number of allogeneic HSCT procedures, and the application of total body irradiation [9].

Table 17.1 Classification of GvHD [2, 7]

	Time of symptoms after HSCT or DLI	Presence of acute GVHD features	Presence of chronic GVH features
Acute GVHD			
Classic	<100 days	Yes	No
Persistent, recurrent, or de novo late acute onset	>100 days	Yes	No
Chronic GVHD			
Classic	No time limit	No	Yes
Overlap	No time limit	Yes	Yes

17.3 Clinical Manifestations

The skin is assessed based on the body surface area of involvement and the type of lesions/rash noted. The mouth, eyes, gastrointestinal tract, liver, lungs, genital tract, joints, and fascia can also be involved.

17.3.1 Acute GvHD

aGvHD develops in 20–50% of patients who receive stem cells from an HLA-identical sibling donor and in 60–80% where there is an HLA mismatch or the HLA-identical donor is not a sibling of the patient [1]. The hallmark cutaneous presentation of aGvHD manifests as a symmetrical morbilliform or macular exanthem, displaying a predilection for the palms, soles, and face. This distinctive rash typically emerges 2–6 weeks post-transplantation. Initial lesions predominantly localize around hair follicles, gradually progressing to involve the entire body, often meeting criteria for erythroderma. In severe cases, manifestations may escalate to epidermal and mucosal sloughing, blistering, and erosions. The onset of the rash may be heralded by sensations of itchiness and burning (Fig. 17.1).

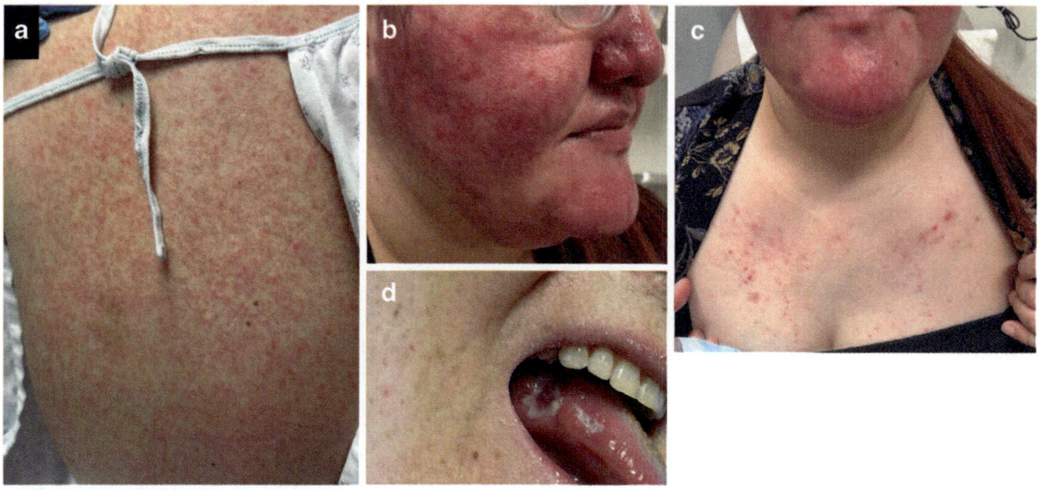

Fig. 17.1 Acute GvHD. (**a**) Extensive, exanthematous papular rash, (**b, c**) severe facial rash resembling rosacea and a more moderate papular eruption on the chest, and (**d**) reactivation of herpes virus (HSV1) mucositis in a patient with acute GhVD

17.3.2 Chronic GvHD

Chronic graft-versus-host disease (cGvHD) impacts a substantial proportion, approximately 60–80%, of patients following allogeneic HSCT, with the skin being affected in over 90% of cases [10]. Notably, cGvHD may manifest without preceding aGvHD in 25–35% of patients, and approximately 20–30% of those who experienced aGvHD do not progress to cGvHD [11].

Several factors contribute to the development of cGvHD, including the age of the recipient (with a higher risk if >20 years old) or the origin of the stem cells (higher for peripheral blood, lower for umbilical cord). T-cell depletion from the bone marrow transplant lowers the risk whereas the risk is increased by the administration of donor lymphocytes post-transplantation [2].

cGvHD exhibits diverse clinical presentations, affecting various systems and organs, more recently proposed to be classified as either sclerotic or non-sclerotic in nature [7]. Diagnostic signs encompass poikiloderma (characterized by hypopigmentation, hyperpigmentation, telangiectasia, and atrophy), lichen planus-like or sclerodermoid skin lesions, dyspigmentation (vitiligo), ichthyosis, keratosis pilaris-like, psoriasiform, and annular erythema (Fig. 17.2). Mucous membranes, hair, and nails are commonly involved (Table 17.2).

In the lichenoid variant of cGvHD, patients present with violaceous or erythematous papules and plaques with fine scale, affecting areas like palms, soles, genitals, and nails. Sclerodermoid cGvHD often initiates on the trunk, becoming generalized over weeks, resembling morphea and/or lichen sclerosus. Joint involvement may lead to contractures and reduced mobility.

cGvHD extends beyond the skin, simulating autoimmune connective tissue diseases. Sicca syndrome is frequent and may lead to significant functional impairment of the vision (eye sicca),

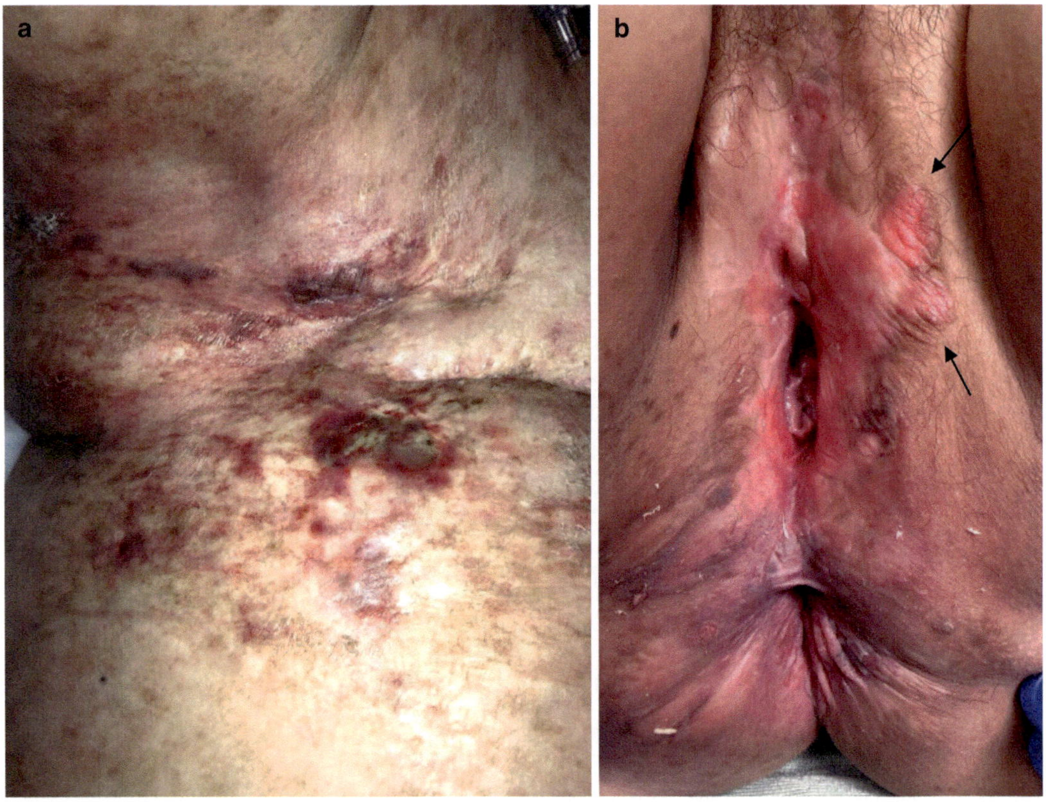

Fig. 17.2 Chronic GvHD. (**a**) Atrophic, fibrotic, sclerodermoid lesions on the trunk and (**b**) vulval atrophy, fibrosis, and treatment-resistant genital warts (highlighted with arrows)

Table 17.2 Clinical features of cGvHD (modified from [12])

Diagnostic features	Lichen-planus like features (lichenoid GvHD) Sclerotic features (sclerodermoid GvHD) Poikiloderma Morphea-like features Lichen sclerosus-like features
Distinctive features	Depigmentation Papulosquamous lesions Nail dystrophy New onset of scarring or non-scarring scalp alopecia Mucosal lesions: xerostomia, mucosal atrophy, ulcers, pseudomembranes
Other	Keratosis pilaris Hypo- or hyperpigmentation Ichthyosis Sweat impairment Pruritus Maculo-papular exanthem/morbilliform eruption Gingivitis Mucositis

disturbances of masticatory function, and precipitate dental pathology due to dryness and oral microbiome imbalance. Gastrointestinal involvement manifests as esophageal dysmotility and diarrhea. Liver cholestasis is observed, and bronchiolitis obliterans may affect the lungs.

Patients face immunodeficiency risks, leading to opportunistic infections and an elevated risk of malignancy. While the risk of non-melanoma skin cancer moderately increases, it is linked to the cutaneous effects of total body irradiation often used in conditioning regimens [13].

17.4 Diagnosis and Severity Assessment

17.4.1 Skin Biopsy

The histopathological features characterizing aGvHD are marked by vacuolar degeneration of the basal cell layer, dyskeratotic keratinocytes, and a mild mononuclear superficial perivascular infiltrate. Initial epithelial damage is localized at the tips of rete ridges and hair follicles. Severe damage may lead to subepidermal clefts emerging from confluent vacuolar degeneration. Mild spongiosis with exocytosis of lymphocytes is a common observation, and lymphocytes tend to surround necrotic keratinocytes, forming a distinctive “satellite sign.”

The histology of lichenoid cGvHD mirrors classic lichen planus, characterized by hyperkeratosis, hypergranulosis, acanthosis, and dyskeratotic keratinocytes with basal layer vacuolization. Saw-tooth rete ridges are evident, accompanied by dermal melanophages. A crucial diagnostic criterion is the presence of a band-like infiltrate along the dermo-epidermal junction, considering that vacuolar degeneration of the basal cell layer is a frequent post-HSCT finding.

Sclerodermoid cGvHD histology reveals epidermal atrophy, edema, and homogenization of collagen in the upper dermis, resembling features seen in lichen-sclerosus-like cGvHD. In cases resembling morphea, collagen sclerosis manifests as pan-dermal, patched, or deep dermal changes, occasionally involving the panniculus and fascia.

17.4.2 Severity Scoring

To gauge the severity of skin involvement, a classification into four stages is employed, contingent on the affected body surface area and the occurrence of epidermolysis. This staging system facilitates a comprehensive understanding of the extent and intensity of cutaneous manifestations in the context of aGvHD. The Mount Sinai Acute GvHD International Consortium (MAGIC) criteria and NIH consensus are commonly used in practice for aGvHD and cGvHD (Tables 17.3 and 17.4) [12, 14].

Table 17.3 Skin scoring of aGvHD

Stage	Cutaneous findings	Grade	Histopathology
0	No rash related to GvH	0	Normal epidermis
1	Macules/papules <25% BSA (body surface area) without associated symptoms	1	Focal or diffuse vacuolar alteration of the basal cell layer
2	Macules/papules or erythema with pruritus or associated symptoms covering <25 and <50% BSA, or localized desquamation	2	Grade 1 plus dyskeratotic squamous cells in the epidermis and/or hair follicle
3	Generalized erythroderma or symptomatic macular, papular, or vesicular eruption with bullae and desquamation covering >50% BSA	3	Grade 2 plus subepidermal vesicle formation
4	Generalized exfoliative dermatitis, ulcerative dermatitis, or bullae	4	Complete separation of the epidermis from dermis

Table 17.4 Skin scoring of chronic GvHD [12]

Score	0	1	2	3
Rash, included are: Maculopapular rash, erythema, skin sclerosis, papulosquamous eruption, ichthyosis, keratosis pilaris-like lesions	No involvement	1–18% BSA (body surface area)	19–50%	>50% BSA
Presence of sclerotic features	Absent	–	Superficial sclerosis (able to pinch the skin)	Deep sclerosis (unable to pinch, ulceration, impaired body mobility)
Mouth (lichen planus-like lesions)	Absent	Mild symptoms not limiting food intake	Moderate symptoms, partially limiting food intake	Major symptoms severely limiting food intake

17.5 Differential Diagnosis

Both aGvHD and cGvHD pose significant difficulties regarding differential diagnoses. The most common problems are drug reactions and skin rashes due to infectious causes, which may even coexist with GvHD and further blur the clinical characteristics of the lesions. Table 17.5 summarizes the most relevant differential diagnoses.

The morbilliform exanthems in GvHD may be clinically indistinguishable from those caused by drugs. It has been argued that in cases where the face, ears, palms, and soles are affected, it tends to lean the differential diagnosis towards aGvHD rather than drug hypersensitivity [15]. However, it is important to note that this manifestation is not always definitive and several drug-induced reactions, e.g., DRESS (drug rash with eosinophilia and systemic symptoms) and toxic erythema resulting from chemotherapy may present similarly, with a distinct emphasis on the face, hands,

Table 17.5 Differential diagnosis of cutaneous aGvHD

aGvHD	cGvHD
Drug-induced exanthem	Drug-induced exanthem
Toxic epidermal necrolysis (TEN)	Toxic epidermal necrolysis (TEN)
Toxic erythema of chemotherapy	Viral exanthems
Viral exanthems	Systemic sclerosis (sclerodermoid GvDH)
Radiation dermatitis	Morphea (sclerodermoid GvDH)
Neutrophil engraftment syndrome	Lichen planus (lichenoid GvHD)
Photosensitivity reactions (especially voriconazole)	Lichen sclerosus et atrophicus (lichenoid GvHD)

and feet, respectively. Toxic erythema of chemotherapy, also known as palmoplantar erythrodysesthesia, is most commonly associated with doxorubicin, docetaxel, fluorouracil, and cytarabine. It manifests as acral dysesthesia followed by tender erythematous swelling of the palms and soles. Histology demonstrates a toxic keratinocyte reaction with subepidermal edema and mild perivascular lymphocytic infiltration.

Toxic epidermal necrolysis (TEN) and grade IV aGvHD pose significant challenges in differentiation, particularly considering the initiation of numerous potential culprit medications around the time of transplantation. Sometimes, the differentiation based on the clinical features and histopathology is not possible, and in those instances, the discontinuation of potential TEN-associated drugs should be considered.

Cutaneous manifestations of viral infections pose a challenge in distinguishing from GvHD due to their variability. Findings include a morbilliform eruption, petechiae, vesiculobullous lesions, and mucocutaneous involvement in the oropharynx, esophagus, and genital tract. Viral reactivation (e.g., Epstein-Barr virus, cytomegalovirus, or human herpesvirus 6) is common after allogeneic HSCT, and viral exanthems may overlap with those of GvHD [16].

Radiation dermatitis, resulting from total body irradiation, can cause inflammation of the skin, adnexal structures, and subcutaneous tissue. Typically, this condition develops 7–14 days after radiation. Chronic radiodermatitis, however, may manifest months to years after radiation exposure, with cutaneous manifestations encompassing telangiectasia, atrophy, sclerosis, dyspigmentation, ulcerations, and both pre-malignant and malignant lesions.

Engraftment syndrome, characterized by fever, rash, and pulmonary injury, shares clinical similarities with aGvHD. Bone marrow engraftment typically occurs between days 12 and 13 after the infusion of donor cells, with pulmonary involvement (edema, hypoxia, pulmonary infiltrates) serving as a helpful clue in differentiation. Other clinical manifestations favoring engraftment syndrome are: fever >38.2°C, weight gain >2.5% of the baseline, and transient encephalopathy [17]. A therapeutic trial with corticosteroids can prove beneficial, with the majority of patients with engraftment syndrome typically experiencing rapid improvement. However, caution is advised as rapid tapers may occasionally result in a flare of the rash and the emergence of refractory aGVHD.

To distinguish systemic sclerosis from cGvHD, certain clinical features should be absent in the latter. Specifically, there should be no presence of sclerodactyly, nail fold capillary changes, or Raynaud's phenomenon in cGvHD. Additionally, cGvHD typically does not exhibit an edematous phase, and there are no positive autoantibodies commonly observed in diffuse or localized systemic sclerosis.

17.6 Therapy [12, 18, 19]

17.6.1 aGvHD

Therapy for aGvHD is employed both prophylactically in the post-transplant period and as a standard treatment once aGvHD has manifested. In the presence of aGvHD, the initial approach involves enhancing immunosuppression, with systemic corticosteroids, such as oral prednisone or intravenous methylprednisolone, being the first-line agents. Response to corticosteroid administration is observed in approximately 50% of patients. The shorter duration of steroid taper (12 weeks) is non-inferior to longer tapers (22 weeks) in aGvHD.

If the disease progresses over 3 days, shows no improvement at 7 days, or the response is incomplete at 14 days, second-line treatments or salvage therapy are initiated. The options are numerous and comprise anti-TNFα agents, anti-IL2 receptor drugs (e.g., daclizumab, basiliximab), lymphodepleting agents (alemtuzumab, anti-thymocyte globulin, rituximab), mycophenolate mofetil, methotrexate, JAK 1/2 inhibitors (ruxolitinib), tyrosine kinase inhibitors (e.g., imatinib), among others. Extracorporeal photopheresis (ECP) has shown promise in aGvHD as well.

17.6.2 cGvHD

General measures. Due to the prevalent dry skin in patients affected by cGvHD, the application of topical moisturizers can be beneficial for alleviating itching and preventing skin cracking. However, it is important to note that the effects are temporary, necessitating regular use.

Patients with cutaneous GVHD should be aware of the potential for photosensitivity, a well-known complication post-transplant that may be exacerbated by certain drugs like voriconazole. It is prudent for patients to avoid exposure to natural sunlight and apply physical or chemical protection.

For those experiencing pruritus, whether from GVHD or other causes, the use of topical or oral antipruritic agents, including antihistamines, can be helpful.

Notably, patients should also be connected to wound care, physiotherapy for joint mobility, nutrition, and psychosocial support [20].

Skin-directed therapy is effective for mild-to-moderate cutaneous cGvHD and comprises topical corticosteroids and topical calcineurin inhibitors (topical tacrolimus). The overall response rate of topical tacrolimus is approximately 70%. Additionally, topical ruxolitinib shows promise for GVHD.

Phototherapy, encompassing PUVA (psoralen plus ultraviolet A), nb-UVB (narrowband ultraviolet B), and UVA (ultraviolet A), is a viable treatment option. While PUVA has demonstrated efficacy, it comes with an increased risk of cutaneous malignancy, requiring careful consideration in treatment decisions. Narrowband UVB is considered a safer option in terms of malignancy risk.

Systemic corticosteroids stand as the first-line treatment for patients with Grade 2–4 chronic cutaneous GvHD. Currently, no other agents have definitively demonstrated superiority over corticosteroid monotherapy or their combination with steroids for the initial treatment of either disease.

As with aGvHD, the first line with cGvHD is systemic corticosteroids. Second-line options are similar to those used in aGvHD and include mycophenolate mofetil, hydroxychloroquine, imatinib mesylate, rituximab, and ruxolitinib. Novel agents targeting STAT signaling (ROCK inhibitors) and Bruton's tyrosine kinase are being studied [20].

Another treatment option for steroid-refractory cGvHD is extracorporeal photopheresis (ECP), a leukapheresis-based photochemotherapy, also used for Sézary syndrome. In this process, leukocytes collected ex vivo are exposed to ultraviolet-A (UV-A) light along with 8-methoxy psoralen (8-MOP), a photosensitizer, and then infused back into the patient. ECP has demonstrated an overall response rate (ORR) ranging from 50% to 91%, with a skin-specific ORR of 64% to 83% across various phase I/II studies. Although ruxolitinib demonstrated superiority to ECP in the REACH-2 trial, ECP was the most common best available therapy [21]. A meta-analysis including 595 steroid-refractory cGVHD patients in 18 studies supports these findings, reporting pooled response rates for skin, liver, ocular, oral, lung, gastrointestinal, and musculoskeletal involvement of 74%, 68%, 60%, 72%, 48%, 53%, and 64%, respectively [22].

References

1. Cho A, Just U, Knobler R. [Cutaneous graft-versus-host disease]. Hautarzt. 2018;69:109–115.
2. Hymes SR, Alousi AM, Cowen EW. Graft-versus-host disease: part I. Pathogenesis and clinical manifestations of graft-versus-host disease. J Am Acad Dermatol. 2012;66:515.e1–18. quiz 533–4
3. Zeiser R. Advances in understanding the pathogenesis of graft-versus-host disease. Br J Haematol. 2019;187:563–72.
4. Teshima T, Reddy P, Liu C, Williams D, Cooke KR, Ferrara JLM. Impaired thymic negative selection causes autoimmune graft-versus-host disease. Blood. 2003;102:429–35.
5. Shimabukuro-Vornhagen A, Hallek MJ, Storb RF, von Bergwelt-Baildon MS. The role of B cells in the pathogenesis of graft-versus-host disease. Blood. 2009;114:4919–27.
6. Filipovich AH, Weisdorf D, Pavletic S, Socie G, Wingard JR, Lee SJ, et al. National Institutes of Health consensus development project on criteria for clinical trials in chronic graft-versus-host disease: I. diagnosis and staging working

group report. Biol Blood Marrow Transplant. 2005;11:945–56.
7. Baumrin E, Loren AW, Falk SJ, Mays JW, Cowen EW. Chronic graft-versus-host disease. Part I: epidemiology, pathogenesis, and clinical manifestations. J Am Acad Dermatol. 2024;90(1):1–16.
8. DiRienzo CG, Murphy GF, Jones SC, Korngold R, Friedman TM. T-cell receptor valpha spectratype analysis of a CD4-mediated T-cell response against minor histocompatibility antigens involved in severe graft-versus-host disease. Biol Blood Marrow Transplant. 2006;12:818–27.
9. Vargas-Díez E, Fernández-Herrera J, Marin A, Cámara R, García-Díez A. Analysis of risk factors for acute cutaneous graft-versus-host disease after allogeneic stem cell transplantation. Br J Dermatol. 2003;148:1129–34.
10. Johnson ML, Farmer ER. Graft-versus-host reactions in dermatology. J Am Acad Dermatol. 1998;38:369–92; quiz 393–6.
11. Lee SJ. New approaches for preventing and treating chronic graft-versus-host disease. Blood. 2005;105:4200–6.
12. Jagasia MH, Greinix HT, Arora M, Williams KM, Wolff D, Cowen EW, et al. National Institutes of Health consensus development project on criteria for clinical trials in chronic graft-versus-host disease: I. The 2014 diagnosis and staging working group report. Biol Blood Marrow Transplant. 2015;21:389–401.e1.
13. Omland SH, Gniadecki R, Hædersdal M, Helweg-Larsen J, Omland LH. Skin cancer risk in hematopoietic stem-cell transplant recipients compared with background population and renal transplant recipients: a population-based cohort study. JAMA Dermatol. 2016;152:177–83.
14. Harris AC, Young R, Devine S, Hogan WJ, Ayuk F, Bunworasate U, et al. International, multicenter standardization of acute graft-versus-host disease clinical data collection: a report from the Mount Sinai Acute GVHD International Consortium. Biol Blood Marrow Transplant. 2016;22:4–10.
15. Byun HJ, Yang JI, Kim BK, Cho KH. Clinical differentiation of acute cutaneous graft-versus-host disease from drug hypersensitivity reactions. J Am Acad Dermatol. 2011;65:726–32.
16. Düver F, Weißbrich B, Eyrich M, Wölfl M, Schlegel PG, Wiegering V. Viral reactivations following hematopoietic stem cell transplantation in pediatric patients—a single center 11-year analysis. PLoS One. 2020;15:e0228451.
17. Spitzer TR. Engraftment syndrome: double-edged sword of hematopoietic cell transplants. Bone Marrow Transplant. 2015;50:469–75.
18. Hymes SR, Alousi AM, Cowen EW. Graft-versus-host disease: part II. Management of cutaneous graft-versus-host disease. J Am Acad Dermatol. 2012;66:535.e1–16; quiz 551–2.
19. Hong J, Fraebel J, Yang Y, Tkacyk E, Kitko C, Kim TK. Understanding and treatment of cutaneous graft-versus-host-disease. Bone Marrow Transplant. 2023;58:1298–313.
20. Baumrin E, Loren AW, Falk SJ, Mays JW, Cowen EW. Chronic graft-versus-host disease. Part II: disease activity grading and therapeutic management. J Am Acad Dermatol. 2024;90(1): 19–36.
21. Zeiser R, Polverelli N, Ram R, Hashmi SK, Chakraverty R, Middeke JM, et al. Ruxolitinib for glucocorticoid-refractory chronic graft-versus-host disease. N Engl J Med. 2021;385:228–38.
22. Savani BN, Tichelli A. Blood and marrow transplantation long term management: survivorship after transplant. Wiley; 2021.

Dermatological Clues to Benign and Malignant Blood Diseases

18

Robert Gniadecki, Minakshi Taparia, Jean Deschenes, Jori Hardin, and Etienne Mahe

In the preceding chapters, we approached dermatological signs starting from their associated hematological conditions. Here we adopt an inverse perspective, beginning with the skin manifestations and tracing back to potential hematological origins. For the dermatologist, recognizing these clues paves the way to consider possible systemic involvement. Conversely, hematologists will find value in this perspective; while the primary focus might be a known hematological condition, skin manifestations might offer clues pointing towards a coexisting or alternative diagnosis.

R. Gniadecki (✉)
Division of Dermatology, University of Alberta, Edmonton, AB, Canada
e-mail: r.gniadecki@ualberta.ca

M. Taparia
Division of Hematology, University of Alberta Hospital, Edmonton, AB, Canada
e-mail: mtaparia@ualberta.ca

J. Deschenes
Department of Pathology and Laboratory Medicine, Cross Cancer Institute, Edmonton, AB, Canada
e-mail: Jean.Deschenes@albertaprecisionlabs.ca

J. Hardin
Division of Dermatology, University of Calgary, Calgary, AB, Canada
e-mail: Jori.hardin@albertahealthservices.ca

E. Mahe
Department of Pathology & Laboratory Medicine, and Hematology & Hematological Malignancies, University of Calgary, Calgary, AB, Canada
e-mail: etienne.mahe@albertaprecisionlabs.ca

The first part of this chapter describes paraneoplastic skin diseases, highlighting their potential role as harbingers of hematological malignancies. Early recognition of these dermatological signs is paramount, as they might be the initial indicators of an underlying malignancy. Being alert to these signs ensures timely interventions and prevents diagnostic delays.

The subsequent segment delves into benign hematological conditions. Diseases such as anemias, hemoglobinopathies, and disorders of coagulation often manifest as nuanced skin signs. Whether these signs accompany a malignancy or merely hint at an additional diagnosis, their recognition remains crucial for a comprehensive clinical assessment. Finally, we address the cutaneous extramedullary hematopoiesis, which is a rare entity most often associated with primary myelofibrosis, chronic myeloproliferative neoplasms, chronic hemolytic states, such as thalassemia, sickle cell anemia and certain solid tumors [1].

18.1 Paraneoplastic Skin Diseases as Clues to Hematological Cancers

18.1.1 Practice Essentials

- Numerous skin conditions have been reported to be associated with hematological malignancies, but only a few have a strong correlation

R. Gniadecki et al. (eds.), *Diseases of Blood and Skin*, https://doi.org/10.1007/978-3-031-65292-9_18

and can be considered paraneoplastic diseases.
- Paraneoplastic skin diseases fall into the following broad categories: neutrophilic dermatoses, eosinophilic dermatoses, depositional diseases, bullous diseases (paraneoplastic pemphigus), paraneoplastic pruritus, and miscellaneous.
- Although some paraneoplastic diseases may occur spontaneously in an otherwise healthy individual, the diagnosis usually warrants further screening to rule out an underlying hematological malignancy.

Paraneoplastic syndromes comprise a myriad of dermatological conditions that coexist with hematological malignancies [2]. However, in most cases, the correlation between skin and blood diseases is not firmly established, and the evidence is based on case reports or case series. This section spotlights only those skin diseases with well-documented links to hematological disorders. When confronted with paraneoplastic manifestations, clinicians should actively pursue the possibility of an underlying hematological malignancy. Remarkably, these syndromes can emerge in certain instances well before the hematological neoplasm becomes clinically evident, underscoring the significance of a thorough medical history in bridging dermatological manifestations with potential malignant hematological underpinnings. Moreover, it's pivotal to elucidate a drug history around the disease's onset since specific drug-induced phenomena can closely resemble paraneoplastic presentations.

It is not an uncommon clinical scenario for dermatologists to encounter a patient presenting with conditions suggestive of paraneoplastic syndromes [3]. The pivotal question is whether to delve deeper with diagnostic evaluations to decisively exclude an underlying hematological malignancy. This decision not only weighs heavily in terms of medical implications but also factors in patient anxiety, economic considerations, and potential therapeutic interventions.

The diagnostic toolkit for such scenarios includes the presence of other systemic symptoms (weight loss, chronic fatigue, night sweats, generalized pruritus), unusual clinical presentation of skin disease (recalcitrant course, deviations from the usual clinical appearance of the lesions), clinical evaluation of peripheral lymph nodes, and the presence of hepatosplenomegaly. Laboratory assessments encompass a detailed peripheral complete blood count, lactate dehydrogenase levels, immunoglobulin quantification, and serum electrophoresis with free light chains to rule out monoclonal gammopathy. In circumstances where leukemia looms as a possible diagnosis, a bone marrow biopsy becomes indispensable. Combined ^{18}F fluorodeoxyglucose positron emission and computed tomography (FDG-PET/CT) scanning serve as invaluable tools, especially when delineating entities like lymphomas and leukemias [4, 5]. Nevertheless, a word of caution is due: certain hematological neoplasms, notably indolent low-grade lymphomas, might elude detection by this modality [6].

Paraneoplastic conditions described in this chapter are listed in Table 18.1.

18.1.2 Neutrophilic Dermatoses

18.1.2.1 Practice Essentials

- Sweet's syndrome and pyoderma gangrenosum are strongly associated with myeloid malignancies and plasma cell disorders and may be the first manifestation of hematological malignancy.
- Other less common paraneoplastic neutrophilic diseases are erythema elevatum diutinum, neutrophilic eccrine hidradenitis, and subcorneal pustular dermatosis.

18.1.2.2 Sweet's Syndrome

Sweet's syndrome (acute febrile neutrophilic dermatosis) can manifest as idiopathic, drug-induced, or paraneoplastic forms. Notably, about 20% of all cases are paraneoplastic, most linked to hematological malignancies like myeloid leukemias and myelodysplasias [7]. Intriguingly, the appearance of Sweet syndrome might be an early indicator, sometimes even a decade before the detection of a hematological malignancy [8].

Table 18.1 Skin diseases strongly associated with malignant hematological disease

Skin disease	Most common association
Neutrophilic dermatoses	Myeloid leukemias and myelodysplasias
Sweet's syndrome	Monoclonal gammopathies, predominantly of the IgA type
Pyoderma gangrenosum	
Neutrophilic eccrine hidradenitis	
Erythema elevatum diutinum	
Subcorneal pustular dermatosis	
Eosinophilic dermatosis of hematological malignancy	Chronic lymphocytic leukemia
Depositional diseases	Monoclonal gammopathies
Scleromyxedema	
Scleredema	
Necrobiotic xanthogranuloma	
Normolipemic xanthomas	
Bullous diseases	Castleman disease
Paraneoplastic pemphigus	Thymoma
	Non-Hodgkin lymphoma
Paraneoplastic pruritus	Lymphomas
Other	Any hematological malignancy
Vasculitis	
Autoimmune, connective tissue diseases	
Trichodysplasia spinulosa	

The exact cause behind paraneoplastic Sweet's syndrome remains ambiguous. However, theories posit a potential hypersensitivity to cancer cell antigens or an autoinflammatory process, possibly mediated by interleukin-1 (IL-1) [9, 10]. Supporting this hypothesis, mutations in the *MEFV* gene, typically responsible for familial mediterranean fever (FMF), have been identified in patients exhibiting both Sweet's syndrome and myelodysplastic syndrome [11].

Clinically, paraneoplastic Sweet's syndrome has an expansive range of manifestations. While the prototypical presentation includes sudden fever, joint pain, and the emergence of tender, red or purplish skin nodules that may appear blistered, patients with the paraneoplastic type might exhibit additional extracutaneous complications (Fig. 18.1). For instance, manifestations such as mucosal lesions, neurological diseases like parkinsonism, and eye complications, including optic neuritis or chorioretinitis, are more prevalent in those with underlying myeloproliferative disorders than in cases of idiopathic Sweet's syndrome [8].

Diverse clinical subtypes have also been identified (Fig. 18.1). The acute necrotizing variant displays a swift onset of swollen red patches on the skin, leading to skin and soft tissue necrosis [12]. The isomorphic variant of Sweet syndrome is seen at trauma sites, be it prior radiation exposure or surgical scars. The subcutaneous type, which shares similarities with pyoderma gangrenosum, tends to be closely related to myeloproliferative diseases, revealing tender skin nodules, especially on the buttocks and legs, without the presence of tissue death and often resolving on its own [13]. Furthermore, the neutrophilic dermatosis of the dorsal hands is a localized form of Sweet's syndrome and has been documented in patients with various cancers, including hematological malignancies [14].

The so-called histiocytoid Sweet's syndrome represents a unique variant of the disease, often associated with myelodysplastic syndromes (MDS) [15, 16]. Rather than neutrophils found in skin infiltrates of classic Sweet's syndrome, the dermal infiltrate in histiocytoid Sweet's syndrome consists of mononuclear cells that can be demonstrated to represent immature myeloid cells (immature neutrophils) that morphologically resemble histiocytes. Patients may experience systemic symptoms such as fever, night sweats, and joint pain. The skin presentation ranges from papulovesicular eruptions to erythematous plaques

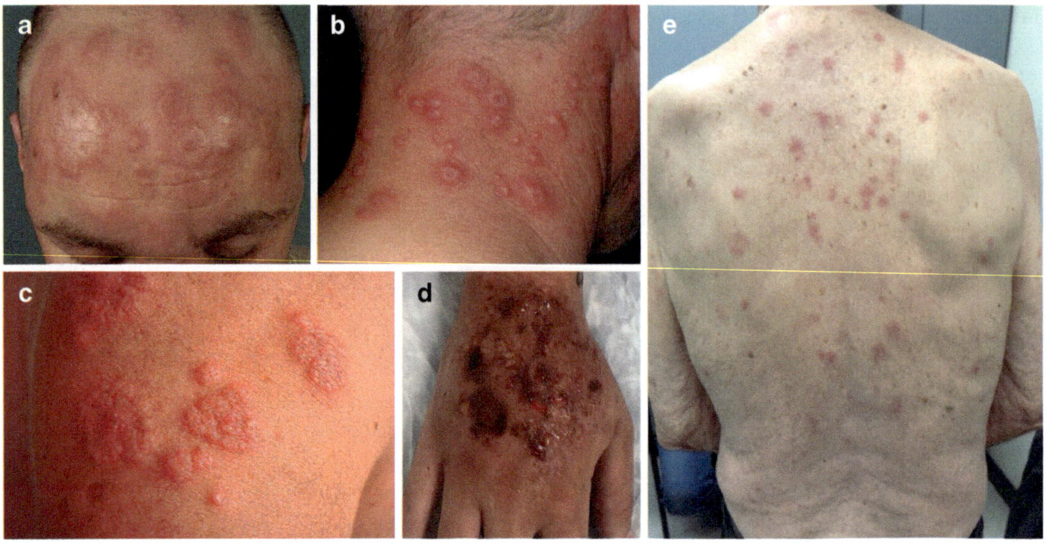

Fig. 18.1 Acute neutrophilic dermatoses. (**a–c**) Sweet's syndrome. Non-scaly round to oval, edematous plaques. Some lesions may show pseudovesiculation (**c**) due to dermal edema. (**d**) Neutrophilic dermatosis of dorsal hands, (**e**) histiocytoid Sweet's syndrome in a patient with myelodysplastic syndrome

and nodules, similar to the lesions of Sweet's syndrome. There is a debate about whether histiocytoid Sweet's syndrome should be classified as a paraneoplastic disease or whether it rather represents myeloid leukemia cutis (see Chap. 2).

Distinguishing paraneoplastic Sweet's syndrome from other neutrophilic paraneoplastic conditions such as neutrophilic eccrine hidradenitis and pyoderma gangrenosum should be considered, but this is not always possible. Neutrophilic dermatoses produce a clinical continuum, e.g., severe, recalcitrant Sweet's syndrome, which may be interpreted as pyoderma gangrenosum. Additionally, vasculitis, erythema elevatum diutinum (EED), infectious neutrophilic panniculitis, panniculitic id reaction, early presentations of erythema nodosum, and leukemia cutis can all mimic the clinical presentation of Sweet's syndrome. This differential diagnosis can be intricate, especially considering that paraneoplastic Sweet's syndrome may concurrently manifest with other neutrophilic paraneoplastic conditions in the same individual [8].

Furthermore, it's crucial to consider drug-induced Sweet's syndrome. Various medications utilized in managing hematological malignancies can trigger the onset of Sweet's syndrome (Table 18.2). As such, a thorough review of the patient's medication history, alongside clinical evaluations, can guide clinicians in making an accurate diagnosis and formulating an appropriate management strategy.

Table 18.2 Drugs associated with sweet syndrome

Cytotoxic anticancer agents	Proteasome inhibitors (bortezomib)
	Mitoxantrone
	Cytarabine
Other anticancer drugs and biological response modifiers	Tyrosine kinase inhibitors (imatinib mesylate)
	Lenalinomide
	Granulocyte colony-stimulating factor (G-CSF)
	All-trans-retinoic acid
	Interferon α
Antibiotics	Clindamycin
	Tetracyclines
	Quinolones
	Trimethoprim with sulfamethoxazole
Antivirals	Abacavir
	Aciclovir

18.1.2.3 Pyoderma Gangrenosum

Pyoderma gangrenosum, a distinct neutrophilic dermatosis, is categorized into four clinical forms: the classic (ulcerative) variety, as well as

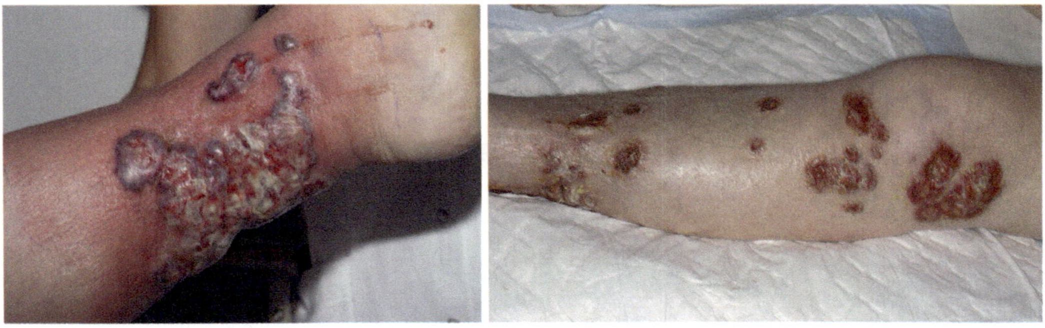

Fig. 18.2 Pyoderma gangrenosum. Chronic, painful ulcerations, often on the lower legs, with a characteristic raised, undermined border

bullous, pustular, and vegetative presentations. Between 20% and 60% of pyoderma gangrenosum cases are associated with a hematological malignancy [17–19]. Among these, the nonclassical manifestations are notably predominant in paraneoplastic presentations [18]. Strikingly, the bullous subtype is correlated with hematological neoplasms in over 70% of instances [20, 21] (Fig. 18.2).

Hematological conditions such as MGUS, myelodysplastic syndromes, and myeloid leukemias are frequently observed as the underlying disorders [19]. Intriguingly, it's not uncommon for both pyoderma gangrenosum and Sweet syndrome to manifest concurrently in a patient affected by a myeloproliferative disorder, supporting the concept that these conditions represent different points on a spectrum of a shared pathogenic process [22].

When pyoderma gangrenosum surfaces in an individual diagnosed with a myeloproliferative disorder, it can potentially signify an adverse prognosis. To underscore this point, data reveals a considerable 1-year mortality rate of 75% in patients with acute myeloid leukemia who subsequently develop pyoderma gangrenosum skin lesions [19].

18.1.2.4 Neutrophilic Eccrine Hidradenitis

Neutrophilic eccrine hidradenitis stands as the most uncommon entity within the spectrum of paraneoplastic neutrophilic dermatoses. The hallmark of this condition is the presence of neutrophilic infiltrates surrounding eccrine sweat glands and their coils. Its correlation with underlying malignancies is profound, as around 90% of individuals with neutrophilic eccrine hidradenitis are found to have an underlying hematological malignancy, primarily acute myelogenous leukemia [23]. Cases have also been documented in association with chronic lymphocytic leukemia, Hodgkin lymphoma, and an array of nodal non-Hodgkin lymphomas. The debate about whether the condition is drug-induced versus truly paraneoplastic persists. Nevertheless, in approximately one-fifth of patients, neutrophilic eccrine hidradenitis presents even before any therapeutic intervention and occasionally even before the diagnosis of the hematological malignancy, suggesting a genuine paraneoplastic nature for these cases.

Interestingly, in about 80% of cases, there's a discernible association between the onset of neutrophilic eccrine hidradenitis and drug administration. The drugs in question mirror those associated with Sweet syndrome, as outlined in Table 18.2. Typically, symptoms arise roughly 9 days post-drug exposure [23].

Clinically, patients often present with infiltrated erythematous papules and plaques, exhibiting a predilection for facial involvement. However, the clinical spectrum is broad. Lesions might also manifest on the upper trunk, arms, and thighs, occasionally appearing annular or linear, bearing resemblance to conditions like erythema multiforme or Sweet's syndrome. Such similarities necessitate careful differentiation and an evaluation of possible infectious causes (Fig. 18.3).

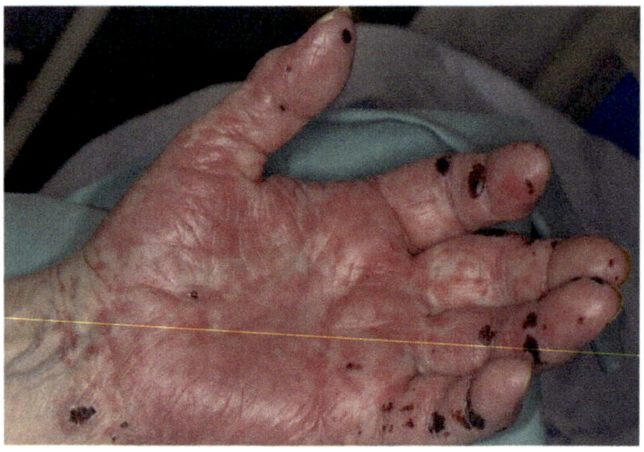

Fig. 18.3 Neutrophilic eccrine hidradenitis in a patient with CLL

18.1.2.5 Erythema Elevatum Diutinum

Erythema elevatum diutinum (EED) is a chronic neutrophilic, leukocytoclastic vasculitis characterized by the appearance of reddish-purple papules, nodules, or plaques, predominantly found on the extensor limbs [24, 25]. EED may appear as an idiopathic condition but has also been linked with various hematological malignancies, notably with monoclonal gammopathies, predominantly of the IgA type, as well as with myelodysplastic syndromes [26]. Less commonly, it has been associated with multiple myeloma, chronic lymphocytic leukemia, and non-Hodgkin's lymphomas. In many cases, the dermatological signs appear several years ahead of the HM diagnosis [26, 27].

18.1.2.6 Subcorneal Pustular Dermatosis

Subcorneal pustular dermatosis is a rare disease distinguished by superficial fragile pustules with characteristic hypopyon (purulent, yellow fluid in the bottom half of the vesicle, with clear fluid in the top half) [28]. A notable association exists between SPD and monoclonal gammopathies, particularly IgA type, making it the most frequently linked hematologic malignancy [29]. Interestingly, the skin manifestations in subcorneal pustular dermatosis can emerge several years before the hematologic malignancy is diagnosed and may show improvement upon treating the associated malignancy [28].

18.1.3 Eosinophilic Dermatosis of Hematological Malignancy (EDHM)

18.1.3.1 Practice Essentials

- Eosinophilic dermatosis associated with hematological malignancies manifests as an itchy, papular rash reminiscent of insect bites.
- It should be differentiated from EBV-related hypersensitivity to insect bites.
- Associated with chronic lymphocytic leukemia.

Eosinophilic dermatosis associated with hematological malignancies represents diverse cutaneous manifestations that predominantly manifest in patients with indolent lymphoproliferative disorders, primarily chronic lymphocytic leukemia [2, 30]. The disease overlaps with the phenomenon of atypical, delayed hypersensitivity reactions to mosquito bites but may also occur in the absence of a clear insect bite history. However, insect bite hypersensitivity should be separated from EDHM as a condition connected to EBV infection, whereas EDHM does not seem to be associated with this virus.

The most common association is chronic lymphatic leukemia where it may be detected in 6–8% of its patients, but it can also develop in the context of leukemias and lymphomas. Skin manifestations might appear well before (in some instances, up to a decade prior) or after the diagnosis of the associated malignancy [2, 31].

Clinically, EDHM can manifest as varied lesions—from papules and blisters to plaques or nodules—often developing against a backdrop of erythematous urticarial skin (Fig. 18.4). Intense itching is a universal complaint. Three primary clinical patterns emerge from a review of published cases: a bullous pattern resembling bullous pemphigoid, an insect bite-like pattern reminiscent of papular urticaria, and a cellulitis-like pattern with similarities to Wells syndrome [24]. Histological examinations consistently reveal inflammation dominated by lymphocytes and eosinophils.

The differential diagnoses are broad and comprise other itchy skin diseases exhibiting eosino-

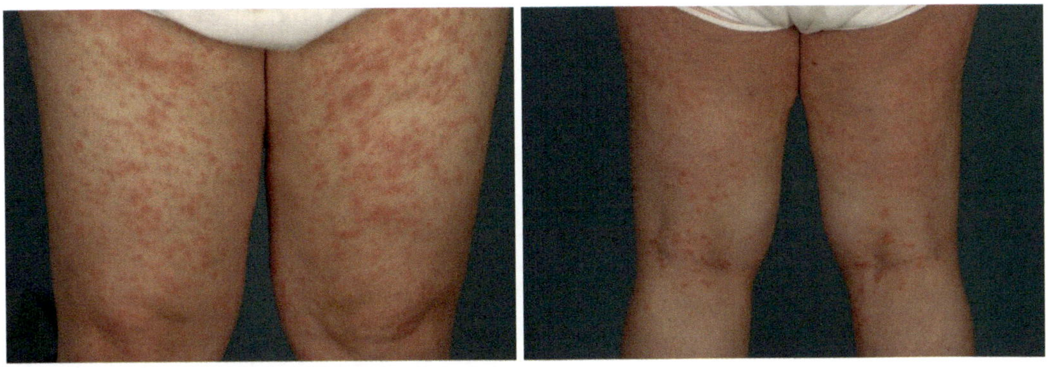

Fig. 18.4 Eosinophilic dermatosis of hematological malignancy (EDHM). Intensely pruritic rash in a patient with CLL

phil infiltration: insect bites, drug reactions, bullous pemphigoid, eosinophilic folliculitis, and Wells syndrome. Moreover, EDHM should be differentiated from other hematological diseases with eosinophilia, such as Kimura disease, hypereosinophilic syndrome (HES), and hyper IgE syndrome.

18.1.4 Depositional Diseases

18.1.4.1 Practice Essentials

- Scleromyxedema and scleredema are strongly associated with monoclonal gammopathies, and those diagnoses should trigger further evaluation to rule out underlying hematological pathology.
- Necrobiotic xanthogranuloma and normolipemic xanthoma may be associated with histiocytoses, monoclonal gammopathies, multiple myeloma, and lymphocytic leukemias.

18.1.4.2 Scleromyxedema

Scleromyxoedema is an uncommon generalized cutaneous mucinosis characterized by elevated mucin production and accumulation, which stems from the proliferation of fibroblasts (refer to Chap. 4). Excluding thyroid-related conditions, scleromyxoedema typically presents in individuals with monoclonal gammopathies, often linked to MGUS, multiple myeloma, or plasmacytomas [32, 33]. A notable majority, exceeding 80% of patients, display IgGλ paraproteinemia.

Clinically, patients often exhibit widespread papular and sclerodermatous skin conditions, with a marked inclination towards facial, auricular, and dorsal hand regions. The papules manifest as firm, semi-transparent, and wax-like (Fig. 18.5). Inflammatory signs are typically minimal or nonexistent, and there's a lack of epidermal alterations. Hardening of the skin may be especially prominent on the extremities, where it may resemble systemic sclerosis, morphea, or eosinophilic fasciitis. Upon histological examination, mucin deposits extensively separate dermal collagen fibers, and there's a notable presence of increased numbers of fibroblast counts and fibrosis.

Systemic manifestations are diverse and play a significant role in the morbidity associated with scleromyxoedema. Prominent symptoms encompass dysphagia, vocal hoarseness, aspiration due to laryngeal complications, generalized or proximal myopathy, polyarthritis, central nervous system disturbances (ranging from encephalopathy and seizures to vertigo and psychosis), cardiac arrhythmias or myocardial infarctions stemming from myocardial complications, and respiratory difficulties due to pulmonary involvement.

The progression of scleromyxedema is relentless, with mortality rates fluctuating between 15% and 50% [34]. The primary causes of fatality are either the advancement of the hematological condition or complications related to the central nervous system.

18.1.4.3 Scleredema

Scleredema is an uncommon condition of skin thickening and non-pitting edema. It often presents with a firm and rigid texture, primarily affecting the facial and neck regions, with potential extension to the scalp and upper torso; the

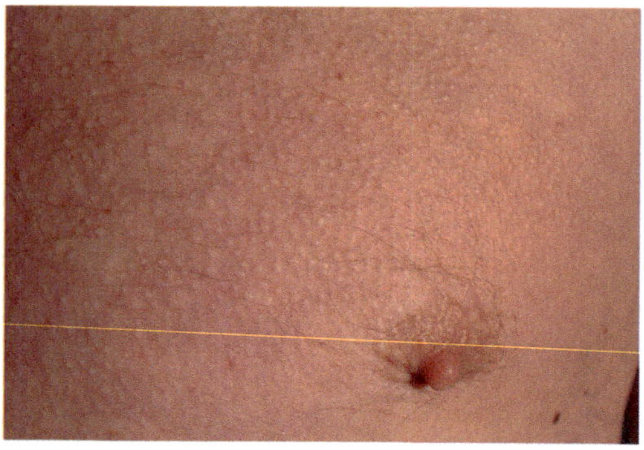

Fig. 18.5 Scleromyxedema in a patient with MGUS

extremities, notably hands and feet, are typically unaffected. Clinically, scleredema is categorized into three subtypes: a classical form (seen in 55% of cases) triggered by fever-related illnesses, the diabetes-associated variant, and the paraneoplastic scleroderma, which constitutes approximately 25% of cases. Like scleromyxedema, paraneoplastic scleredema is associated with monoclonal gammopathies or B-cell lymphomas [35]. Scleredema emerges in conjunction with IgG2/IgG3-κ or IgA-κ paraproteins rather than IgG1-λ in scleromyxedema.

Unlike scleromyxedema, scleredema doesn't display mucin protein deposits, but there's a notable thickening of the dermis and subcutaneous layers, attributed to augmented glycosaminoglycans that intersperse collagen fibers. It's worth noting that the paraneoplastic variant doesn't exhibit spontaneous resolution, a characteristic seen in the classical type. Furthermore, scleredema has the potential to involve internal organs, with specific predilections towards the heart, joints, and ocular structures, and is associated with the POEMS syndrome [36, 37] (Fig. 18.6).

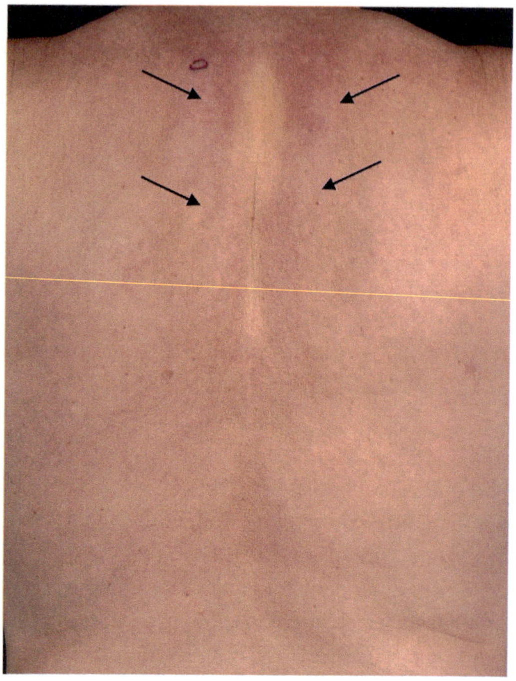

Fig. 18.6 Scleredema Buschke in a patient with MGUS. Note the thickening of the skin in the middle back with a change in skin color (arrows)

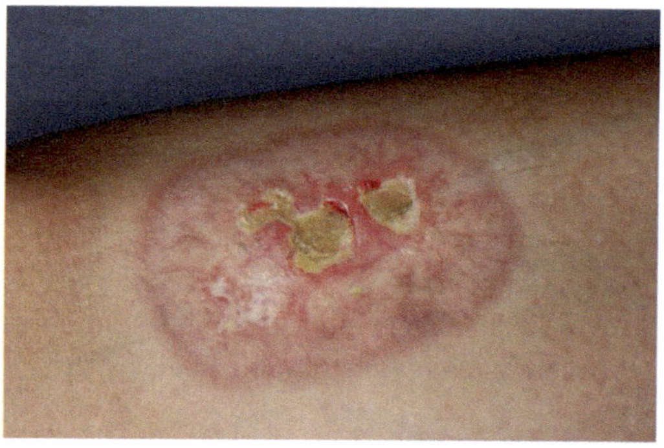

Fig. 18.7 Necrobiotic xanthogranuloma on the upper arm of a patient with MGUS. Note yellow hue, telangiectasias and central ulceration

18.1.4.4 Necrobiotic Xanthogranuloma and Normolipemic Xanthoma

Diffuse normolipemic xanthoma and necrobiotic xanthogranuloma are manifestations of histiocytoses (see Chap. 12) but can also emerge as paraneoplastic conditions [38]. Necrobiotic xanthogranuloma represents the majority, approximately two-thirds, of such paraneoplastic xanthomas. Normolipaemic xanthomas, in their clinical presentation, mirror the manifestations of classical hyperlipaemia xanthomas. Conversely, necrobiotic xanthogranulomas present as firm papules, nodules, or plaques, primarily around the eyes, often accompanied by ulceration, crusting, or telangiectasia (Fig. 18.7). In rare scenarios, lesions can extend to extracutaneous regions, encompassing sites like the oral cavity, eyes, bones, liver, or lungs.

In the context of their association with monoclonal gammopathies, both necrobiotic xanthogranuloma and normolipemic xanthoma are implicated in 80–90% of cases. Most cases, about 80%, are tied to IgG paraproteinaemias. This includes predominantly MGUS (around 50%) and multiple myeloma (roughly 40%). The residual associations include Waldenström macroglobulinemia, chronic myelomonocytic leukemia, chronic lymphocytic leukemia, and non-Hodgkin lymphoma. Notably, in most situations, the xanthomas predate the identification of the hematological condition.

Differential diagnosis of eyelid xanthomas in the context of hematological disease is further discussed in Chap. 12.

18.1.5 Bullous Diseases

18.1.5.1 Paraneoplastic Pemphigus (PNP)

Practice Essentials

- PNP is a severe, potentially fatal blistering disease of the mucosa and the skin associated with Castleman disease, thymoma, or non-Hodgkin lymphoma.
- Bronchiolitis obliterans and respiratory insufficiency is the most common cause of death.

This debilitating disease is an infrequent but severe autoimmune blistering disorder affecting the skin and mucosa. PNP most commonly correlates with hematologic malignancies, non-Hodgkin lymphoma (approximately 40%), followed by chronic lymphocytic leukemia (20%), Castleman disease and thymoma (20%) [39] (see Chap. 15).

Historically, PNP has been identified as a unique type within the pemphigus spectrum but it is now clear that PNP differs from other pemphigus variants in several ways. The mucosal manifestations in PNP tend to be more intense and less responsive to immunosuppressive interventions. Erosive involvement of the vermillion border is mentioned as a typical feature of PNP, but it is not diagnostically discriminative and can also be seen in pemphigus vulgaris. Additionally, the cutaneous lesions in PNP can mimic multiple conditions, from pemphigus and bullous pemphigoid to erythema multiforme, toxic epidermal necrolysis, lichen planus, and even graft versus host disease. Histological examinations typically reveal a lichenoid lymphocytic infiltration at the dermal-epidermal junction, in addition to acantholysis [39, 40]. PNP doesn't always display the same IgG antibodies against desmogleins and therefore the direct immunofluorescence test, which is conclusive in relation to pemphigus vulgaris, may be difficult to interpret in PNP patients. Ultimately, the diagnosis of PNP relies on clinicopathological correlations (Fig. 18.8).

18.1.6 Paraneoplastic Pruritus

Prolonged itchiness, lasting beyond 6 weeks, has frequently been linked with hematological malignancies, especially malignant lymphomas [41]. Paraneoplastic pruritus can sometimes manifest before any evident signs of lymphoma, often lingering for several weeks or even months. Its severity can range from mild discomfort to severe irritation, with a tendency to worsen during nighttime. In some cases, the skin on the limbs may display ichthyosiform alterations alongside the itch. Hodgkin lymphoma has a notable 30% incidence rate of associated paraneoplastic pruritus. Other hematological malignancies with associated pruritus include non-Hodgkin lymphomas (with a 10–20% incidence rate), multiple myelomas, and chronic lymphocytic leukemia. Additionally, aquagenic pruritus is predominantly found in individuals with myelodysplastic syndromes, especially polycythemia vera, and in cases of T-cell lymphomas.

18.1.7 Other Paraneoplastic Conditions (Table 18.3)

Classical syndromes such as erythema gyratum repens and paraneoplastic acanthosis nigricans are occasionally linked to hematological cancers,

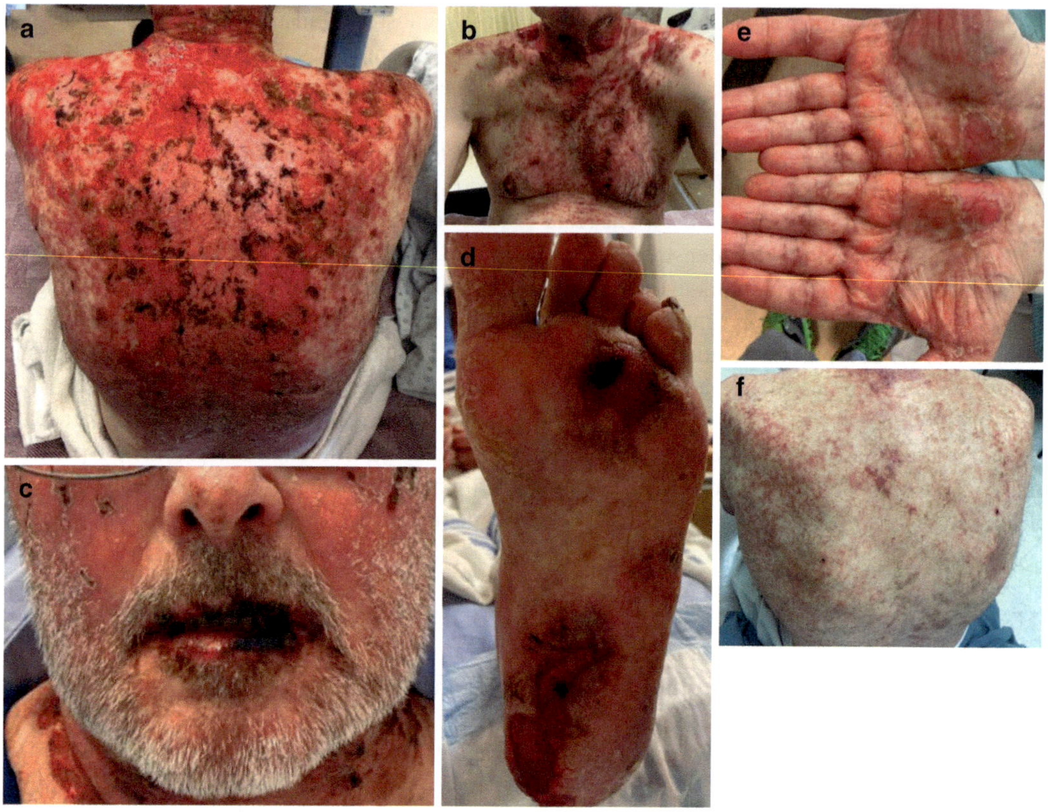

Fig. 18.8 Paraneoplastic Pemphigus in a male patient with stage IV diffuse large B-cell lymphoma. Note severe ulcerative lesions on the trunk (**a, b**), oral mucosa involving the vermillion border (**c**), plantar and palmar surfaces (**d, e**). (**f**) Beneficial effect of therapy with anti-CD20 agent

Table 18.3 Less common paraneoplastic diseases associated with hematological neoplasms

Hematological neoplasm	Skin disease
Myeloid neoplasms	Vasculitis
	Relapsing polychondritis
	Vitiligo
	Dermatomyositis
	Linear IgA dermatosis
	Acquired angioedema
	Behçet disease
Chronic lymphocytic leukemia	Leukocytoclastic vasculitis
	Paraneoplastic lymphocytic vasculopathy
	Trichodysplasia spinulosa
Waldenström macroglobulinemia	Cutaneous small vessel vasculitis
Immunosuppressed patients	Trichodysplasia spinulosa

but the association is very uncommon and almost never seen in the clinic.

There's a substantial correlation between hematological malignancies and various autoimmune conditions. For instance, conditions like myelodysplastic syndrome, myeloid leukaemias, and chronic lymphocytic leukemia have shown coexistence with autoimmune diseases in about 10–15% of patients [42, 43]. In several instances, autoimmune symptoms manifest before the detection of the underlying hematological condition.

Vasculitis is probably the most common association with a hematological malignancy. Although only 5% of cutaneous vasculitis is paraneoplastic, 90% of those patients have an underlying leukemia, lymphoma, or a myeloid neoplasm.

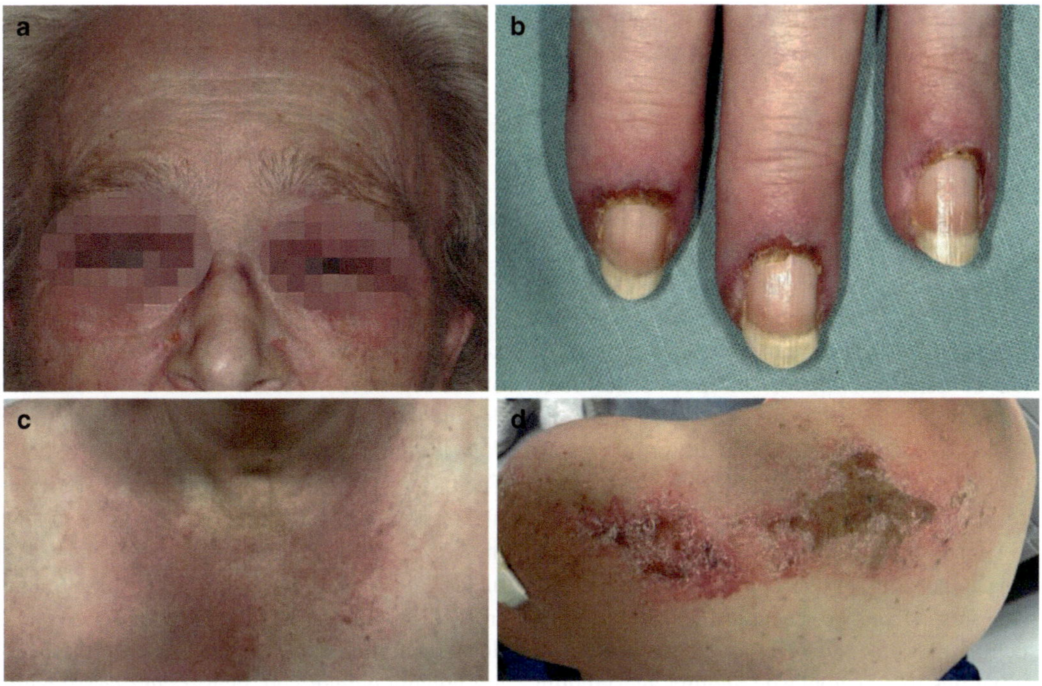

Fig. 18.9 Paraneoplastic, amyopathic dermatomyositis in a patient with diffuse large B-cell lymphoma. Note the characteristic heliotrope rash and swelling of the eyelids (**a**), periungual erythema and necrosis (**b**), and erythema on the upper chest (**c**). Some patients may develop painful, necrotic skin lesions on the upper trunk (**d**)

Connective tissue diseases may coexist with hematological malignancies (Fig. 18.9). An association between lupus erythematosus and diffuse large B-cell lymphoma has been well documented [44]. Marginal zone lymphomas are associated with Sjogren's syndrome [45, 46]. Dermatomyositis, once considered to be mainly associated with solid tumors, is now known to be a paraneoplastic disease in relation to non-Hodgkin lymphomas, Hodgkin disease, and myeloid cancers [47, 48]. Amyopathic and erythrodermic forms might have a higher association with hematological malignancy [47, 49] (Fig. 18.9).

Trichodysplasia spinulosa is a rare but clinically distinctive condition characterized by the emergence of keratin spines from hair follicles, often referred to as spicules. While the nose is most commonly impacted, spicules can arise anywhere on the skin or even be widespread. Trichodysplasia spinulosa seems to be exclusive to patients with compromised immune systems, typically those who have undergone organ transplantation or those undergoing treatment for leukemia [50] and is attributed to the polyomavirus [51]. Skin biopsy shows enlarged and widened hair follicles with keratin obstructing the follicular openings and a conspicuous absence of hair shafts. Moreover, the inner root sheath epithelium shows signs of dystrophy, characterized by deposits of eosinophilic trichohyalin protein. The disease is resistant to treatment, but in cases related to iatrogenic immunosuppression, spontaneous regressions were observed [51].

18.2 Skin in Benign Hematological Diseases

18.2.1 Skin Manifestations in Anemia

18.2.1.1 Practice Essentials

- Skin signs in patients with anemia are related to iron deficiency rather than being a result of low concentration of hemoglobin.

- Hair loss, pruritus, ulcerative stomatitis, candidiasis, and intolerance to cold are the most common signs.
- Skin pallor is an unreliable sign of anemia in adults.

One of the signs of anemia is a noticeable pallor in the skin and mucosal tissues. This pallor arises from peripheral vasoconstriction as the body responds to a decreased oxygen supply reaching the skin and not from the low concentration of hemoglobin. For children under five, assessing palmar pallor serves as a valuable method to identify anemia at the primary care level [52]). Distinct pallor within the palmar creases becomes apparent when hemoglobin levels fall below 70 g/L. Pruritus is more common in females, seen in 15%, as opposed to 5% in males with iron-deficiency anemia [53]. Conditions such as glossitis and ulcerative stomatitis have strong ties to megaloblastic anemia and vitamin B12 deficiency, with oral mucosal symptoms presenting in up to 65% of those with megaloblastic anemia [53, 54]. While glossitis and ulcerative stomatitis do not correlate with other forms of anemia, a higher prevalence of oral candidiasis is evident in those with iron-deficiency anemia [53–55].

Cold intolerance has been linked to iron deficiency [56]. Cold intolerance might be linked to iron deficiency alone, because the intracellular activity of thyroid hormones is contingent upon adequate iron stores. Consequently, an iron deficiency can diminish the thyroid hormone efficacy [57].

Hair loss is a common and frustrating problem in iron-deficient women. Diffuse non-scarring alopecia can develop at the levels of ferritin <100 ng/dL, which are high enough to ensure normal hemoglobin biosynthesis but not always sufficient to maintain hair growth [58].

Fingernail abnormalities and conditions like trachyonychia and koilonychia have been historically connected to iron deficiency anemia. However, newer studies have not definitively confirmed this link [52].

18.2.2 Hemoglobinopathies

18.2.2.1 Practice Essentials

- Chronic, painful leg ulcers, resembling venous ulcers, are the primary manifestations of hemoglobinopathies.

Sickle cell anemia and thalassaemias, both classified as hemoglobinopathies, present with a notable skin manifestation: ulceration in 10–20% of affected individuals, but the prevalence depends on geographic location varying from 75% in Jamaica to only 10% in the UK [59, 60]. These ulcers, mirroring the appearance of venous ulcers, predominantly arise in the gaiter region of the lower limbs, at medial malleoli [61]. The underlying cause of these ulcerations likely stems from microvascular blockages and tissue hypoxia due to abnormal erythrocytes. These erythrocytes are notably dehydrated, denser, and less flexible than their normal counterparts. Hydroxyurea, a drug used in the treatment of sickle cell anemia was believed to aggravate leg ulcerations, but this connection has been disproved [62].

Livedoid vasculopathy is a microvascular disorder which has also been linked to hemoglobinopathies [60]. It is recognized clinically by the distinctive "atrophie blanche" – a lace-like, reticulated white scar of the skin.

18.2.3 Skin in the States of Hypercoagulation

18.2.3.1 Practice Essentials

- Livedoid vasculopathy and livedo reticularis are often associated with inherited and acquired hypercoagulable states.
- Other less specific skin manifestations are petechiae, purpura, ulcerations, and skin necrosis.
- Protein C and/or S deficiency, factor V Leiden mutation, and prothrombin gene variant (20210A) are inherited coagulation disorders

with the highest risk of thrombosis and skin involvement.

- Warfarin-induced skin necrosis and heparin-induced thrombocytopenia have severe, necrotic skin manifestations and are associated with high mortality.

Hypercoagulable states are characterized by an increased tendency to form clots, even if preventive measures are employed. Importantly, dermatological manifestations can sometimes serve as the initial indicator of an underlying hypercoagulable condition.

States of increased coagulation can be inherited or acquired (Table 18.4).

Table 18.4 Common causes of hypercoagulation (modified from [63])

Inherited	Acquired
Antithrombin deficiency	**Drug induced**
Protein C and/or S deficiency	Warfarin
Factor V Leiden mutation	Heparin
Prothrombin gene variant (20210A)	Oral contraceptives
Heparin cofactor II deficiency	**Concomitant diseases**
Hyperhomocystinemia	Diabetes mellitus
Dysfibrinogenemia	Hyperlipidemia
Increased factor VIII	Polycythemia vera
Abnormal plasminogen	Hyperfibrinogenemia
Decreased plasminogen activator	Nephrotic syndrome
Increased plasminogen activator inhibitor	Malignancy
Increased factor XI	Thrombocythemia
Sticky platelet syndrome	Homocystinemia
	Sepsis
	Antiphospholipid syndrome
	Other factors
	Surgery
	Smoking
	Pregnancy
	Obesity
	Trauma
	Immobility
	Cold

18.2.3.2 Skin Manifestations of Hypercoagulable States

Livedoid Vasculopathy

Beyond the traditional large vessel thromboses, hypercoagulation can precipitate microvascular clot formations. Livedoid vasculopathy is a notable dermatological marker in hypercoagulable states characterized by painful ulcers in the lower extremities and feet, presenting in distinct, punched-out patterns amidst livedo reticularis or retiform purpura. As these ulcers heal, they leave behind atrophic, star-shaped white scars surrounded by telangiectasia and evidence of hemosiderin accumulation, often referred to as atrophie blanche [64] (Fig. 18.10). Histological examination of nonulcerated skin typically reveals intravascular thrombi and marked hyalinization of vessel walls with minimal surrounding inflammation, but unlike vasculitis there is no destructive inflammatory process in the vessel wall [65].

Livedoid vasculopathy can be seen in any disease of hypercoagulation, but the most common conditions are inherited coagulopathies (factor V Leiden mutation, prothrombin G20210A mutation, protein C and protein S deficiency, antithrombin III deficiency, hyperhomocysteinemia), cryoglobulinemias, and antiphospholipid syndrome [64].

Livedo Reticularis and Livedo Racemosa

Livedo reticularis is characterized by a reddish-purple, net-like, accentuated venous pattern often visible during episodes of slowed venous blood flow. This pattern predominantly manifests on the lower extremities and can intensify in colder environments. While initially, it may disappear upon warming the affected region, this discoloration tends to become persistent over time. The decision to conduct a systemic

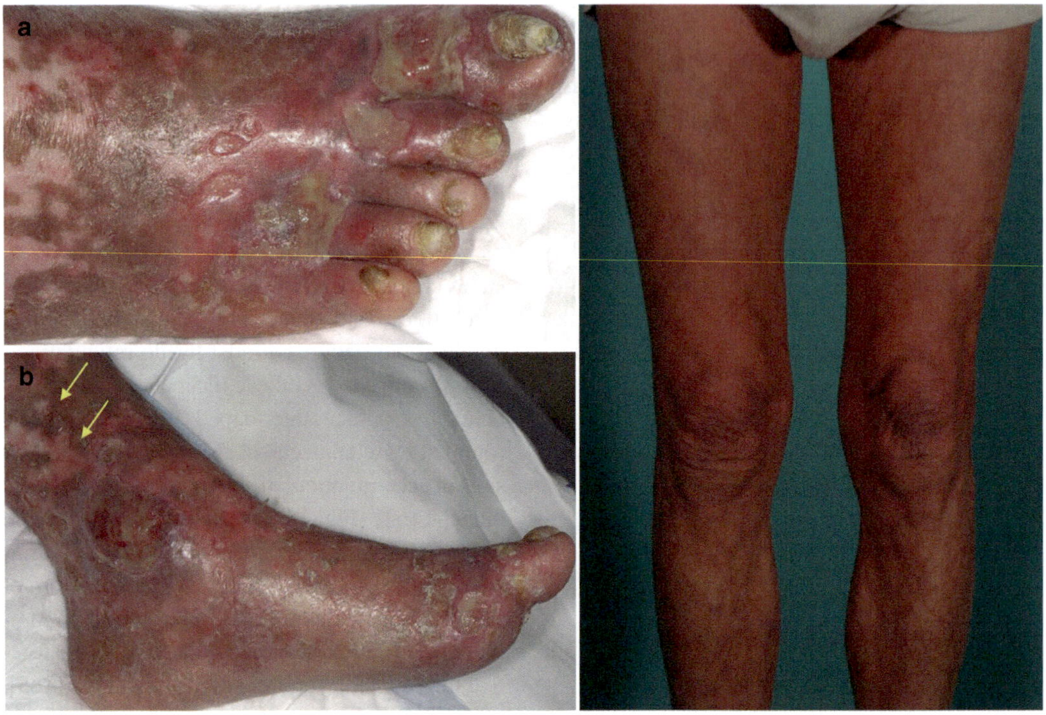

Fig. 18.10 (**a, b**) Severe livedoid vasculopathy in a patient with protein C and S deficiency. Note areas of atrophie blanche (arrows) and skin necrosis. (**c**) Livedo racemosa in a patient with antiphospholipid syndrome

investigation in patients presenting with livedo reticularis is largely influenced by their clinical history and physical examination findings [66]. If the venous patterns are permanent, display irregularities, and don't diminish upon warming, it's referred to as livedo racemosa, which often hints at an underlying systemic ailment. When a skin biopsy is taken from the slightly discolored area surrounding the lesion, it can unveil features of vasculopathy or vasculitis, depending on the underlying conditions. Thus, the biopsy should also be taken from the central area of pallor.

Livedo reticularis/racemosa is particularly characteristic for antiphospholipid syndrome, cryoproteinemias, and polycythemia vera. However, livedo reticularis is not specific to hypercoagulable states and is seen in a variety of unrelated conditions, such as neurologic disease, large vessel occlusions, medium vessel vasculitis (e.g., polyarteritis nodosa), as a drug reaction or reaction to infections, among other numerous conditions [67].

Non-specific Lesions: Petechiae, Purpura, Ulcers

Petechiae are small (≤3 mm), non-fading, red-purple macules that arise due to the escape of erythrocytes from minor skin vessels. In the absence of injury, these lesions can be indicative of underlying thrombocytopenia, vascular fragility (senescence, vitamin C deficiency), or mild vasculitis. When trauma-induced, the prominence of petechiae can be disproportionate to the extent of the injury, especially if there's a deficiency of platelets or an anomaly in blood clotting. Typically, no supplementary diagnostic evaluations are required for pinpoint petechiae.

Purpura are characterized by red to purple-colored macules or papules that arise due to the spillage of erythrocytes from the dermal vasculature. The presence of palpable purpura is a hallmark of vasculitic conditions. Notably, the retiform variant of purpura, which exhibits a star-shaped or irregular pattern, often signifies an obstruction in vessels larger than capillaries. Such obstruction can be a result of vasculitis, vasculopathy, or blockage within the lumen due to thrombosis or atherosclerotic changes.

Development of an ulcer in the context of hypercoagulable state is the further progression of livedoid vasculopathy. Ulcerations are commonly seen in a myriad of other diseases (most commonly venous ulcers, arterial ulcers, diabetic ulcers, hypertensive ulcer of Matorell, etc.) and hypercoagulable states contribute only to a minority of cases. Ulcers associated with hypercoagulation are similar to venous ulcers: are localized in the malleolar region of the lower extremity and may even be associated with signs of venous insufficiency due to previous venous thrombosis phenomena. Unusual persistent wounds, particularly lower extremity ulcers that don't fit the pattern of venous or arterial causes, should raise suspicion for an underlying coagulation disorder. The most common diseases associated with ulceration are cryoglobulinemia and antiphospholipid syndrome [66].

18.2.3.3 Skin Signs of Inherited Hypercoagulable States

Most inherited hypercoagulable states present with livedoid vasculopathy. Skin lesions are mostly found in patients with Protein C/S deficiency, factor Leiden mutation and 20210A prothrombin gene, who are also prone to the development of chronic leg ulcers that may be difficult to differentiate from common venous leg ulcers or even from pyoderma gangrenosum. Generally, leg ulcers or livedoid vasculopathy in individuals younger than 50 years should trigger further investigations to rule out hypercoagulability (Table 18.5).

Table 18.5 Skin signs of common inherited hypercoagulable states [66]

Disease	Typical skin findings
Antithrombin deficiency	Livedoid vasculopathy Skin lesions are uncommon
Protein C and/or S deficiency	Livedoid vasculopathy Calciphylaxis Venous thrombosis and leg ulcers Risk of warfarin-induced skin necrosis
Factor V Leiden mutation	Deep venous thrombosis Skin ulcers
Prothrombin gene variant (20210A)	Ulcerated papules on the lower leg Livedoid vasculopathy Leg ulcers
Hyperhomocystinemia	Livedoid vasculopathy Malar rash Livedo reticularis due to associated cryoglobulinemia

Table 18.6 Skin signs of common inherited hypercoagulable states [66]

Disease	Typical skin findings
Warfarin-induced skin necrosis	Ecchymoses, blistering, hemorrhagic skin necrosis in the areas of abundant fat.
Heparin-induced thrombocytopenia	Hemorrhagic skin necrosis at the site of heparin injection.
Thrombotic thrombocytopenic purpura	Petechiae and purpura
Cryoglobulinemia and cryofibrinogenemia	Raynaud phenomenon Purpura Livedo reticularis Ulcerations

18.2.3.4 Skin Signs of Acquired Hypercoagulable States

The acquired states of hypercoagulation represent a very wide and heterogeneous category, but from the clinical point of view, the most significant are those caused by the administration of anticoagulants. While intended to prevent clot formation, those drugs can paradoxically instigate a hypercoagulable state, further leading to skin necrosis. The mechanism is most probably the rapid depletion of protein C by the anticoagulant, creating a transient hypercoagulable state. Thus, patients with protein C and S deficiency have an increased risk of warfarin-induced skin necrosis and heparin-induced thrombocytopenia [68–70].

Skin signs of other acquired hypercoagulable states are summarized in Table 18.6 (Fig. 18.11).

Warfarin-Induced Skin Necrosis

Warfarin-induced skin necrosis often emerges between the third and fifth day following the commencement of warfarin treatment, particularly if initiated with a sizable loading dose or in the absence of simultaneous heparin therapy. Predominantly, regions with an abundance of adipose tissue and compromised blood flow, such as the breasts, buttocks, abdomen, thighs, and calves, are most susceptible [71]. Initial symptoms manifest as pain and purpura, which can escalate to dramatic and extensive full-thickness skin necrosis, often with hemorrhagic blisters [66, 72] (Fig. 18.11). A preventive approach involves initiating anticoagulation via heparin for a span of 4 to 5 days prior to commencing warfarin therapy. If warfarin-induced skin necrosis develops, immediate interventions include halting warfarin, transitioning to heparin-based anticoagulation, and administering vitamin K or fresh frozen plasma to counteract the effects of warfarin. The role of local wound management is paramount, and in severe cases, surgical interventions, extending to amputation, might become necessary.

Warfarin-induced skin necrosis should be differentiated from other conditions with ecchymoses and skin necrosis, especially calciphylaxis, microembolic events (septic, cholesterol), heparin-induced thrombocytopenia, and infections (bullous erysipelas, necrotizing fasciitis).

Heparin-Induced Thrombocytopenia

Heparin-induced thrombocytopenia (HIT) is characterized by thrombocytopenia, resistance to anticoagulation with heparin, and/or arterial or venous thromboses. The predominant clinical manifestation of HIT is skin necrosis that typically develops between 6 and 13 days post-initiation of therapy [63, 66, 71] (Fig 18.11). The lesions appear at the injection site but can occasionally manifest elsewhere. There are two types of HIT—the non-immune driven thrombocytopenia and the immune-mediated HIT in which heparin-associated antibodies lead to a hypercoagulable state by activating both platelets and the vascular endothelium. Scoring systems have been developed to facilitate the diagnosis of HIT [73]. The differential diagnoses of HIT are similar to those of warfarin-induced skin necrosis.

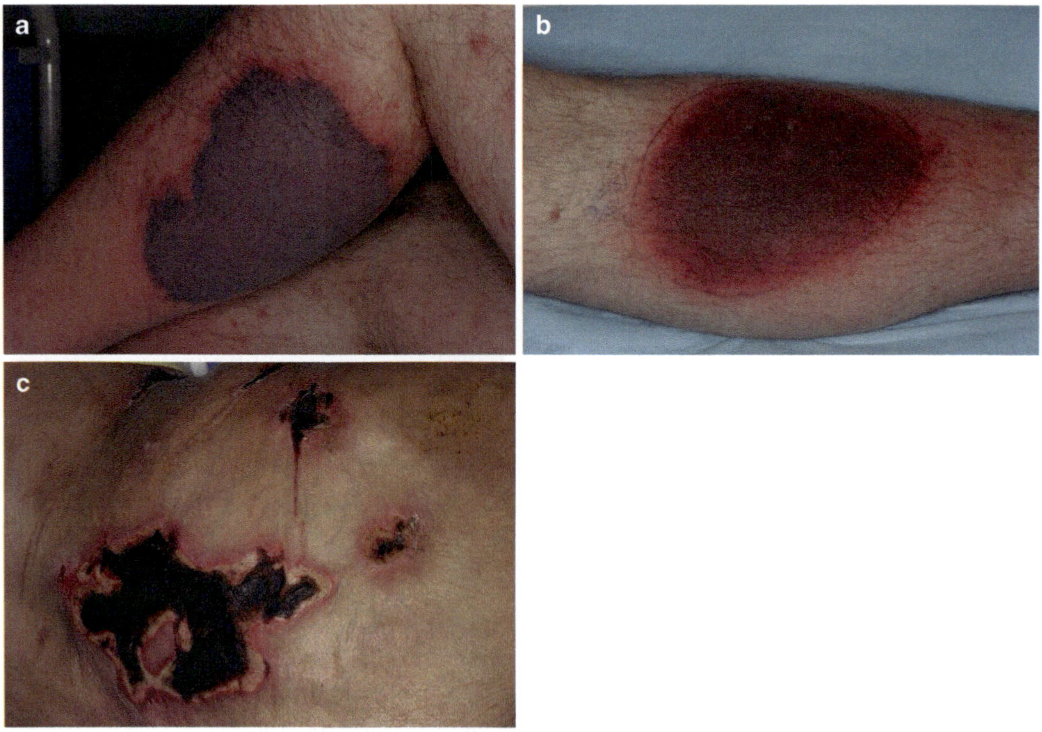

Fig. 18.11 Skin necrosis in different acquired hypercoagulable states. (**a**) Warfarin-induced skin necrosis, (**b**) Heparin necrosis developing at a site of venipuncture due to heparin-induced thrombocytopenia, (**c**) calciphylaxis

18.2.4 Transfusion-Related Dermatologic Manifestations

18.2.4.1 Practice Essentials

- Transfusion-induced dermatologic reactions comprise acute allergic reactions, transfusion-associated graft-versus-host disease (GvHD), and post-transfusion purpura.
- Transfusion-related GvHD can be very severe and presents as morbiliform rash up to 1 month after transfusion.
- Post-transfusion purpura is a thrombocytopenic purpura within 2 weeks after transfusion.

18.2.4.2 Acute Allergic Responses to Transfusion

The likelihood of allergic reactions following platelet or red blood cell transfusion stands at 3.7% and 0.15%, respectively [74]. Interestingly, only a subset of these reactions manifest dermatologically as acute urticaria or erythema. Predominant allergens include plasma proteins, notably IgA and haptoglobin. It's pertinent to note that individuals with IgA deficiency (having IgA levels <0.5 mg/L) are more susceptible (see also Chap. 16). Populations in South-East Asia, where haptoglobin deficiency is more prevalent, may be particularly at risk. Additionally, certain chemical and food allergens have been implicated in such reactions, with methylene blue (used for inactivating viruses in fresh plasma) and inadvertently transferred peanut allergens serving as prime examples [74].

18.2.4.3 Transfusion-Related GvHD

Transfusion-associated GvHD emerges due to the transfusion product containing alloreactive donor leukocytes. Typically, the presentation includes an erythematous maculopapular rash 2–30 days post-transfusion, often coexisting with systemic symptoms like liver enzyme anomalies, jaundice, and gastrointestinal symptoms such as diarrhea [75, 76]. Unfortunately, the prognosis is often poor, especially if gastrointestinal GvHD is present. Risk is accentuated in immunocompromised patients or those receiving transfusions from related donors.

18.2.4.4 Post-Transfusion Purpura

Post-transfusion purpura is an uncommon adverse event following the transfusion of platelet-containing products such as packed red blood cells or granulocyte infusions. Its pathogenesis lies in the generation of antibodies against the transfused platelet alloantigens, often seen in females sensitized previously during pregnancy [77]. Remarkably, the patient's immune response not only targets the transfused platelets but also their native platelets, the exact mechanism of which remains elusive. This culminates in abrupt thrombocytopenia and thrombocytopenic purpura 4–11 days post-transfusion [78].

18.3 Cutaneous Extramedullary Hematopoiesis

18.3.1 Practice Essentials

- Extramedullary hematopoiesis (EMH) refers to the production of blood cellular components outside their usual site in the bone marrow.
- Cutaneous EMH in adults is very rare and is mostly associated with chronic myeloproliferative syndromes.

Cutaneous extramedullary hematopoiesis (CEMH) presents a well-defined clinicopathological entity, characterized by hematopoietic activity occurring outside its canonical medullary milieu and manifesting within the dermis and subdermis. While the neonatal form, exemplified by the "blueberry muffin baby" syndrome, is documented extensively, this discourse will deliberate upon the relatively esoteric adult-onset CEMH tethered to myeloid malignancies or other hematological diseases, like thalassemia. Hence EMH may represent a clonal process or be a nonclonal reactive phenomenon secondary to marrow insufficiency in the setting of serious hematological stress, such as thalassemia. Systemic work-up, including bone marrow biopsy, is required in cases where the underlying causes are not obvious.

18.3.2 Clinical Manifestations

The spectrum of extramedullary hematopoiesis predominantly spans visceral organs, with the liver and spleen being paramount, followed by the lymphatic domain, notably the lymph nodes and the retroperitoneal space. Cutaneous involvement is an exceptional rarity, with a documented incidence of less than 0.5% among all presentations [79, 80]. This limited prevalence underscores the importance of clinical acumen when encountering potential cutaneous manifestations. Clinically, the skin may exhibit erythematous to violaceous nodules or plaques, varying in dimension and distribution [81, 82]. Often truncal in localization, these lesions might manifest solitarily or in clusters. Ulceration is a potential sequela, with affected sites eliciting symptoms such as pruritus, tenderness, and localized pain. A notable clinical simulacrum is leukemia cutis, necessitating astute differentiation, a challenge further compounded by the potential presence of mutated myeloid cells within CEMH lesions [83].

The prognostic implications associated with CEMH remain shrouded in uncertainty. While the extant literature underscores a somewhat grim prognosis for hepatosplenic and non-hepatosplenic EMH [79, 84], the limited documentation specific to CEMH obfuscates any definitive prognostic delineation.

18.3.3 Diagnosis

Histopathological evaluation remains the cornerstone of CEMH diagnosis. Cutaneous biopsies often reveal perivascular dermal infiltrates comprising an assemblage of hematopoietic cells, reflecting varied maturation stages. The histological tableau usually captures the triad of cell lineages: erythroid, myeloid granulocytic, and megakaryocytic, but predominantly unilineage cases have been described, especially with erythroid mature terminally differentiated cells.

Critical diagnostic markers include dysplastic megakaryocytes, abnormal and/or dysplastic myeloid maturation, and increased numbers of immature cells or blast cells. Given the potential implications of atypical cytomophological features or increased, often aggregated immature cells, these findings signal a broader underlying pathology, potentially pointing towards myeloproliferative disorders or other marrow insufficiencies (myelofibrosis). It is recognized that, in rare instances, myeloid sarcomas can simulate EMH, and these cases will often feature prominent immature erythroid or megakaryocytic precursors. Many useful IHC stains may be used in cases where the trilineage features need to be demonstrated and scrutinized, and the reader is referred to Chap. 2. dealing with myeloid sarcomas. CD34, although imperfect, will enable a better assessment of the immature blastic population. Other immunohistochemical markers include glycophorin A, CD43, lysozyme, CD68, CD117, E-cadherin, MPO, CD61, among others.

18.3.4 Therapy

Symptomatic CEMH lesions necessitate therapeutic intervention. The therapeutic armamentarium is diverse, ranging from low-dose radiation and electron beam therapy to strategies specifically targeting the etiological myeloid neoplasm [79, 85, 86]. Topical corticosteroids have been used on deposits of cutaneous EMH without effect.

References

1. Gupta S, Krishnan AS, Singh J, Gupta A, Gupta M. Clinicopathological characteristics and management of extramedullary hematopoiesis: a review. Pediatr Hematol Oncol J. 2022;7:182–6.
2. Maglie R, Genovese G, Solimani F, Guglielmo A, Pileri A, Portelli F, et al. Immune-mediated dermatoses in patients with haematological malignancies: a comprehensive review. Am J Clin Dermatol. 2020;21:833–54.
3. Fogo A, du Vivier A. The cutaneous manifestations of haematological malignancy. Clin Med. 2009;9:366–70.
4. Krug B, Sonet A, Pirson A-S, Mahy N, Bosly A, Borght TV. FDG PET utility in paraneoplastic sweet syndrome. Clin Nucl Med. 2004;29:91–2.
5. Linke R, Voltz R. FDG-pet in paraneoplastic syndromes. Recent Results Cancer Res. 2008;170:203–11.

6. Wu L-M, Chen F-Y, Jiang X-X, Gu H-Y, Yin Y, Xu J-R. 18F-FDG PET, combined FDG-PET/CT and MRI for evaluation of bone marrow infiltration in staging of lymphoma: a systematic review and meta-analysis. Eur J Radiol. 2012;81:303–11.
7. Raza S, Kirkland RS, Patel AA, Shortridge JR, Freter C. Insight into Sweet's syndrome and associated-malignancy: a review of the current literature. Int J Oncol. 2013;42:1516–22.
8. Anzalone CL, Cohen PR. Acute febrile neutrophilic dermatosis (Sweet's syndrome). Curr Opin Hematol. 2013;20:26–35.
9. Kluger N, Gil-Bistes D, Guillot B, Bessis D. Efficacy of anti-interleukin-1 receptor antagonist anakinra (Kineret®) in a case of refractory Sweet's syndrome. Dermatology. 2011;222:123–7.
10. Delluc A, Limal N, Puéchal X, Francès C, Piette JC, Cacoub P. Efficacy of anakinra, an IL1 receptor antagonist, in refractory Sweet syndrome. Ann Rheum Dis. 2008;67:278–9.
11. Jo T, Horio K, Migita K. Sweet's syndrome in patients with MDS and MEFV mutations. N Engl J Med. 2015;372:686–8.
12. Kroshinsky D, Alloo A, Rothschild B, Cummins J, Tan J, Montecino R, et al. Necrotizing Sweet syndrome: a new variant of neutrophilic dermatosis mimicking necrotizing fasciitis. J Am Acad Dermatol. 2012;67:945–54.
13. Chan MP, Duncan LM, Nazarian RM. Subcutaneous Sweet syndrome in the setting of myeloid disorders: a case series and review of the literature. J Am Acad Dermatol. 2013;68:1006–15.
14. Galaria NA, Junkins-Hopkins JM, Kligman D, James WD. Neutrophilic dermatosis of the dorsal hands: pustular vasculitis revisited. J Am Acad Dermatol. 2000;43:870–4.
15. Ghoufi L, Ortonne N, Ingen-Housz-Oro S, Barhoumi W, Begon E, Haioun C, et al. Histiocytoid Sweet syndrome is more frequently associated with myelodysplastic syndromes than the classical neutrophilic variant: a comparative series of 62 patients. Medicine. 2016;95:e3033.
16. Chow S, Pasternak S, Green P, Tremaine R, Reardon M, Murray S, et al. Histiocytoid neutrophilic dermatoses and panniculitides: variations on a theme. Am J Dermatopathol. 2007;29:334–41.
17. Motta A, González LF, García G, Guzmán J, Prada L, Herrera H, et al. Atlas of dermatology: inflammatory, infectious and tumoral skin diseases. Springer Nature; 2022.
18. Bennett ML, Jackson JM, Jorizzo JL, Fleischer AB Jr, White WL, Callen JP. Pyoderma gangrenosum. A comparison of typical and atypical forms with an emphasis on time to remission. Case review of 86 patients from 2 institutions. Medicine. 2000;79:37–46.
19. Duguid CM, O'Loughlin S, Otridge B, Powell FC. Paraneoplastic pyoderma gangrenosum. Australas J Dermatol. 1993;34:17–22.
20. Koester G, Tarnower A, Levisohn D, Burgdorf W. Bullous pyoderma gangrenosum. J Am Acad Dermatol. 1993;29:875–8.
21. Su WPD, Davis MDP, Weenig RH, Powell FC, Perry HO. Pyoderma gangrenosum: clinicopathologic correlation and proposed diagnostic criteria. Int J Dermatol. 2004;43:790–800.
22. Caughman W, Stern R, Haynes H. Neutrophilic dermatosis of myeloproliferative disorders. Atypical forms of pyoderma gangrenosum and Sweet's syndrome associated with myeloproliferative disorders. J Am Acad Dermatol. 1983;9:751–8.
23. Bachmeyer C, Aractingi S. Neutrophilic eccrine hidradenitis. Clin Dermatol. 2000;18:319–30.
24. Qiao J, Sun C-E, Zhu W, Zhu D, Fang H. Flame figures associated with eosinophilic dermatosis of hematologic malignancy: is it possible to distinguish the condition from eosinophilic cellulitis in patients with hematoproliferative disease? Int J Clin Exp Pathol. 2013;6:1683–7.
25. Momen SE, Jorizzo J, Al-Niaimi F. Erythema elevatum diutinum: a review of presentation and treatment. J Eur Acad Dermatol Venereol. 2014;28:1594–602.
26. Queipo de Llano M, Yebra M, Cabrera R, Suarez E. Myelodysplastic syndrome in association with erythema elevatum diutinum. J Rheumatol. 1992;19:1005–6.
27. Yiannias JA, el-Azhary RA, Gibson LE. Erythema elevatum diutinum: a clinical and histopathologic study of 13 patients. J Am Acad Dermatol. 1992;26:38–44.
28. Watts PJ, Khachemoune A. Subcorneal pustular dermatosis: a review of 30 years of progress. Am J Clin Dermatol. 2016;17:653–71.
29. Kasha EE Jr, Epinette WW. Subcorneal pustular dermatosis (Sneddon-Wilkinson disease) in association with a monoclonal IgA gammopathy: a report and review of the literature. J Am Acad Dermatol. 1988;19:854–8.
30. Gulati A, Puttanniah V, Bruel BM, Rosenberg WS, Hung JC. Essentials of interventional cancer pain management. Springer; 2018.
31. Visseaux L, Durlach A, Barete S, Beylot-Barry M, Bonnet N, Chassine A, et al. T-cell papulosis associated with B-cell malignancy: a distinctive clinicopathologic entity. J Eur Acad Dermatol Venereol. 2018;32:1469–75.
32. Cokonis Georgakis C-D, Falasca G, Georgakis A, Heymann WR. Scleromyxedema. Clin Dermatol. 2006;24:493–7.
33. Heymann WR. Scleromyxedema. J Am Acad Dermatol. 2007;57:890–1.
34. Rongioletti F, Merlo G, Cinotti E, Fausti V, Cozzani E, Cribier B, et al. Scleromyxedema: a multicenter study of characteristics, comorbidities, course, and therapy in 30 patients. J Am Acad Dermatol. 2013;69:66–72.
35. Beers WH, Ince A, Moore TL. Scleredema adultorum of Buschke: a case report and review of the literature. Semin Arthritis Rheum. 2006;35:355–9.

36. Rimon D, Lurie M, Storch S, Halon D, Eisenkraft S, Laor A, et al. Cardiomyopathy and multiple myeloma. Complications of scleredema adultorum. Arch Intern Med. 1988;148:551–3.
37. Curtis AC, Shulak BM. Scleredema adultorum. Not always a benign self-limited disease. Arch Dermatol. 1965;92:526–41.
38. Szalat R, Arnulf B, Karlin L, Rybojad M, Asli B, Malphettes M, et al. Pathogenesis and treatment of xanthomatosis associated with monoclonal gammopathy. Blood. 2011;118:3777–84.
39. Frew JW, Murrell DF. Paraneoplastic pemphigus (paraneoplastic autoimmune multiorgan syndrome): clinical presentations and pathogenesis. Dermatol Clin. 2011;29:419–25, viii.
40. Solimani F, Maglie R, Pollmann R, Schmidt T, Schmidt A, Ishii N, et al. Thymoma-associated paraneoplastic autoimmune multiorgan syndrome-from pemphigus to lichenoid dermatitis. Front Immunol. 2019;10:1413.
41. Yosipovitch G. Chronic pruritus: a paraneoplastic sign. Dermatol Ther. 2010;23:590–6.
42. Saif MW, Hopkins JL, Gore SD. Autoimmune phenomena in patients with myelodysplastic syndromes and chronic myelomonocytic leukemia. Leuk Lymphoma. 2002;43:2083–92.
43. Cristiano A, Belardi R, Hajrullaj H, Fabiani E, Falconi G, Galossi E, et al. Correlation analysis between auto-immunological and mutational profiles in myelodysplastic syndromes. Inflamm Res. 2023;72:1695–707.
44. Klein A, Polliack A, Gafter-Gvili A. Systemic lupus erythematosus and lymphoma: Incidence, pathogenesis and biology. Leuk Res. 2018;75:45–9.
45. Vasaitis L, Nordmark G, Theander E, Backlin C, Smedby KE, Askling J, et al. Population-based study of patients with primary Sjögren's syndrome and lymphoma: lymphoma subtypes, clinical characteristics, and gender differences. Scand J Rheumatol. 2020;49:225–32.
46. Sebastian A, Madej M, Sebastian M, Butrym A, Woytala P, Hałoń A, et al. Prevalence and clinical presentation of lymphoproliferative disorder in patients with primary Sjögren's syndrome. Rheumatol Int. 2020;40:399–404.
47. Park JK, Subhawong AP, Ziminski CM, Grader-Beck T. Dermatomyositis as the initial presentation of a large anaplastic T-cell lymphoma. J Clin Oncol. 2011;29:e378–80.
48. Marie I, Guillevin L, Menard J-F, Hatron PY, Cherin P, Amoura Z, et al. Hematological malignancy associated with polymyositis and dermatomyositis. Autoimmun Rev. 2012;11:615–20.
49. Ledwich LJ, Olenginski TP. A rare lymphoma in a patient with amyopathic dermatomyositis. Am J Clin Dermatol. 2010;11:151–5.
50. Choi R, Bhullar S, McNiff J, Persico J, Leventhal J. A rare case of viral-associated trichodysplasia spinulosa in a patient with chronic lymphocytic leukemia. Int J Womens Dermatol. 2023;9:e069.
51. Curman P, Näsman A, Brauner H. Trichodysplasia spinulosa: a comprehensive review of the disease and its treatment. J Eur Acad Dermatol Venereol. 2021;35:1067–76.
52. Dawson AA, Ogston D, Fullerton HW. Evaluation of diagnostic significance of certain symptoms and physical signs in anaemic patients. Br Med J. 1969;3:436–9.
53. Takkunen H. Iron-deficiency pruritus. JAMA. 1978;239:1394.
54. Piskin S, Sayan C, Durukan N, Senol M. Serum iron, ferritin, folic acid, and vitamin B12 levels in recurrent aphthous stomatitis. J Eur Acad Dermatol Venereol. 2002;16:66–7.
55. Lu S-Y, Wu H-C. Initial diagnosis of anemia from sore mouth and improved classification of anemias by MCV and RDW in 30 patients. Oral Surg Oral Med Oral Pathol Oral Radiol Endod. 2004;98:679–85.
56. Brigham D, Beard J. Iron and thermoregulation: a review. Crit Rev Food Sci Nutr. 1996;36:747–63.
57. DeLoughery TG. Iron deficiency anemia. Med Clin North Am. 2017;101:319–32.
58. Anastassakis K. Androgenetic alopecia from A to Z: Vol. 2 drugs, herbs, nutrition and supplements. Springer Nature; 2022.
59. Bartolucci P, Brugnara C, Teixeira-Pinto A, Pissard S, Moradkhani K, Jouault H, et al. Erythrocyte density in sickle cell syndromes is associated with specific clinical manifestations and hemolysis. Blood. 2012;120:3136–41.
60. Dick A, Schwartzman G, Khachemoune A. Cutaneous manifestations of sickle cell disease: an updated review. Arch Dermatol Res. 2023;315:729–34.
61. Gniadecka M, Gniadecki R, Serup J, Søndergaard J. Microvascular reactions to postural changes in patients with sickle cell anaemia. Acta Derm Venereol. 1994;74:191–3.
62. Wong TE, Brandow AM, Lim W, Lottenberg R. Update on the use of hydroxyurea therapy in sickle cell disease. Blood. 2014;124:3850–7; quiz 4004.
63. Johnson CM, Mureebe L, Silver D. Hypercoagulable states: a review. Vasc Endovasc Surg. 2005;39:123–33.
64. Alavi A, Hafner J, Dutz JP, Mayer D, Sibbald RG, Criado PR, et al. Livedoid vasculopathy: an in-depth analysis using a modified Delphi approach. J Am Acad Dermatol. 2013;69:1033–1042.e1.
65. Hairston BR, Davis MDP, Pittelkow MR, Ahmed I. Livedoid vasculopathy: further evidence for procoagulant pathogenesis. Arch Dermatol. 2006;142:1413–8.
66. Dabiri G, Damstetter E, Chang Y, Baiyee Ebot E, Powers JG, Phillips T. Coagulation disorders and their cutaneous presentations: diagnostic work-up and treatment. J Am Acad Dermatol. 2016;74:795–804; quiz 805–6.
67. Fleischer AB Jr, Resnick SD. Livedo reticularis. Dermatol Clin. 1990;8:347–54.
68. Aronson JK. Side effects of drugs annual: a worldwide yearly survey of new data and trends in adverse drug reactions. Elsevier; 2011.

69. Rose VL, Kwaan HC, Williamson K, Hoppensteadt D, Walenga J, Fareed J. Protein C antigen deficiency and warfarin necrosis. Am J Clin Pathol. 1986;86:653–5.
70. Gailani D, Reese EP Jr. Anticoagulant-induced skin necrosis in a patient with hereditary deficiency of protein S. Am J Hematol. 1999;60:231–6.
71. Nazarian RM, Van Cott EM, Zembowicz A, Duncan LM. Warfarin-induced skin necrosis. J Am Acad Dermatol. 2009;61:325–32.
72. Kakagia DD, Papanas N, Karadimas E, Polychronidis A. Warfarin-induced skin necrosis. Ann Dermatol. 2014;26:96–8.
73. Cuker A, Gimotty PA, Crowther MA, Warkentin TE. Predictive value of the 4Ts scoring system for heparin-induced thrombocytopenia: a systematic review and meta-analysis. Blood. 2012;120: 4160–7.
74. Hirayama F. Current understanding of allergic transfusion reactions: incidence, pathogenesis, laboratory tests, prevention and treatment. Br J Haematol. 2013;160:434–44.
75. Fast LD. Developments in the prevention of transfusion-associated graft-versus-host disease. Br J Haematol. 2012;158:563–8.
76. Six CK, Haught JM, Safyan EL, Patton T, Stahlfeld K. Transfusion-associated graft-versus-host disease: a case report and review of literature. J Am Acad Dermatol. 2012;66:e141–3.
77. DeVirgilio C, Grigorian A. Review of surgery for ABSITE and Boards E-book. Elsevier Health Sciences; 2017.
78. Waters AH. Post-transfusion purpura. Blood Rev. 1989;3:83–7.
79. Koch CA, Li C-Y, Mesa RA, Tefferi A. Nonhepatosplenic extramedullary hematopoiesis: associated diseases, pathology, clinical course, and treatment. Mayo Clin Proc. 2003;78:1223–33.
80. Haniffa MA, Wilkins BS, Blasdale C, Simpson NB. Cutaneous extramedullary hemopoiesis in chronic myeloproliferative and myelodysplastic disorders. J Am Acad Dermatol. 2006;55:S28–31.
81. Mizoguchi M, Kawa Y, Minami T, Nakayama H, Mizoguchi H. Cutaneous extramedullary hematopoiesis in myelofibrosis. J Am Acad Dermatol. 1990;22:351–5.
82. Patel BM, Su WP, Perniciaro C, Gertz MA. Cutaneous extramedullary hematopoiesis. J Am Acad Dermatol. 1995;32:805–7.
83. LeBlanc RE, Lester L, Kwong B, Rieger KE. JAK2-positive cutaneous myelofibrosis presenting as sclerosing extramedullary hematopoietic tumors on the scalp: case presentation and review of the literature. J Cutan Pathol. 2015;42:858–62.
84. Tefferi A. The forgotten myeloproliferative disorder: myeloid metaplasia. Oncologist. 2003;8:225–31.
85. Hocking WG, Lazar GS, Lipsett JA, Busuttil RW. Cutaneous extramedullary hematopoiesis following splenectomy for idiopathic myelofibrosis. Am J Med. 1984;76:956–8.
86. Bakst RL, Tallman MS, Douer D, Yahalom J. How I treat extramedullary acute myeloid leukemia. Blood. 2011;118:3785–93.

Index

R. Gniadecki et al. (eds.), *Diseases of Blood and Skin*, https://doi.org/10.1007/978-3-031-65292-9

GPSR Compliance

The European Union's (EU) General Product Safety Regulation (GPSR) is a set of rules that requires consumer products to be safe and our obligations to ensure this.

If you have any concerns about our products, you can contact us on ProductSafety@springernature.com

In case Publisher is established outside the EU, the EU authorized representative is:

Springer Nature Customer Service Center GmbH
Europaplatz 3
69115 Heidelberg, Germany

Batch number: 10732801

Printed by Printforce, the Netherlands